Equine Exercise Physiolog

David Marlin
Animal Health Trust

Kathryn Nankervis
Hartpury College

Blackwell
Science

Blackwell Science, a Blackwell Publishing company
Editorial offices:
Blackwell Science Ltd, 9600 Garsington Road, Oxford OX4 2DQ, UK
Tel: +44 (0) 1865 776868
Blackwell Publishing Professional, 2121 State Avenue, Ames, Iowa 50014-8300, USA
Tel: +1 515 292 0140
Blackwell Science Asia Pty Ltd, 550 Swanston Street, Carlton, Victoria 3053, Australia
Tel: +61 (0)3 8359 1011

First published 2002
15   2015

ISBN 978-0-6320-5552-4

Library of Congress Cataloging-in-Publication Data
Marlin, David
Equine exercise philosophy/David Marlin, Kathryn Nankervis.
p.   cm.
1. Horses—Training.   2. Horses—Exercise.   I. Nankervis, K.J.   II. Title.
SF287 M34 2003
636.1′0835—dc21

2002026041

A catalogue record for this title is available from the British Library

Set in 9.5/12 pt Times by SNP Best-set Typesetter Ltd., Hong Kong

The publisher's policy is to use permanent paper from mills that operate a sustainable forestry
policy, and which has been manufactured from pulp processed using acid-free and elementary
chlorine-free practices. Furthermore, the publisher ensures that the text paper and cover board
used have met acceptable environmental accreditation standards.

For further information on Blackwell Publishing, visit our website:
www.blackwellpublishing.com

Foreword

The training of competition horses has changed a great deal over the last few decades, for example with the introduction of the all weather gallop and the 'interval' method of training for staying horses.

This book explains the scientific reasoning behind the training of horses for competition in a manner that those working with horses will comprehend. It explains why training methods succeed and, just as importantly, if your horse is over stressed why those methods might fail.

The trainer of today's horse is presented with a different set of problems from those of yesteryear. Arguably the competition is now tougher, which puts a horse under greater stress, and trainers are presented with ever more information about the condition of their horses – blood tests, food analysis and so on. We need to have at the very least a basic understanding of these factors if we are to make rational decisions about what is best for our horses. This book will help you understand how to manage your competition horse in today's environment.

Equine Exercise Physiology is a readable, up-to-date account of how to achieve the highest standards in your competition horses. It will suit all horse enthusiasts and students, as well as experienced trainers.

Peter Scudamore

Acknowledgements

The authors would like to thank the following friends and colleagues for comments on various chapters within this book: Rachel Neville (Chapters 2 and 20), Dr Stephanie Valberg (Chapters 3 and 7), Dr Rachel Murray (Chapters 4 and 8), Dr Bob Colborne (Chapters 4, 8 and 13), Dr Colin Roberts (Chapters 5, 9 and 18), Dr Lesley Young (Chapters 6 and 10), John Robertson and Rod Fisher (Chapter 14), Dr Catherine Dunnett (Chapter 20), Matthew French at Hartpury College for assistance in the production of the figures and Dr David Evans, Equine Performance Laboratory, University of Sydney, for providing Fig. 18.10.

Cover photo: Courtesy of Dr D.J. Marlin.

To Roma and George (DM)

To Tom (KN)

Contents

Part I
The Raw Materials

Chapter 1

Introduction

Why train?

In theory and in practice, the horse must surely be considered the best all round athlete of the animal kingdom. Horses are not great thinkers or fighters, they are runners. Whatever the breed or type of horse, they are all blessed with the same basic structure and the same basic physiological mechanisms; therefore they all have the potential to respond favourably to training. A horse's performance, i.e. how fast it runs, how high it jumps, is largely determined by its natural ability, and to a lesser extent by its level of training. Natural ability is determined mainly by the genes the horse inherits from its parents (Fig. 1.1). We can't do anything about the genes an individual horse has once it has been born, but we can do something about the training. To reach a horse's genetic potential for performance, whether it is aimed at local riding club events or the Derby, it must be fit! From the unfit to fit state the horse undergoes a metamorphosis and its shape, its gaits, its looks, often even its attitude to life, are altered. Whatever we strive to achieve with our horses, there is much to be gained by making sure that they are fit enough for the task. To compete on an unfit horse puts both you and your horse at risk, quite apart from decreasing your chances of success and also the likelihood of the two of you going on to compete year after year.

Horses are always huge investments in terms of both time and money. If you aim to compete at any level, it pays to improve the horse's chances of completing the work goals without risking mechanical breakdown and so incurring large veterinary bills, long periods of rehabilitation at best and destruction at worst. There is no doubt that training is an art, but a little understanding of the physiology of the horse can help anyone perfect their own art.

Much of what we currently understand about equine exercise physiology has been established in the last 20 to 30 years, largely as a result of an increased scientific and veterinary interest in exercise physiology, improvements in technology, and availability of equipment such as high speed treadmills. High speed treadmills enable vets and scientists to study the horse in controlled situations where the speed, distance, slope, going and environmental conditions can all be closely regulated. In addition, with a horse exercising on a treadmill it is a very simple matter to collect a blood sample from a catheter in an artery or vein, or to measure how much oxygen the horse is using. Procedures such as these are either difficult or at present not possible to undertake in the field. Inevitably, running on treadmills is not the same as running round a racetrack or a cross-country course, but it has enabled scientists to make great advances in the study of the horse's responses to exercise and training. Many of these advances can now easily be applied to the management and training programmes of our own competition horses with a good degree of success. Whilst science cannot guarantee a winner, it may well shorten the odds in our favour.

What are the aims of a training programme?

What exactly are we trying to achieve as a result of training? The fundamental purposes of any training programme are to:

(1) Increase the horse's exercise capacity
(2) Increase the time to the onset of fatigue
(3) Improve overall performance, by increasing:
   — Skill
   — Strength

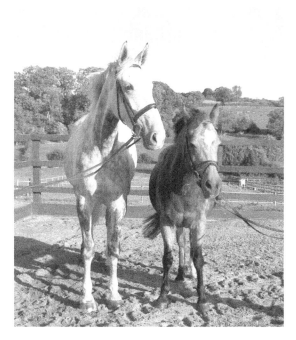

Fig. 1.1   A horse's performance is largely determined by the genes the horse inherits from its parents.

— Speed
— Endurance
or all four of these
(4) Decrease the risk of injury.

By analysing the adaptations the horse makes in the short term (during exercise) and in the long term (throughout training) we can begin to understand how to design the horse's work programme to achieve these aims (Fig. 1.2).

Exercise, work, training, fitness and performance

First of all, let's tackle the vocabulary of 'exercise physiology'. Being associated with horses entitles you to become a member of a club that has its own language, a language which is only understood by those 'in the know'. Consider some of our expressions: we talk about grey when we mean white; we 'break' horses when we are introducing them to being ridden; a three-day event can be held over 4

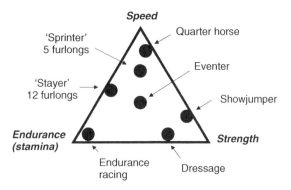

Fig. 1.2   Requirements for speed, strength and endurance in a range of equestrian sports.

days. What chance do outsiders have? Scientists also have their own language, one that is universal amongst all sorts of them, such as biochemists, geneticists, physiologists, etc. To be able to translate the results of scientific studies and apply them to real-life training situations we need to become familiar with the scientific vocabulary associated with equine exercise physiology.

Physiology is the study of the function of cells, tissues, organs and whole systems. Exercise physiology is thus the study of all systems involved in exercise. Exercise is a good example of a word commonly used in completely different contexts by scientists and horse people. Horse people often differentiate between lungeing a horse either for exercise or for work. The horse person's interpretation of this is that by lungeing for exercise you are merely allowing the horse to 'stretch its legs' on the end of the lunge line, but it is not asked to do anything too taxing. Lungeing a horse for work means that it would probably wear side reins or maybe a 'gadget', e.g. a pessoa, and would be asked to engage its hindquarters and carry itself in a correct outline. To a scientist, work refers to the energy used up when an object moves a known or fixed distance; the amount of work done is described in terms of the energy used and is commonly measured in units such as joules (J) or kilojoules (kJ), or calories (cal) or kilocalories (kcal). A force has to be applied in order to perform work, and this force requires energy to be expended. Therefore the horse is doing work simply by moving from A to B. In scientific circles, 'work' does not infer anything about the quality of the movement (i.e. speed, distance or direction), simply that something has moved. In fact, in strict scientific terms, it takes the same amount of energy to move a horse from A to B at a walk as it does at the gallop: the difference is in the rate at which energy is used. The same amount of energy is required to move from A to B, regardless of the speed, but when the horse moves at the gallop, the rate of energy utilisation must be greater. The rate of energy usage is referred to in terms of power. Power is measured in terms of the rate of work done (units of energy per unit time), e.g. in joules per second or watts. In galloping from A to B, the horse must generate more power than if he walks from A to B. Exercise refers to any movement or activity, so as soon as the horse moves off from a standstill, it is performing exercise. To use our scientific terms, if the horse is exercising, work is being done.

Training is another term that may have different interpretations depending upon the context in which it is used. To horse people, 'training' often implies that the horse is learning: its 'basic training' is its basic education. To an exercise physiologist, training is a long-term process of repeated bouts of exercise, which results in an improvement in fitness, where fitness refers to a certain capacity for exercise. Training for improvement in fitness is sometimes also referred to as 'conditioning', particularly in the USA.

Throughout exercise and training, the horse's body should make certain physiological adjustments, adaptations or responses. An exercise response is any short-term physiological adaptation that is made as a result of an increase in the level of muscular activity, whilst a training response is a long-term physiological adaptation to repeated bouts of increased muscular activity. Exercise responses tend to return to baseline levels after the work is done. For example, during exercise there is an increase in heart rate, corresponding to the intensity of the work done. When the horse stops exercising, the heart rate will gradually return to resting levels. Training responses are more long lasting and are maintained as long as the horse continues to regularly undertake a certain volume of work. For example, a training response may be an increase in heart mass (weight) or an increase in the

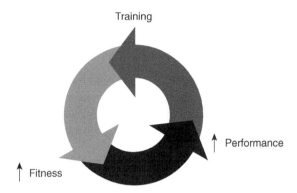

Fig. 1.3 Training leads to an increase in fitness and an improvement in performance.

number of capillaries (small blood vessels) around each muscle fibre. Changes such as these occur over a period of time as the horse responds to a gradual increase in workload, but they do not change throughout the course of an exercise bout. Training changes are mainly mediated through activation of genes that may then 'code' for greater production of an enzyme in an aerobic energy pathway, for example.

The type of work undertaken is particularly important in determining whether or not a training response is induced. For example, walking a horse 16 km (10 miles) a day, 3 days a week for a month may produce a noticeable loss of body mass (bodyweight) as the horse will be using up a considerable amount of energy on each of these walks. However, it may do very little in terms of increasing fitness, i.e. producing a training response. When we think about training it is therefore not simply how much energy we use, i.e. the volume of work, that counts but the way in which that work is done, i.e. the quality of work, to induce appropriate training responses.

In summary, if we want to improve our horse's performance, we would do well to increase their fitness (Fig. 1.3). This can be done by carrying out regular exercise, of progressively increasing workloads, to bring about the necessary training responses. The key is knowing what is the right work for what sport and when to settle for less than 100% fitness to reduce the risk of injury that might come from training very hard for a long time.

KEY POINTS

- Horses are natural athletes.
- Probably the biggest impact we can have on how well a horse performs is through training.
- The aims of training are to increase the time to the onset of fatigue, improve performance and decrease the risk of injury.
- Physiology is the study of the function of cells, tissues, organs or whole systems.
- Exercise means that work is done and so by definition energy is used.
- Exercise responses, e.g. an increase in heart rate, are short term.
- Training is a longer process of many repeated bouts of exercise that brings about an increase in fitness.
- Training responses, e.g. an increase in heart size, occur over a relatively long period of time.

Chapter 2

Energetics of exercise

Introduction

A little knowledge of biochemistry is a powerful thing! When you first become aware of the cellular processes involved in the conversion of nutrients into mechanical energy for muscle contraction it is like an enormous penny dropping, making so much of what the nutritionists tell us fall into place. For performance horses, one of the most important considerations is the energy content of the diet. To make sure our horse has enough energy for exercise, it helps to understand something about the way the horse's muscles obtain energy from nutrients within the diet, and this forms the basis of the study of the energetics of exercise. Awareness of the energetics of exercise can help us formulate a diet to achieve a specific result. As far as interpretation of energetics is concerned, the horse is not dissimilar to a car: we input fuel at great expense and we expect a certain performance in terms of mechanical output. The horse, like the petrol engine in a car, is required to perform mechanical work. Unlike cars, however, the horse can run on a variety of fuels, and we can expect to see a difference in performance depending upon the type of fuel we put in.

Horse diets usually vary from being 100% forage-based to about 80% cereal-based. We should never feed a 100% cereal-based diet to horses, because they need a certain minimum amount of forage for effective functioning of the digestive tract. Consequently, most horses are fed a combination of forage and cereals which has to be broken down by a combination of mechanical, chemical and microbial digestive processes. The products of digestion are then absorbed into the bloodstream mainly from the small and large intestine. Some of these products may be used immediately to supply energy for muscular contraction, but the majority are more likely to be converted to fuel stores within the liver, muscle and adipose tissue (fat) to be used at a later date. Regardless of the type of feed we put into the horse, all the nutrients capable of releasing energy for work (glucose, fatty acids and amino acids) are ultimately converted to just one vital ingredient – ATP or adenosine triphosphate. ATP is our energy 'currency' that is required for normal functioning of all cells both at rest and during exercise.

The resting horse

A certain amount of fuel must be provided within the diet to support the horse's energy requirements at rest and to do so whilst maintaining its body mass. Within 1 or 2 hours of a meal, particularly a cereal meal, the levels of glucose in the horse's blood rise from about 5 millimoles per litre (mmol/l) of blood to about 7 mmol/l of blood. In response to this increase, the pancreas increases the secretion of insulin, a hormone that acts to decrease blood glucose, and several hours later the blood glucose levels are restored to 5 mmol/l. Insulin brings about a lowering of blood glucose by increasing the uptake of glucose into the muscle and liver. In other words, in times of plenty the emphasis is on accumulation of potential fuel sources within the liver and muscle. This ensures that muscle has sufficient fuel stores should there be an increase in muscle activity, and also that the liver has sufficient fuel stores to 'buffer' fluctuations in blood glucose arising as a result of exercise. Whilst glucose has a very important role in providing energy for muscular contraction, it is far more important from a physiological 'housekeeping' perspective to ensure that the brain and the heart are provided with glucose, because glucose is the primary fuel source for these vital organs. One of the most important functions of the liver, aided by a number of hormones, is to act as a 'glucostat', i.e. a regulator of blood glucose, ensuring that blood glucose does not significantly decrease or increase, thereby guaranteeing a constant supply of glucose for the brain and heart, regardless of whether the horse is fed, starved, exercised or rested.

The energy for muscle contraction

Energy cannot be created or destroyed: it is merely converted from one form into another. All animals convert chemical energy from food into mechanical energy of work and heat is given off as a by-product. No process of converting stored or potential energy into work or movement is 100% efficient. In fact, animals (including humans) are rather inefficient energy converters, with only around 20% of the energy obtainable from food being converted into useful work, i.e. used for movement by muscle, and the rest (about 80%) being released as heat. To put this in context of mechanical engines, modern car engines would be able to convert around 20–30% of the potential energy in petrol into movement.

Adenosine triphosphate (ATP) is the universal fuel source: it has to be produced and stored within all cells in the body, whether muscle cells or any other cell, because it cannot be transported around the body. ATP is stored throughout the muscle cell. The structure of ATP is shown in Fig. 2.1. It is made up of adenosine attached to ribose and three phosphate groups. Only a certain amount of ATP can exist within the muscle: this is approximately 6 mmol/kg wet muscle (equivalent to 24 mmol/kg dry muscle) or approximately 700 g throughout all the skeletal muscle in the body of a 500 kg horse.

ATP provides a chemical energy source that is used by all cells, in all animals. Muscles cannot contract or even relax without ATP being present. When muscle cells contract, ATP is broken down into adenosine diphosphate (ADP) and phosphate (see Fig. 2.1), a reaction that is triggered by an enzyme within the muscle cell called adenosine triphosphatase (ATPase). The breakdown of ATP to ADP releases a fixed amount of energy – exactly 1.8 kJ per mole of ATP. To give some idea of the

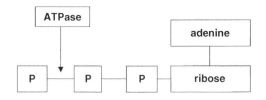

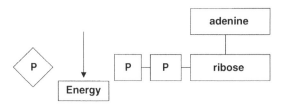

Fig. 2.1 Adenosine triphosphate breakdown to adenosine diphosphate.

enormous rate of ATP regeneration, consider that the average person turns over (breaks down and restores) more than half their own bodyweight in ATP in a day, just at rest. An active horse may actually turn over four times their own bodyweight in ATP per day. The chemical breakdown of fuel stored within the muscle ensures that this enormous demand for ATP is met.

The main fuels used to provide energy are glucose, glycogen (both glucose and glycogen are forms of carbohydrate) and fatty acids (fat). Protein is only used to provide energy in cases of extreme exhaustion, starvation or disease. Glucose and fatty acids both circulate in the bloodstream and can also be easily taken up or released by muscles. Glycogen is the animal equivalent of starch in plants and is simply a long string of glucose units joined together. Because of its structure and size, glycogen in cells cannot leave and enter the bloodstream. The main sites of glycogen storage are within liver and muscle.

The conversion of food into useful energy for exercise

Muscle contractions can only be produced using ATP. Because only a small amount of ATP exists within the muscle and this is rapidly used up during exercise (in fact within one or two muscle contractions), to continue working the muscle must constantly regenerate ATP by phosphorylating ADP to ensure a constant release of energy. The phosphorylation of ADP is achieved by several different biochemical processes or energy pathways within the muscle cell, all of which require the input of nutrients or fuels. One way to look at this would be to think about electricity and gas which are two different forms of energy or fuel. Electricity could be produced from a gas turbine generating station, but we can only light a bulb using electricity not gas. ATP is the equivalent of electricity, whereas gas is the equivalent of all the other potential fuels such as glucose, glycogen and fat. You may wonder why we cannot simply stick the phosphate back on to the ADP to regenerate ATP. To do so would be like trying to send the reaction uphill against an energy gradient: if it were possible to recycle ATP in this fashion, there would be no need to obtain energy from our diet and exercise could continue indefinitely. Simple recycling is not an option, and if we do not want to deplete our stores of ATP, we must utilise fuel supplies. Ideally, we should aim to regenerate ATP as fast as it is being used up by muscular contractions. The faster an animal travels, the greater the rate of ATP consumption by the muscles and the more quickly it needs to regenerate ATP from ADP to match demand to supply. Whilst regeneration of ATP from ADP is important to maintain a high ATP concentration, it is also important to keep the ADP concentration low because an increase in free ADP may contribute to muscle fatigue.

The energy demands of a single bout of exercise can significantly deplete a horse's fuel stores; however, on a day-to-day basis, the food provided in the horse's diet should keep the main carbohydrate and fat stores stocked up. Carbohydrates and fats are stored within the liver, skeletal muscle and adipose tissue. Glucose (a carbohydrate) is stored as glycogen within the liver and skeletal muscle, whilst fatty acids (fat) are stored as triglycerides within liver, muscle and adipose tissue, e.g. around the withers, crest, loins and around internal organs. A certain amount of fuel is available within the bloodstream, in the form of glucose and free fatty acids. The primary fuel supplies for any given piece of exercise are normally provided by glycogen

within the muscle and free fatty acids from the bloodstream. Fuel stores within the liver and adipose tissue are used to top up the muscle stores when demand for energy is substantially increased as a result of exercise of either high intensity or long duration.

Energy pathways

There are several biochemical routes for phosphorylation of ADP, otherwise known as 'energy pathways', and one or more of these pathways will be automatically selected within any particular period of exercise. However, it is important to understand that the pathways available are not used on an all or nothing basis and that a number of different pathways may be used simultaneously for generating energy. The different pathways vary in their fuel economy, i.e. in how much ATP is released per gram of fuel broken down, and also in their 'performance', i.e. how quickly ATP is made available for contraction. There is no one energy pathway that has both a high ATP yield, i.e. is economic, and a high rate of ATP production, i.e. a high performance. The horse will therefore select a particular combination of energy pathways depending on the nature of the exercise and the state of its fuel stores. There are four basic energy pathways, two requiring oxygen (aerobic energy pathways) and two that do not require oxygen (anaerobic energy pathways). It is important to understand that the two anaerobic pathways are not only used in situations when there is no oxygen around. They are called anaerobic because they do not need oxygen, but they may be used when there is a plentiful supply of oxygen to the muscle.

Pathway 1: anaerobic phosphorylation of ADP using high energy phosphate stores in muscle

High energy phosphates include molecules such as phosphocreatine (PCr) that have high energy phosphate bonds. In other words, the energy is bound up in their structure. If these molecules can be broken down, the energy stored within their bonds becomes available for the regeneration of ATP from ADP. The production of ATP from ADP using

PCr is catalysed by creatine phosphokinase (CK or CPK), and is described by the chemical equation

$$PCr + ADP \rightarrow Cr + ATP$$

Phosphocreatine thus provides a quick method of regenerating ATP for use by the muscle. By 'stealing' a phosphate from PCr, ATP is very quickly regenerated within the muscle cell. Phosphocreatine stores can be used in this way to regenerate enough ATP rapidly, but there is only enough stored PCr to last for several seconds' exercise. Earlier we learned that the concentration of ATP in the horse's muscle is around 6 mmol/kg wet muscle, but the amount of stored PCr is around 15–20 mmol/kg wet muscle. However, it is important to emphasise again that the muscle cells cannot use the energy bound in the phosphate bond in PCr directly, but only after it has been transferred to ATP.

In certain circumstances, another reaction known as the myokinase reaction (named after the enzyme catalysing the reaction) may take place. This reaction occurs when the rate of breakdown of ATP is very fast, such as during acceleration or galloping, and the concentration of free ADP within the muscle fibres (cells) starts to increase. In this instance, ADP is the high energy phosphate, but also like PCr, it cannot be used directly by the muscle cells. However, when two ADP molecules are combined, one ADP effectively loses a phosphate (producing a molecule of adenosine monophosphate, AMP) whilst the other ADP gains a phosphate to become ATP. The chemical equation for this reaction is

$$ADP + ADP \rightarrow ATP + AMP$$

The myokinase reaction normally only occurs during high intensity exercise and then primarily in those muscle fibres which are recruited during high speed exercise, acceleration and jumping. Reactions such as this are often self-limiting in that if there is a build up of, in this case, AMP, the reaction from left to right will slow down. Because increases in ADP may be related to the fatigue process in high intensity exercise, the aim would be to try and keep the ADP low by removing it as fast as it appears. To do this, the muscle also needs a way to remove the AMP: this is carried out by the enzyme AMP deaminase. AMP deaminase converts AMP to inosine monophosphate (IMP) and ammonia.

All these reactions regenerate ATP quickly and without the use of oxygen. High energy phosphates such as PCr are used at the onset of exercise or for an explosive effort such as in a jump, or whenever speed of ATP regeneration is the primary requirement. The stores of ATP and PCr are small; therefore to sustain exercise for more than merely a few seconds, the body must switch to other energy pathways to regenerate ATP for muscle contraction. Once other forms of energy production have taken over, the high energy phosphate stores will themselves be replenished if exercise is of low to medium intensity. During higher intensity exercise the muscle ATP and PCr concentrations may be reduced by 50–70% by the end of the exercise bout as a result of decreases in muscle pH consequent to lactic acid production (see later).

The following two energy pathways (see pathways 2 and 3) involve the breakdown of fuel stores to support exercise lasting from several minutes to many hours. Fuel stored in the form of fat and carbohydrate can be broken down aerobically, i.e. in the presence of and requiring oxygen, to produce significant amounts of energy in the form of ATP. Glycogen (a carbohydrate) is a very large polymer (many strings of glucose molecules) of glucose residues and is the animal storage form of glucose (equivalent to starch in plants). By storing glucose in the form of glycogen, energy from glucose is available between meals. The glycogen molecules themselves vary enormously in size, existing in cells in the form of glycogen granules that cannot pass out of the cell into the bloodstream.

Pathway 2: aerobic (oxidative) phosphorylation of ADP using carbohydrate stores

The breakdown of glycogen within the muscle using oxygen involves several stages, with oxygen playing a part only in the final stage. The first stage of the breakdown involves the conversion of glycogen to pyruvate, which occurs in the cytoplasm of the muscle cell and without the involvement of oxygen. The conversion of glycogen to pyruvate involves a specific sequence of phosphorylating reactions known as glycolysis (see Fig. 2.2). Glycolysis itself takes place rapidly but only yields a small amount

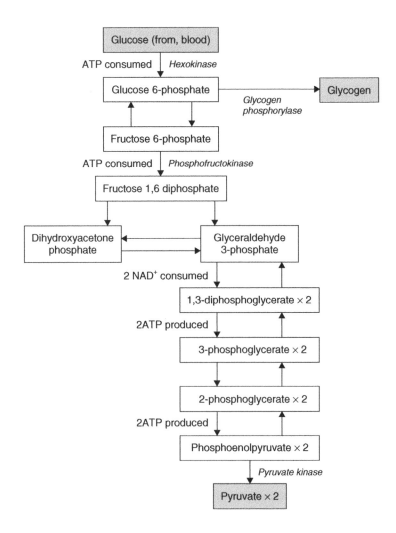

Fig. 2.2 Glycolysis.

of ATP directly (three ATP molecules per glucose unit broken down from carbohydrate stored within the muscle, i.e. from glycogen). However, more importantly, glycolysis produces two molecules of pyruvate that are used to feed into the next stage of the aerobic energy pathway, ultimately yielding considerably more ATP. Up to this stage, all reactions have taken place in the cytoplasm of the muscle cell.

The next stage in the aerobic breakdown of glycogen is the conversion of pyruvate to another three-carbon structure known as acetyl coenzyme A (acetyl CoA). This reaction only occurs inside mitochondria and is catalysed by an enzyme called pyruvate dehydrogenase (PDH). Mitochondria are found throughout the muscle cell, but particularly around the myofibrils (see Chapter 3). Mitochondria are specialised structures with an outer mem-

brane and an inner folded membrane on which the enzymes of oxidative phosphorylation are located. The folding of the membrane increases the surface area available for reactions to take place. The number of mitochondria within a cell or tissue is an indication of its activity. Hence, the density of mitochondria is high in both locomotory muscle and cardiac muscle cells. Acetyl CoA then enters the third stage of the aerobic breakdown of glycogen that occurs within the mitochondria. Acetyl CoA initiates a series of reactions known as the tricarboxylic acid (TCA) cycle (see Fig. 2.3), also sometimes referred to as the Krebs cycle.

The net result of the TCA cycle is the production of two molecules of ATP and two hydrogen ions. Two hydrogen ions are also produced by glycolysis and these hydrogen ions combine with the two coenzymes nicotinamide adenine dinucleotide

(NAD) and flavin adenine dinucleotide (FAD) to produce NADH and FADH$_2$. NADH and FADH$_2$ enter the 'electron transport chain' (see Fig. 2.4) on the inner mitochondrial membrane.

The hydrogen ions are then split into electrons and protons, and through a series of chemical reactions ('electron transport') ADP is regenerated to yield 34 molecules of ATP and the hydrogen ions are eventually combined with oxygen to produce water. Because this process requires oxygen it can be termed aerobic or oxidative phosphorylation. The production of water at the end of the chain has the advantage of 'removing' hydrogen ions from the cell because these would make the inside of the cell acidic. Both glycogen and glucose can be used in glycolysis. Glycogen would be obtained from the muscles' own glycogen stores whilst glucose would be obtained from the bloodstream. The process of glycogen breakdown is known as glycogenolysis and results in the formation of glucose-1-phosphate. The breakdown of glycogen is controlled by an enzyme called glycogen phosphorylase which has both inactive and active forms, termed a and b. Whilst glucose units from glycogen breakdown end up as glucose-1-phosphate and after conversion to glucose-6-phosphate can enter directly into the glycolytic pathway, glucose taken up into the muscle from the blood must first be phosphorylated, i.e. have a phosphate added to make it into glucose-6-phosphate. This reaction is catalysed by an enzyme called hexokinase and requires a molecule of ATP to 'donate' a phosphate. The fact that glucose-1-phosphate is produced directly from glycogen breakdown saves an ATP being expended in the initial stages of glycolysis, and prevents leakage out of the muscle cell, because phosphorylated compounds, including ATP, ADP and AMP, cannot normally cross cell membranes unless these have been damaged. Whether the glucose units come from blood glucose or muscle glycogen, the first stage of glycolysis is therefore considered to be the production of glucose-6-phosphate.

Complete aerobic metabolism (breakdown) of one glucose unit from glycogen to water and carbon dioxide (formed from the TCA cycle) yields 39 molecules of ATP (three ATP from glycolysis, two ATP from the TCA cycle and 34 ATP from the electron transport chain). The complete aerobic breakdown of glucose taken up by the muscle cell from the

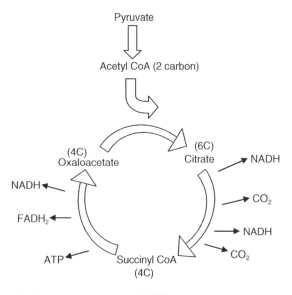

Fig. 2.3 Tricarboxylic acid (TCA) cycle.

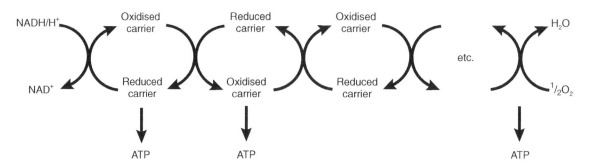

Fig. 2.4 Electron transport chain.

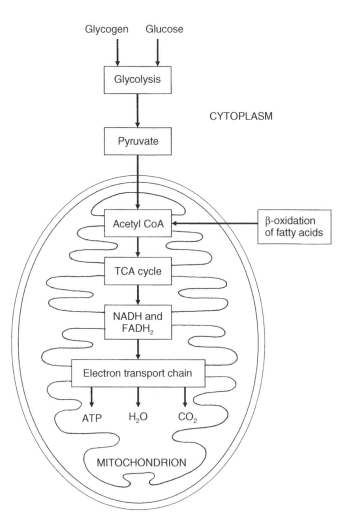

Fig. 2.5 Schematic overview of the stages of glycogen and fat breakdown.

bloodstream yields one less ATP because one ATP molecule is required to convert glucose to glucose-6-phosphate in the first stage of glycolysis. Therefore the net ATP yield from the aerobic breakdown of glucose is 39 − 1 = 38.

Pathway 3: aerobic phosphorylation of ADP using fatty acids

The aerobic breakdown of fat in the form of fatty acids begins with the conversion of 2-carbon chunks of fatty acid being converted to acetyl CoA by a process called beta-oxidation. In the breakdown of fat, acetyl CoA is therefore not produced by glycolysis but by beta-oxidation. The mitochon-

drial stages of the breakdown of fat, i.e. the TCA (Krebs) cycle and the electron transport chain, are thus identical to those of glycogen, but the steps leading to acetyl CoA formation are different. A schematic overview of the stages of glycogen and fat breakdown is shown in Fig. 2.5.

The individual stages involved in the aerobic breakdown of fat (as for carbohydrate) are also known collectively as oxidative phosphorylation. The yield of ATP from fat is always higher than for the same mass of carbohydrate (whether glucose or glycogen) but also varies between different types of fat source. The fats stored within the body are in a form known as triglycerides that consist of one molecule of glycerol and three fatty acid molecules. The

Table 2.1 Power, acceleration, oxygen requirement and capacity of the different sources of energy available to mammals (adapted from Sahlin (1985))

	Maximum power (mmol ATP/kg/s)	Time to reach maximum power	O_2 requirement (mmol O_2/ATP)	Work time to fatigue
Anaerobic				
ATP[a]	11.2	<1 s	0	seconds
PCr[b]	8.6	<1 s	0	seconds
CHO[c] → lactate	5.2	<5 s	0	minutes
Aerobic		2–3 min		
CHO[c] → CO_2 + H_2O	2.7	30 min	0.167	hours
FFA[d] → CO_2 + H_2O	1.4		0.177	days!!

[a] Adenosine triphosphate.
[b] Phosphocreatine.
[c] Carbohydrate.
[d] Free fatty acid.

triglycerides are broken down by enzymes known as lipases and the process is referred to as lipolysis. Once the fatty acids have been separated from their glycerol 'backbone', they are free to move into the bloodstream and be taken up by muscle. In this state they are known as free fatty acids (FFA). Muscle itself also contains small triglyceride stores that can also be broken down to liberate FFA that can be used inside the muscle cell. There are a number of different FFAs found in the body which differ primarily in the number of carbon atoms they contain. Volatile fatty acids (VFAs) are another very important source of fuel, being produced from the fermentation of carbohydrates in the large intestine. Once in the circulation VFAs can be taken up and used immediately to fuel muscle contraction after conversion to ATP; if not, they are stored in adipose tissue as triglycerides.

The complete aerobic metabolism of palmitic acid (a typical 16-carbon fatty acid) with the molecular formula $C_{16}H_{32}O_2$ yields 129 molecules of ATP net per molecule of fatty acid. The total production is 131 molecules of ATP, but two ATPs are used to 'activate' (prepare) the FFA before they can enter the TCA cycle. Activation of FFA takes place on the outer mitochondrial membrane before oxidative phosphorylation within the mitochondria that results in a total of 35 ATP. Every time the fatty acid chain is shortened by two carbons, one $FADH_2$ and one NADH are formed, resulting in the production of five ATP molecules by oxidative phosphorylation. In a 16-carbon fatty acid, the

chain is shortened by two carbons seven times to leave eight two-carbon pieces; hence $5 \times 7 = 35$ ATP. The TCA cycle yields eight ATP molecules directly and 88 by oxidative phosphorylation, totalling 131 ATP minus two ATP for fatty acid activation, giving 129 ATPs.

The fact that oxidative phosphorylation of fat yields about three times as much ATP as the oxidative phosphorylation of carbohydrate explains why fat is referred to as an 'energy-dense' food source. With one molecule of fat yielding three times as much energy as one molecule of carbohydrate, you can begin to see why exercising to lose fat often seems like an uphill struggle as you have to expend considerable amounts of energy at a relatively low intensity, i.e. exercise over a longer time in order to break down excess adipose tissue. On the positive side, the fact that fat is energy-dense is great news for endurance athletes, as a little bit of fat goes a long way. Even a thin horse will only use a small proportion of stored body fat to complete a 100-mile endurance race.

On a mass for mass basis, 1 gram of fat is better than 1 gram of carbohydrate when it comes to ATP yield, but the disadvantages of fat as a fuel are that, firstly, it requires far more oxygen to break down one molecule of fatty acid than it does to break down one molecule of glycogen. Secondly, the speed (rate) of energy release from fat is much slower than from carbohydrate (see Table 2.1). Exercise using fat as the main fuel source is therefore limited to trotting and slow–medium speed cantering. At speeds above this the body must gradually switch to using more and more carbohydrate to match the increased rate of ATP usage by the muscles with the rate of rephosphorylation of ADP. The faster a horse runs the less it is able to use fat as an energy source.

Pathway 4: anaerobic phosphorylation of ADP using carbohydrate

Technically, the conversion of ADP back to ATP using phosphocreatine (pathway 1, described above) is an anaerobic energy pathway, but the overall contribution of this energy pathway to the total energy cost of a bout of exercise is not usually significant because most exercise bouts last more than a few seconds. The most significant anaerobic energy pathway involves the conversion of glycogen or glucose to lactic acid to yield ATP. Only glycogen or glucose can be used to produce energy anaerobically via the glycolytic pathway. The glycolytic pathway involves the production of pyruvate from glucose or glycogen as in aerobic energy production, but this time, instead of the pyruvate being converted to acetyl CoA and entering the mitochondria, the pyruvate is converted to lactic acid by the enzyme lactate dehydrogenase (LDH). Lactic acid immediately dissociates into a free hydrogen ion (with a positive charge) and a lactate ion (with a negative charge). The two terms lactic acid and lactate are often used interchangeably, for example when referring to blood or plasma concentrations. Thus, the reactions involved in the aerobic and anaerobic productions of ATP are identical up to the point at which pyruvate is formed. The net result of the anaerobic breakdown of carbohydrate is the production of a small amount of ATP (three ATP molecules if glycogen is the glucose source and only two ATP molecules if blood glucose is used) and the conversion of NAD to NADH. NADH is an important intermediary in glycolysis and one that would normally be regenerated to NAD following the completion of the electron transport chain in oxidative phosphorylation. Because there is no electron transport chain in the anaerobic pathway, the only way of regenerating NAD from NADH to allow continued production of ATP by glycolysis is as a by-product of the conversion of pyruvate to lactic acid. If all the NAD in

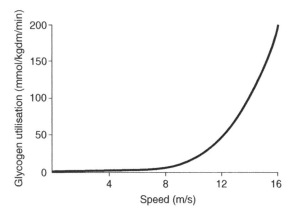

Fig. 2.6 Glycogen utilisation as a function of running speed.

a muscle cell were converted to NADH then glycolysis would stop. The production of lactic acid enables NADH to be regenerated to NAD and allows glycolysis to proceed beyond glyceraldehyde 3-phosphate.

$$Pyruvate + NADH \rightarrow Lactate + H^+ + NAD$$

The anaerobic energy yield from one molecule of 'glucose' from glycogen is three ATP molecules, whereas it is two ATP molecules for one molecule of glucose from blood. Two molecules of lactate are also formed which can be converted back to pyruvate and eventually to glucose by a process known as the Cori cycle. Because the anaerobic production of energy involves the conversion of pyruvate to lactate, it can be seen that it would be impossible to break down fat anaerobically.

Anaerobic energy production is inefficient but fast

When you need energy fast, such as during acceleration, when galloping or jumping, glycogen is broken down anaerobically to lactic acid. A major disadvantage of anaerobic energy production is the low ATP yield per molecule of glycogen or glucose; therefore substantial reliance on anaerobic energy production leads to significant depletion of muscle glycogen stores (Fig. 2.6). Resting muscle glycogen concentrations in the horse are in the region of 100 mmol/kg wet muscle, and up to around 150 mmol/kg wet muscle (600 mmol/kg dry muscle) or more in trained horses. Muscle glycogen concentrations can be reduced by one-third after just a single bout of high intensity exercise. Fine! Go fast, use lots of glycogen, but if you want to do it again in a few hours' time, or tomorrow, and the day after, and the day after that, you may run into trouble. The muscle needs a certain amount of time to restore the glycogen levels to those before exercise. In man, it has been shown that by manipulating the diet it is possible to both increase glycogen storage before exercise (glycogen loading) and to speed up glycogen repletion after exercise. So far, no one has managed to achieve the same in horses and it doesn't matter if after exercise you feed your horse hay, or hay and cereals, or even pure glucose powder, the rate of glycogen repletion appears to be the same.

The duration of exercise that you can undertake when using glycogen alone as the energy source is limited because fatigue is partly related to the acidification of the muscle cells by the free hydrogen ions produced in the conversion of pyruvate to lactic acid. At the sort of rates of glycogen breakdown seen during maximal all-out sprints, muscle glycogen stores can be reduced by around 50%. Even more glycogen can be used by carrying out repeated bouts of short, fast exercise with recovery periods in between (often termed intermittent, high intensity exercise or intermittent, maximal exercise). However, as more and more lactic acid is produced and the muscle pH becomes lower (more acid), a feedback mechanism takes over to prevent complete exhaustion of muscle glycogen stores. The rate of glycolysis slows and therefore so does the rate of glycogen breakdown and lactic acid production. This process of fatigue is actually protective. Whilst it is possible to completely use up all the muscle glycogen present in those cells used the most during high intensity exercise, it is not possible to deplete all cells in a muscle. Glycogen depletion can also occur in endurance exercise, affecting those cells used predominantly during low to medium intensity exercise (see Chapter 3).

Energy partitioning

At the onset of maximal exercise the demand for energy is high, but there is a lag time in reaching maximal aerobic energy production. In other words, anaerobic pathways are often necessary to supply energy for the early stages of exercise (even though there may be no shortage of oxygen in the muscle) whilst the aerobic pathways get up to speed. It can take up to at least a minute to reach maximal aerobic energy production at the start of maximal exercise. Thus the intensity of the exercise and the nature of the onset of the high intensity exercise (gradual increase in speed to maximum or flat out from a standing start) have a bearing on the extent to which aerobic and anaerobic pathways contribute to the overall energy requirement.

During low intensity exercise of long duration (exercise producing heart rates up to around 160 beats/min), energy is provided largely by aerobic pathways because these can produce ATP at a sufficient rate and offer the greatest fuel economy. During high intensity exercise of short duration energy is provided by anaerobic pathways offering high rates of ATP production but low fuel economy. However, there is not a point at which a direct switch from one source to the other occurs. At any point in time, some muscle fibres will be functioning aerobically and some anaerobically, but there is a general increase in the reliance on anaerobic pathways as speed increases. At speeds greater than 8–10 m/s, i.e. 500–600 m/min (around 20 mph), the mitochondria tend to back-up with substrate and there is neither sufficient area of mitochondrial membrane nor aerobic enzymes available to cope with demand. Latterly it was thought that the switch was due to lack of oxygen availability, but this is not usually the case. Oxygen delivery to the working muscles is usually sufficient; the main drive to begin to recruit anaerobic pathways is the point at which the aerobic energy pathways are working at maximum, but demand for ATP is still rising, i.e. the horse is being asked to go faster. The resultant shortfall in ATP supply must be addressed using anaerobic pathways resulting in an increase in blood lactate levels. The point at which lactate levels start to rise in often called the 'anaerobic threshold' (AT). This term is widely used among lay people to describe the point at which anaerobic pathways begin to contribute significantly to total energy requirements, but it is a slightly misleading term in that it implies there is a switch from one form of energy pathway to the other, which is not true, as described above.

The contribution of each energy pathway to the total energy requirement for exercise is known as energy partitioning. Scientists have been able to estimate how much each pathway contributes to the total energy requirements by measuring oxygen uptake and carbon dioxide and lactic acid production at various speeds of exercise. In the UK, the shortest distance raced is 5 furlongs or 1000 metres. In the USA, Quarter horses run over 2 furlongs or 400 m: these are the true sprinters of the horse world, reaching speeds of around 40 m.p.h. During exercise of this intensity and duration, the horse will obtain approximately 60% of its energy anaerobically and 40% aerobically. Compare this to human sprinters who run 100 metres near 100% anaerobically; only taking one or two breaths in 10 seconds. In contrast, the true equine sprinters, the Quarter horses, are running for at least double this time. In a middle distance Thoroughbred horse race such as the Derby run over $1\frac{1}{2}$ miles (2.4 km), the energy partitioning would be approximately 80% aerobic and 20% anaerobic. The anaerobic portion is mainly required for the acceleration at the start and for the last furlong or so.

The true endurance athletes of the horse world are able to complete 100 miles (160 km) in a day, travelling at speeds of 10 m.p.h. (16 km/h). True endurance horses will work about 96% aerobically at this speed. Even the speed and endurance day of a three-day event is predominantly aerobic (about 90%).

Normally, anaerobic energy production begins at a heart rate of around 150–180 beats/min, but there is great individual variation. A heart rate of 150–180 beats/min is the equivalent of a 'good' or three-quarter speed canter. In other words, as soon as the horse starts to really open up the canter stride, it is likely that it is getting some of its energy by anaerobic means, with the resultant appearance of lactic acid in the bloodstream.

Although it is possible to give general guidelines concerning the onset of anaerobic processes in muscle, a number of factors can affect the speed at which anaerobic energy production starts. For example, a horse will start anaerobic energy production at a lower speed when unfit compared to when fit. A horse that has a high proportion of fast-twitch high glycolytic ('sprinting' or type IIB fibres) in its muscles will produce lactate at a lower speed than a horse with few of this type of muscle fibre. Health problems that interfere with oxygen transfer from atmosphere to mitochondria, such as

upper airway obstruction, cardiovascular disease or lower airway disease will also tend to decrease the speed at which anaerobic energy production starts. Even excitement, pain, amount and type of warm-up exercise, time of feeding and environmental conditions can affect the point at which the anaerobic metabolism becomes significant and the concentration of lactic acid in blood begins to increase.

How can we tell what fuels are being used for energy generation? The amounts of oxygen used up and carbon dioxide produced vary according to the energy substrates being used at any point in time. The respiratory exchange ratio (RER) is the ratio of carbon dioxide production ($\dot{V}_{CO_2}$, litres/min) to oxygen consumption ($\dot{V}_{O_2}$, litres/min) measured at the nostril (p. 94). The ratio of carbon dioxide production to oxygen consumption or RER is 1.0 when carbohydrate is the only fuel being used and is being fully oxidised. However, when fat is the sole fuel source a relatively greater amount of oxygen is required and the RER is 0.7. Any RER value between 0.7 and 1.0 either at rest or during exercise therefore indicates that both fat and carbohydrate are being used simultaneously (see Table 2.2). During moderate to intense exercise, the production of lactic acid within muscles causes an increase in the hydrogen ion concentration of blood (blood pH decreases). As a consequence of the mechanism within the blood for buffering hydrogen ions, there is an increase in the amount of exhaled carbon dioxide. Thus, an RER above 1.0 indicates that some of the energy is coming from anaerobic lactic acid production. The higher the RER the greater the contribution from lactic acid to total energy production, with values as high as 1.4 being reached in intense exercise. However, once the RER has risen above 1.0 it is not possible to estimate the

Table 2.2 Approximate percentage contribution of energy from fat and carbohydrate during exercise in relation to respiratory exchange ratio (RER)

RER	% Energy from carbohydrate	% Energy from fat
0.70	0	100
0.80	33	66
0.90	66	33
1.0	100	0
>1.0	100	0

Table 2.3 Estimated times to exhaust each of the main body energy stores of a 500 kg horse if each fuel was used as the only energy source at 60% (endurance), 90% (four-star three-day event steeplechase speed) and 120% $\dot{V}_{O_2 max}$ (1 mile (1.6 km) flat race)

	Total body stores[a] (kJ)	Exercise time at		
		60% $\dot{V}_{O_2 max}$	90% $\dot{V}_{O_2 max}$	120% $\dot{V}_{O_2 max}$
ATP	38	3.3 s	1.8 s	1.1 s
PCr	188	16.3 s	9.0 s	5.7 s
Glycogen	75 300	109 min	60 min	38 min
Fat	640 000	15.4 h	8.5 h	–[b]

[a] From McMiken (1983).
[b] No figure has been calculated for 120% $\dot{V}_{O_2 max}$ because at this intensity no fat would be used.

relative contributions of fat and aerobic and anaerobic carbohydrate metabolism.

RER can be used to determine responses to dietary manipulation, exercise and training, and may also reflect the muscle fibre type composition in horses with very different muscle types. RER in humans can be around 0.7–0.8 at rest but is generally around 0.9 in horses. In a study of Standardbred horses fed different diets for 4 weeks each, RER was about 0.9 on a typical hay and concentrate diet, but was around 0.75 on a high fat diet (containing 15% soyabean oil), indicating that the horses were actually using more fat for energy at rest on the high fat compared to the normal hay–concentrate diet (Pagan *et al.* 1987).

Size of the fuel stores

How much fuel can a 500 kg horse carry? The sum of fat, muscle and liver comes to just over 230 kg, with muscle weighing about 200 kg, liver about 6.5 kg and fat about 25 kg.

The horse has around 95% of its total body glycogen stored in muscle and around 5% in the liver (although the actual concentration of glycogen in the liver is greater than in muscle). In contrast, around 95% of the body's fat is stored in adipose tissue, with only around 5% stored within the muscles.

Approximately ten times as much energy (either in terms of kilojoules or kilocalories) is stored as fat compared with glycogen (see Table 2.3). This means that if you were to oxidise or simply burn (literally

set alight) all the available fuel in the horse's body, the fat stores would give off ten times as much heat energy as glycogen. However, if all the available fuel is respired aerobically, approximately 30 times as much ATP is produced from the oxidative phosphorylation of fat as from the oxidative phosphorylation of glycogen. Remember, in terms of ATP yield, fat is better than glycogen, with over three times as much ATP produced per gram of fat compared with a gram of carbohydrate. Fat is an energy-dense source; literally, a little bit of fat goes a long way. If you were setting out on a day's walking or trekking and you had to carry all your food for the day, you would look to carry those foods which gave you lots of energy, but did not weigh very much; in other words, you would look for energy-dense foods. If you were a horse embarking upon a 100-mile endurance ride, it would pay you to use fat as your fuel source as far as possible because it is so energy-dense. Exercise is rarely, if ever, limited by running out of fat.

Fat is ideal for exercise where the body requires:

- Slow release of energy, i.e. for exercise at low speed
- A large energy reserve, i.e. for exercise of long distance or duration.

Training of low speed and long duration increases the number of enzymes involved in the oxidative phosphorylation of fat, so that the body becomes better at utilising fat, and will tend to rely more on fat as an energy source. This is good news for those of us thinking of training to get rid of unwanted fat: the more you train, the better you are at burning fat, but you must keep the speed and intensity of the exercise sessions low. If, as a rider you want to lose weight, i.e. reduce your body mass, there is no better way to start than by doing plenty of walking and slow jogging. Start to run faster and you will start using more and more carbohydrate up to a point where you won't be using any fat. You can get fit but won't necessarily weigh any less. It is alarming how many people still think that the best way to reduce a horse's waistline is to gallop and 'get a sweat on him'. If you gallop a fat horse, all you will do is:

(1) Risk breakdown of musculoskeletal structures
(2) Make it sweat and lose body mass (due to loss of fluid) in the short term which it will put back on as soon as it can drink
(3) Use up muscle glycogen
(4) Give it an appetite!

You will not encourage utilisation of fat stores. It is also worth being aware that when you train your horse, although its shape and appearance may change, its body mass may not change dramatically. This doesn't mean that you aren't working it hard enough. Fat is less dense than muscle. The density of fat is $0.9007 \, \text{g/cm}^3$ ($1 \, \text{cm}^3 = 1 \, \text{ml}$), whilst the density of muscle is $1.065 \, \text{g/cm}^3$, i.e. 20% more dense than fat. That means that the same volume of fat weighs less than the same volume of muscle. Therefore, if you replace 1 kg of body fat by 1 kg of muscle, it will take up less space but you will have the same body mass. This is why dieting combined with exercise may mean your shape changes as you lose fat but your body mass may stay the same or even increase as a result of muscle development from the exercise.

Running out of energy

Fatigue during exercise is almost never caused by running out of fat because the fat stores through-out the body are so plentiful, but is commonly due to running out of muscle and/or liver glycogen. Depletion of muscular glycogen leads to muscular fatigue. Depletion of liver glycogen and as a consequence low blood glucose may make you feel light headed and tired. Human athletes competing in long duration events use a technique called glycogen loading or carbohydrate loading to try and offset fatigue. It involves either exercising to fatigue or fasting in order to deplete the existing glycogen stores, and then eating large quantities of a high carbohydrate meal. Depletion before loading seems to increase the amount of glycogen that it is possible to store. Glycogen loading is not recommended in horses because it would require the feeding of large, high carbohydrate meals, when we know that high energy feeds should be split up into several small meals to avoid conditions such as colic or azoturia (tying-up).

Whilst we should not attempt to strategically glycogen load our horses, it is likely that a horse in hard regular work that is not provided with sufficient energy in its diet will be at a disadvantage. Following a hard piece of work that significantly reduces muscle glycogen, such as a short fast gallop, it may take 2 days for the horse to fully replenish the glycogen stores. This should be remembered when planning a training programme that involves fast work. You cannot expect a horse to perform intense work, e.g. maximal sprint or interval work, well more than two or three times a week or on consecutive days, because glycogen stores will not be fully replenished before the next bout of intense work. In addition, the rate at which glycogen can be broken down in glycolysis to yield ATP has been shown to be dependent on its concentration. If the concentration is high, the rate of breakdown will be high and vice versa. This is likely to be an advantage in high intensity sprint or jumping events.

KEY POINTS

- Energy that is used each day for exercise must be replaced by energy obtained from the diet.

- Glycogen (the animal form of starch) and fat represent the two main sources and body stores of energy.

- Cells cannot use glucose, glycogen or fat directly, only the energy released from the breakdown of ATP to ADP.
- At rest, food is converted via digestion to stores of glycogen (liver and muscle) and fat (adipose tissue).
- Energy cannot be created or destroyed, only changed from one form to another.
- The efficiency of conversion of energy into useful, mechanical work is only around 20%.
- Stores of ATP within the body are only sufficient for several seconds of exercise; for continued exercise ADP must be regenerated to ATP by two anaerobic (PCr and glycolysis to lactic acid) or aerobic pathways (oxidative phosphorylation of glucose or glycogen or fatty acids).

- PCr and metabolism of glucose or glycogen to lactic acid regenerate ADP fast without the need for oxygen but inefficiently, i.e. only a small amount of ADP is regenerated.
- Aerobic oxidation of carbohydrate and fat require oxygen and are much more efficient but regenerate ADP to ATP more slowly.
- Energy partitioning describes the relative contribution of different pathways of ADP regeneration at different stages of exercise and during different types of activity.
- The respiratory exchange ratio (RER) indicates what fuels are being used at any point in time.
- Fat stores almost never limit exercise capacity, but carbohydrate (glycogen) stores can become significantly depleted by repeated bouts of high speed exercise or prolonged endurance exercise.

Chapter 3

Muscles

Introducing skeletal muscle

Muscles are what make the skeleton move. When stimulated by their associated nerve supply muscles contract and exert forces on joints. As well as bringing about movement, skeletal muscles also enable the animal to maintain its posture. There are around 700 skeletal muscles in the horse making up 40–50% of the total body mass. In Thoroughbreds, the muscles may constitute as much as 55% of the body mass, giving a greater power-to-body mass ratio than many other breeds of horse. In comparison, skeletal muscle only makes up around 40% of the body mass of an average man. Muscle is a form of excitable tissue, so called because electrical impulses can be transmitted along its cell membranes in much the same way as nerve impulses are transmitted. Skeletal muscle operates under what is known as voluntary or conscious control. There are muscles within the body that cannot be influenced by conscious control, such as the muscle lining the airways, blood vessels or gastrointestinal tract, and these are known as involuntary muscles. In fact there are three basic types of muscle within the body:

(1) Smooth (or involuntary) muscle
(2) Cardiac (or heart) muscle
(3) Skeletal (striated or voluntary) muscle.

Skeletal muscle is made up of numerous muscle bundles and each muscle bundle is made up of hundreds of individual muscle fibres (Fig. 3.1). A muscle fibre is actually an elongated single muscle cell. The blood supply for muscle fibres is supplied by an extensive capillary network that runs between the fibres. In horse muscle, there are from 200 to 1000 capillaries per mm^2. Skeletal muscle contracts under the control of motor nerves. Each individual motor nerve fibre terminates at its branched end on several muscle fibres. A nerve fibre plus the muscle fibres it supplies (innervates) is called a motor unit. One motor nerve will supply anywhere from 10 to 2000 muscle fibres, often widely distributed throughout a region of muscle. Where fine precise movements are required, the number of muscle fibres served by one nerve fibre is small, perhaps as few as ten per nerve. Such motor units are found within the eye muscle and the muscles of the lips and ears. Less precise but more powerful movements are brought about by motor units where the number of muscle fibres served by one nerve fibre is greater with up to around 2000 muscle fibres per nerve fibre. Large motor units like this are found in the *gastrocnemius* muscle of the hind limb and the *longissimus dorsi* muscle along the back.

All skeletal muscles receive a certain amount of nerve impulses, even when the muscles are not being used. This 'baseline' stimulation may amount to only a few impulses per second and is known as tone. Tone exists to prepare muscle for contraction and to maintain posture. Immobilisation or nerve damage as a result of injury that prevents this baseline electrical activity can lead to muscle wastage (atrophy). Atrophy can be corrected by increasing the level of activity of the muscle and improving its blood supply, for example by using specific exercises, massage, or controlled muscle stimulation using electrotherapy techniques.

An adequate blood supply is also essential for normal muscle function. In practice, this means that a horse should be warmed up thoroughly before performing any strenuous activity. Not only does this allow sufficient time for the blood supply to the muscle to be increased to meet the increased demand for oxygen, but also it literally increases the temperature within the muscles by about 1°C, bringing them to their optimum working temperature.

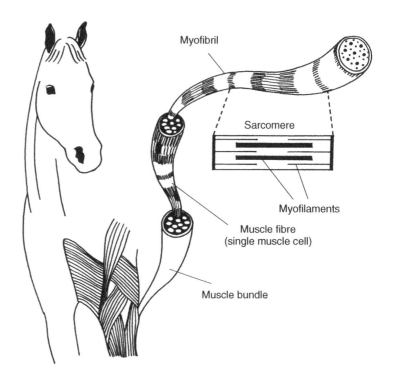

Fig. 3.1   Structure of skeletal muscle.

Inside the muscle cell

A single muscle may contain up to one million muscle fibres. Each individual muscle fibre is simply a single muscle cell. Each muscle fibre is approximately 30–100 μm in diameter, but individual fibres can vary in length from a few millimetres to several centimetres. The muscle fibre consists of:

- An outer cell membrane called a sarcolemma
- Nuclei (squeezed to edge of cell)
- Glycogen granules
- Fat droplets
- Red muscle pigment (myoglobin) that stores oxygen and helps with its movement across the cell
- Mitochondria (the aerobic power station of the cell)
- Hundreds of myofibrils made up of myofilaments, which consist of contractile proteins.

The repeating unit of organisation within the muscle fibre is called the sarcomere (see Fig. 3.2).

The sarcomere is also the functional unit of contraction and is made up largely of special contractile proteins. Muscle contraction is brought about by these contractile proteins moving across one another and exerting a force that acts to shorten the sarcomere by pulling the Z lines closer towards the centre. Closer examination of these contractile proteins and their structural arrangement enables us to understand the process of muscle contraction. Under a microscope, bands within the sarcomere can be identified as follows:

- *I band* This corresponds to the area within the sarcomere containing only thin myofilaments. The thin filaments are made up of a protein called actin. These filaments are approximately 5 nm in diameter and 10 000 nm long. They extend from the Z line towards the centre of the sarcomere. Actin is a polymer of G-actin that forms an alpha helix. In the groove of the alpha helix lies another protein called tropomyosin (see Fig. 3.3). A further protein, troponin is attached to tropomyosin. There are three troponin subunits, T, C and I.
- *H band* This consists of thick myofilaments which have a diameter of 12 nm and are 1600 nm in length. Each thick filament is surrounded by a

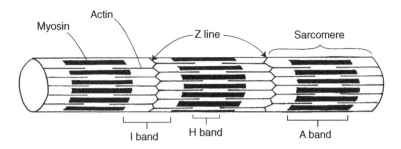

Fig. 3.2 A section of the myofibril showing the repeating unit of organisation – the sarcomere.

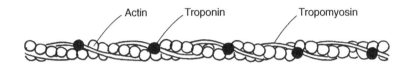

Fig. 3.3 The actin polymer, showing the position of tropomyosin and troponin.

hexagonal array of thin filaments, and helically arranged cross-bridges extend towards the thin filaments.

* *A band* This includes the H band and the region of overlap of myosin and actin fibres. It is the length of the myosin filaments.

Muscle contraction is brought about by the shortening of individual sarcomeres in sequence in response to a nerve impulse arriving at a specialised area of the muscle membrane known as the motor end-plate. Sarcomere shortening occurs as a result of the movement of the contractile proteins, myosin and actin within it, a process known as excitation–contraction coupling.

How does the nerve impulse make the muscle contract?

The incoming electrical signal alters the electrical charge on either side of the muscle membrane and causes a small electrical charge to 'flow' along the membrane. The flow of charge is carried deep within the muscle fibre along transverse tubules which are invaginations of the muscle cell membrane.

The transverse tubules are in close proximity to specialised areas of the sarcoplasmic reticulum (SR). The SR serves to sequester intracellular calcium. The arrival of the electrical impulse at the SR causes calcium ion channels to open within the SR membrane. Calcium ions are then able to leave the SR and enter the muscle cytoplasm.

Sequence of events in muscular contraction

The arrival of an electrical impulse causes the release of calcium ions into the cytoplasm of the muscle cell; this raises the concentration of free calcium ions within the muscle cell cytoplasm about 1000-fold. Calcium ions then bind to troponin C, which has four calcium binding sites. The binding of calcium ions to troponin C causes a configurational change in troponin I. This change in troponin I lifts tropomyosin off the binding sites on actin and allows the myosin head to bind to the actin. Effectively, the binding site on actin is protected by troponin until the concentration of calcium is increased. The myosin head contains an ATPase that is able to split a phosphate from ATP to provide the energy for the binding of myosin to actin. Having bound to actin, the myosin head moves through 90°, pulling the actin filament along with it towards the centre of the sarcomere (see Fig. 3.4). The H band, which was made up of myosin filaments, disappears as the filaments slide over each other. A process of binding and release, binding and release then follows, with the actin filaments moving over one another in a ratchet-like fashion.

Both the process of contraction and the process of release require ATP. If no ATP was available and calcium ion concentrations remained high in the muscle cell, the muscle cell could not relax. After an animal dies, the ATP in the muscle cells is gradually used up, because there is no longer a supply

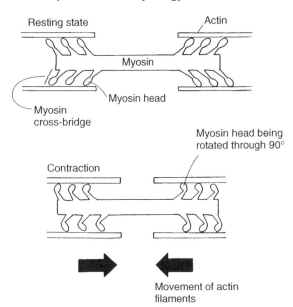

Fig. 3.4 Rotation of the myosin head during muscle contraction.

of oxygen to keep the mitochondria functioning, and glycolysis will eventually stop as muscle cell pH falls to around 5. At some point in time there will be no ATP left to provide the energy to uncouple actin and myosin, and so the muscle is unable to relax, and the body is in *rigor mortis*. Relaxation only occurs when enzymes known as proteases that are released after death start to break down the proteins forming the muscle cross-bridges.

Following a contraction, ATP is needed to pump calcium back into the SR. The ability to do so may become impaired when the muscle ATP stores become reduced, as is often the case towards the end of a piece of hard, fast work. Measurements of ATP concentration in muscle samples containing several thousand individual muscle fibres taken by muscle biopsy show that after such work, the average concentration may have fallen from the resting value of around 6 mmol/kg wet muscle to 2–3 mmol/kg wet muscle. However, studies of the ATP content of single muscle fibres show that rather than all fibres showing a similar decrease in ATP, some fibres may have virtually no ATP left whilst others have a near resting concentration. The ATP content of an individual muscle fibre after exercise will probably therefore reflect the extent

to which it was recruited (used) during the preceding exercise.

Properties of muscular activity

Whilst the characteristics of the nerve impulse do not change, i.e. the nerve impulse is an 'all or nothing' event – the nerve either fires or doesn't fire, the characteristics of the associated muscle response must vary considerably by selective motor unit activation in order to be able to produce an almost infinite series of responses, graded according to the strength of the muscle action that is required. We need to be able to produce muscle actions that are finely controlled in terms of strength of response and speed of contraction. Much of the voluntary motor control originates in a part of the brain called the basal ganglia. The knowledge of the involvement of the basal ganglia in motor function comes mainly from observations of motor function abnormalities occurring as a result of damage or degeneration in these areas, e.g. in Parkinson's disease (producing tremor) and choreas (producing rapid, jerky and involuntary movements). The strength of a motor response depends on how many motor units are activated at any one time. Narrow diameter nerves have a low threshold for stimulation and generally supply motor units with few muscle fibres, whilst larger diameter nerves (which require a greater stimulus to make them fire) supply motor units with larger numbers of muscle fibres. The narrow diameter nerves have what is known as a low threshold potential; in other words, they respond to very low levels of sensory stimuli. The greater the magnitude of the incoming stimuli, the more nerve fibres and consequently the more muscle fibres that will be recruited, i.e. will contract. The maximum strength of a muscle is realised when all nerve fibres, even those of the highest threshold, are stimulated. It is not possible to recruit all muscle fibres under voluntary control, but this can be achieved using involuntary electrical stimulation. An increase in the number of muscle fibres stimulated with increasing strength of the stimulus is known as recruitment. This is one of the fundamental ways in which different grades of muscular response are brought about. Just as different numbers and types of muscle fibres are recruited at various stages of exercise, so they will fatigue at different stages. This explains why you can often delay fatigue by alternating between types of exercise, such as in circuit training, or 'Fartlek' training. Fartlek training is a type of exercise regime that involves short bursts of high intensity work superimposed on a background of low intensity continuous exercise. As the slow and fast work will use slightly different numbers and types of muscle fibres and the horse's muscle switches between using different groups of muscle fibres throughout the exercise period, fatigue can be delayed.

The type of response elicited from a muscle depends not only on the number of nerve fibres stimulated, but also on the frequency with which the nerve impulses arrive at the motor end-plate. The application of a single nerve impulse to a muscle fibre leads to a single contraction and re-laxation within the muscle fibre known as a single twitch (see Fig. 3.5). This is the mechanical response to an electrical stimulus.

In a single twitch, the mechanical event (the contraction) lasts longer than the electrical event (the nerve impulse). There is a delay of about 3 milliseconds between the start of the action potential and the start of the muscular contraction. This delay represents the time it takes for the electrical charge to spread through the T-tubule system and for the subsequent release of calcium from the SR. As a result of one nerve impulse, a certain amount of calcium is released that diffuses through the cytoplasm to be pumped back into the SR after the nerve impulse has passed. If another nerve impulse arrives before the calcium has been pumped back into the SR, further calcium ions are released, adding to the quantity of calcium within the cytoplasm. The greater the concentration of calcium within the cytoplasm, the more binding sites will be exposed to allow actin–myosin interaction. In this situation, a second twitch occurs before the first has completely finished and, as a result, the second twitch will have a peak tension greater than the first. This is a phenomenon known as summation. So, if a second nerve impulse follows hot on the heels of the first, a second and stronger contraction occurs.

If a whole series of nerve impulses are received by the muscle membrane in quick succession, the tension developed is greater still, with only some

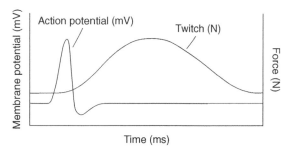

Fig. 3.5 Relationship between the electrical and mechanical events in a single twitch.

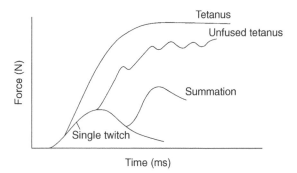

Fig. 3.6 Summation and tetanus.

relaxation between successive stimulations. This is known as an unfused tetanus (see Fig. 3.6). A fused tetanus is where there is not time for the muscle to relax at all, and the individual responses fuse into one contraction. The tension developed can be four times that of a single twitch. The stimulation frequency at which summation occurs depends on the duration of the twitch of a muscle fibre. If a muscle fibre has a twitch duration of 10 milliseconds and is stimulated at a frequency of less than one every 10 milliseconds (equivalent to less than 100 times per second or 100 Hz), discrete muscular contractions would be brought about. At frequencies greater than 100 Hz, summation would occur. If all muscular contractions were brought about by discrete, single twitches, the resulting muscular movements would be jerky and abrupt. Summation is used to bring about muscular contractions that are smooth as a result of the superimposition of summated responses from various motor units within a muscle. Contraction of various motor units is asynchronous (not all contracting at exactly the same time), so whilst certain fibres are relaxing others are

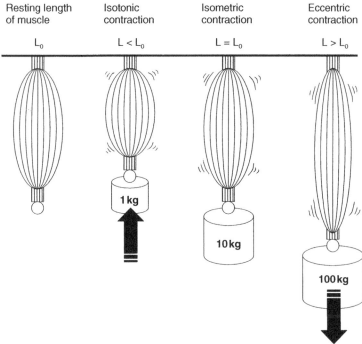

Fig. 3.7 Isotonic, isometric and eccentric muscular contractions.

contracting, but the net result is a smooth muscular movement.

Isotonic and isometric activity

When muscles contract, they exert a force on whatever they are attached to, and if the force developed by the muscle fibre is greater than the force against which it acts shortening of the muscle will occur. In certain situations, for example if you were trying to pick up a very heavy object, the force developed within the muscle may not be sufficient to actually move the object. In this situation, the muscle is contracted, but is unable to actually shorten. When considering types of muscle contractions, there are two measurable variables: length and tension (where tension is the force developed within the muscle).

In an isotonic (i.e. same tension) contraction, the tension is constant and the length of the muscle changes. The muscle actively shortens, bringing about visible movement of the joint. This can also be referred to as a concentric contraction. Another type of isotonic contraction would be where the muscle actively contracts against an external passive stretching force. Such a contraction would occur when a muscle was acting in an antagonistic fashion to its partner on the opposite side of a joint to regulate joint movement and is thus known as an eccentric, rather than a concentric, contraction. In an isometric (same length) contraction, the length is constant and the tension changes. There is no visible shortening, although there is an increase in tension, as cross-bridges between myosin and actin form and are recycled, but the external force is too great for actin filaments to be moved (Fig. 3.7).

Passive tension

Every muscle will withstand a certain amount of force being applied before it actually lengthens in response to passive stretching. This property is due to the presence of what is known as series elastic (SE) components. These consist of tendons, sarcolemma (the membrane surrounding each individual muscle fibre), connective tissue fibres and the hinges at the myosin heads, all of which resist stretching. In an isometric contraction the contractile machinery shortens, but the passive parts, i.e. the SE components, are stretched and therefore

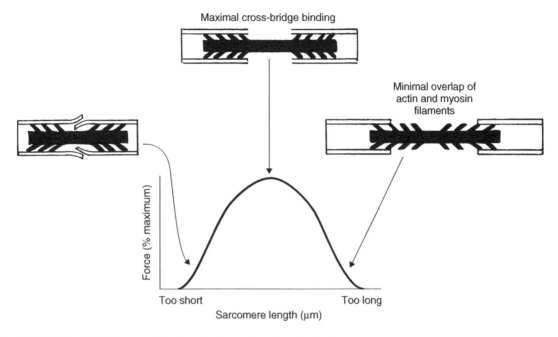

Fig. 3.8 Relationship between original length of muscle and contractile force.

there is no net movement. The SE components are stretched a little during isotonic contractions. At the beginning of contraction, the SE components are slack; as the contractile machinery shortens, slack is taken up, until the SE components can support the load that is to be moved.

Specific passive stretching exercises are often used as a form of therapy or for 'routine care' of muscles. It can also be carried out by horse owners once they have learnt the simple techniques and can be incorporated into the horse's daily routine.

Length–tension relationship

All voluntary muscles in the body are under slight tension. If one or other tendon inserting into the muscle at opposite ends is cut, the muscle shortens. The relaxed length is the length of the muscle before contraction with the SE components under slight tension. Stretching of the muscle (as in passive stretching) pulls the muscle beyond this 'initial length' and tension starts to increase due to stretching of the SE components. If a muscle is stimulated isometrically starting with various known lengths, it is seen that maximum active tension occurs when we start with natural or resting

(relaxed) length. The total tension developed by a muscle is the summation of active tension and passive stretch, both of which vary with fibre length. The fact that the muscle is under slight tension means that it is primed and ready to respond when an electrical stimulus arrives.

At the optimum muscle length, muscle fibres and thus sarcomeres are at a length that gives maximum overlap between actin and myosin filaments. If the muscle is pulled out too far, the fibres are stretched beyond their optimum length. This means that there is less overlap of myosin and actin filaments, fewer cross-bridges can be formed and therefore less tension develops (see Fig. 3.8).

If the muscle fibres are shorter than their optimal length when the contraction begins, the actin filaments begin to overlap each other as the muscle shortens during contraction. This also means that fewer cross-bridges can be formed, and again less tension is developed. Think about weightlifters: their first job is to get the weight and their arms into a position where the muscles are not being actively stretched by the weight hanging down around their knees. Only when their arms are in flexion can they apply maximum force. The key point of this example is that the degree of flexion or extension of a joint has a bearing on the power that can be developed by any given contraction; to expect maximum power from the muscle requires that the muscle should be literally 'in a position' to respond. Many of the subtle stride-by-stride adjustments made by the dressage rider or showjumper are placing the horse's body in such a way that the muscles are able to respond to best effect.

Muscle fibre types and distribution

Classification of muscle fibre types

Muscles are made up of different fibre types. Meat, i.e. muscle, from different animals, or even cuts of meat from the same animal, often look different in colour. Think of the colour of cooked chicken breast and cooked chicken leg: the difference in visual appearance reflects the differences in fibre types within these muscles.

We have learnt a lot about muscle fibre types and muscle function over the last 25 years as a result of the introduction and application of the muscle needle biopsy technique. Muscle biopsies are normally taken from large locomotory muscles such as the middle gluteal muscle of the hindquarters of the horse, because this is one of the major retractors of the hind limb and is therefore responsible for developing much of the driving force for forward movement. It is also a large muscle group and it is relatively easy to select a standardised site to collect the sample from simply on the basis of visual observation and external measurement. One approach attempting to standardise where samples are collected is to take the sample at a point one-third of the distance along a line running from the point of the hip (tuber coxae) to the root of the tail. Once the area for sampling has been selected, the area of skin overlying the muscle is shaved, disinfected and local anaesthetic is injected under the skin using a fine needle. A muscle biopsy needle (usually around 6 mm diameter) is used to take a very small sample of muscle (up to about 200 mg). The biopsy needle has a small window at the bottom and surrounds an inner cutting cylinder. When the needle is at the chosen depth within the muscle (usually somewhere between 2 and 8 cm deep), the cutting cylinder is raised to expose the window and then

pushed down again to cut a piece of muscle out. Local anaesthetic is only used to anaesthetise the skin because muscle does not contain nerves that would react to 'pain'. The sensation of a muscle biopsy, according to people who have had this done, is of pressure. The muscle should heal by regeneration of muscle tissue with minimal deposition of scar tissue, and so taking a biopsy should not affect the muscle in the long term.

Muscle fibres are classified according to their contractile properties, i.e. how fast they are able to contract and relax, which depends on the type of myosin and myosin-ATPase present, and also according to their oxidative capacity (ability to use oxygen). The faster a fibre contracts, the more it will rely on anaerobic pathways and the less on oxidative capacity. Using histochemical techniques, transverse (across, i.e. with all the fibres approximately vertical) sections of the muscle biopsy sample around 10 μm thick are cut and stained to show the activity of ATPase present in the different fibres. Dark staining reflects high myosin ATPase activity and light or no staining reflects low myosin ATPase activity. When the staining is carried out at pH 10.3 (alkaline conditions), two different fibre types are apparent. Light staining fibres are classified as type I and have low myosin-ATPase activity at pH 10.3; these fibres are also referred to as slow twitch fibres. Dark staining fibres are classified as type II and have high myosin-ATPase activity at pH 10.3; these fibres are also referred to as fast twitch fibres. The type II fibres can be further divided into two subtypes if the muscle sections are incubated in an acid solution of around pH 4.4–4.6 before they are stained for ATPase activity at pH 10.3. With this staining procedure, the type I fibres which previously stained light at pH 10.3 without acid pre-incubation now stain dark. The type II fibres now stain either very light and are classified as type IIA whilst fibres that stain intermediate in colour between types I and IIA are classified as type IIB (see Fig. 3.9). Whilst the IIA and IIB fibres are still both fast twitch fibres, the type IIB fibres are able to contract faster than the IIA fibres. Although in most cases nearly all fibres in a muscle biopsy section will clearly stain as types I, IIA or IIB using this technique, sometimes fibres are seen which seem to fall between a IIA and a IIB. These are often referred to as type IIAB fibres. Its possible that these are fibres that

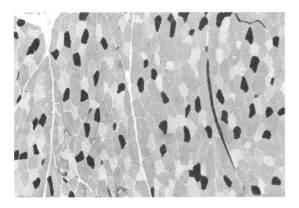

Fig. 3.9 Staining of muscle fibres according to myosin ATPase activity at pH 10.3 after acid pre-incubation at pH 4.4–4.6. Black = type I; white = type IIA; grey = type IIb.

are borderline in ATPase activity between types IIA and IIB that have been 'caught' whilst changing, probably as a result of training or ageing. A further fibre type, the IIC, is often found in regenerating muscle and contains both fast twitch and slow twitch myosin. The method of identifying IIC fibres is to cut two serial (one directly above the other) sections from the muscle biopsy and incubate one section at pH 4.4–4.6 (acid pre-incubation) and the other at pH 10.3 (alkali pre-incubation) before staining for myosin-ATPase activity at pH 10.3. Because two thin serial sections have been cut one after each other from the same sample of muscle and the fibres are generally longer than $20\,\mu m$, the stained sections will represent the same fibres. When both sections are viewed side by side it will then be possible to identify the same fibre, because while types I and II fibres reverse dark/light staining in acid/alkali pre-incubation, the type IIC fibre does not.

A more recent and precise approach to categorising muscle fibres according to their contractile function has been to use antibodies to myosin heavy chain (MHC) protein. Myosin cross-bridges are made up of different forms (isomers) of myosin heavy chain protein, and it is the form of MHC protein that confers the myosin ATPase activity of the fibre. These studies were initially carried out in rats, so the classification of horse MHC follows the rat classification system. The horse types I and IIA fibres are both the same as the type I MHC and type IIA MHC identified in rats. However, the

horse IIB fibre corresponds to the rat IIX MHC fibre, not the rat IIB MHC fibre. This approach seems to have a great advantage in that the classification of fibre types is more definitive and without the overlap seen in the myosin-ATPase approach; however, it is currently very expensive. Those laboratories working with horses and using the myosin-ATPase staining procedure will probably continue to use the I, IIA, IIB, IIAB and IIC nomenclature, whilst those using the MHC antibodies will use the I, IIA and IIX classification.

Type I fibres (red endurance muscle)

These are characterised by having high myosin-ATPase activity after acid pre-incubation. They are slow twitch fibres, meaning that they are slow to contract and to relax. They are usually the narrowest in diameter of all the fibres, and because fibre diameter is proportional to power developed they are not capable of generating as much power as IIA and IIB fibres. However, they can work for long periods aerobically without fatiguing and so are ideal in muscles used for maintaining posture.

They have the highest oxidative, i.e. aerobic, capacity of all the muscle fibre types because they contain a very high number of mitochondria. This can be demonstrated with techniques similar to those used to identify the fibre types: very thin $(5–10\,\mu m)$ sections of muscle are stained for succinate dehydrogenase (SDH) activity, an enzyme within the TCA cycle. Measuring muscle SDH activity is commonly used as an estimate of the aerobic capacity of a muscle. Type I fibres also have the lowest anaerobic (glycolytic) capacity. The nerve supply to type I fibres is via small diameter nerves with a low threshold potential, which means that they will respond to a relatively low level stimulus. The muscle fibre to motor nerve ratio is low, i.e. 20–30 muscle fibres per nerve; in other words, the motor unit is small. Smaller motor units tend to produce more precise, but less powerful contractions. The lipid content within these fibres is high, and the glycogen content is lower than that of type IIA and IIB fibres, reflecting the role of these fibres in posture and prolonged, sub-maximal exercise, relying mainly on aerobic energy pathways.

Type II fibres
(white sprint muscle)

These are the 'sprint' or 'jumping' fibres: they are more powerful than type I fibres but much less resistant to fatigue. There are two types of type II fibres, IIA and IIB. Type IIA are 'middle of the road' fibres in terms of their aerobic/anaerobic characteristics in that they show none of the extremes of type I or IIB. Type IIB fibres are the true sprint fibres with low aerobic capacity and high glycolytic capacity. They are characterised by low-medium myosin-ATPase activity after acid pre-incubation.

Type IIA fibres contract four times as fast and type IIB fibres contract ten times as fast as type I fibres, the contraction speed of type I fibres being 0.33 mm/s. Type II fibres are of greater diameter than type I fibres and therefore develop more power.

In man, the diameter of type IIB and type IIA fibres is generally similar as is, therefore, their power, whereas in horses type IIB fibres are often considerably larger than type IIA so there is a greater power differential between them. This is usually the case in the untrained horse or horses trained for sprinting; however, after primarily aerobic training, both type IIA and IIB fibres tend to decrease to become a similar size.

Type II fibres are supplied by large diameter nerves with a high threshold potential and as such are activated in response to large stimuli. Type IIB fibres have a relatively poor capillary supply because they do not need to rely on a good oxygen supply; they have a low density of mitochondria and generate ATP during exercise primarily by anaerobic glycolysis. Their high glycolytic capacity is also reflected in the nature of the fuel stores within them, with low lipid but high glycogen content. The muscle fibre to motor nerve ratio is very high (up to 2000 fibres to one nerve) so they bring about very powerful contractions when stimulated.

Type II fibres also have a more prominent sarcoplasmic reticulum than type I fibres, reflecting their requirement for fast calcium ion turnover associated with rapid contraction and relaxation.

Muscle capillary supply

There are a number of different ways to describe the capillary supply in a muscle sample. Whilst the overall capillary density in terms of capillaries per mm^2 gives some information, it doesn't tell us anything about the relationship between capillaries and fibres. If we count both the capillaries and the fibres we can express the mean number of capillaries per muscle fibre. In a study in Standardbreds by Karlstrom et al. (1991) the average number of capillaries in contact with each fibre type was 5.0 (type I), 5.6 (type IIA) and 5.9 (type IIB). This seems at odds with what we have learnt about type IIB fibres in that they have the lowest oxidative capacity, i.e. few mitochondria. However, describing the number of capillaries in contact with each fibre type does not take into account differences in fibre size and therefore the diffusion distance for oxygen. Remember that oxygen has to reach all parts of the muscle fibre and not just the edge, so fibre size must come into the equation as well, because oxygen will have further to diffuse from the capillary inside larger fibres. In general terms, type IIB fibres are usually the largest in cross-sectional area, followed by type IIA and then type I. In Karlstrom et al.'s study, when the fibre area was taken into account by expressing the number of capillaries in contact per unit of fibre area, the values were 2.6 capillaries in contact per μm^2 of type I fibre area, 2.3 for type IIA and 1.5 for type IIB. This makes more sense in relation to what we know about how each of the fibre types functions metabolically.

Muscle fibre recruitment

In general terms, muscle fibres are recruited in the following order: type I, type IIA, type IIB. To maintain posture and at low speeds, primarily type I and type IIA fibres are recruited; for rapid acceleration or for jumping, large numbers of type IIB fibres are recruited. Type IIA fibres can be thought of as the 'Jack of all trades' fibres, as they enable the horse to have the best of both worlds – speed and stamina together.

In endurance events, although initially types I and IIA fibres would be used, in the latter stages these may start to run out of glycogen and become fatigued so type IIB fibres would then be recruited. If you think about running at a medium pace yourself, you will note that however tired you are, you can usually always manage a short sprint, even for 15 metres or so before you finally collapse! This is because you are using different muscle fibres for the sprint to those that you were previously using to maintain a steady and slower pace. Similarly, when sprinting, you get to a point when you absolutely cannot continue at top speed, but would be quite comfortable at a lower speed for another couple of miles. In this case at a slower speed you are using fibres you were not using during flat-out running.

Distribution of muscle fibre types

The number and type of muscle fibres that are found in an individual is genetically determined. It seems likely that individuals who have a high percentage of fast twitch fibres will be naturally good sprinters and those with a large percentage of slow twitch fibres will have more stamina or endurance capacity. In man, with the exception of elite athletes, there are approximately equal numbers of slow and fast twitch fibres in common locomotor muscles; however, even in the average horse, the gluteal muscles have considerably more type II than type I fibres. Basically, this means that horses are born with a greater natural aptitude for sprinting than for endurance, and their endurance capacity has to be increased by training throughout their lifetime. Our knowledge of the distribution of fibre types within an individual, and indeed between individuals, is still increasing. The following variations are known to exist.

Variations between breeds

The breed or type of a horse may influence the proportions of different muscle fibre types that are present. The percentages of slow twitch (type I) fibre (the remainder being fast twitch) found within the middle gluteal muscle by Snow and Guy (1981) are reported in Table 3.1. Further studies have shown fairly broad fibre type variation within breeds.

Table 3.1 Fibre composition in middle gluteal muscle of various breeds of horse (adapted from Snow & Guy 1981)

Breed	Type I (%)
Quarter horse	9
Thoroughbred	11
Arab	14
Standardbred	18
Shetland pony	21
Pony	23
Donkey	24
Heavy hunter	31

To a certain extent, breed or type determines for what sort of disciplines horses are suitable. Coupled with the conformation typical of the breed, the fibre type characteristics determine the suitability of the breeds or types to certain disciplines. Whilst Arabs can race over relatively short distances and Thoroughbreds can do well in endurance, Arabs naturally perform better in endurance and Thoroughbreds are faster. This is obviously not solely due to their muscle fibre characteristics; however, inherent muscular characteristics will contribute to performance in a particular discipline.

Variations between individual muscles

Throughout the horse's body, different muscles have different fibre composition reflecting their role. Generally, the hindquarter muscles have a higher percentage of type II fibres, reflecting the fact that they are primarily responsible for generating locomotory force. Forelimb muscles have a higher percentage of type I fibres than the hind limbs, reflecting their role in supporting the weight of the horse during locomotion.

Variations within individual muscles

In an individual muscle, the distribution of fibre types is not uniform. There are more type II fibres on the outside than inside the muscle belly (see Table 3.2). By having type II fibres concentrated on the outside of the muscle, it is shortened relatively more when the type II fibres contract than if they were deep within the muscle belly. This contributes to greater generation of force because the effectiveness of a muscle is determined by the amount of leverage it can exert. By having the most powerful muscle fibres on the outside, the distance through which they can exert their force is maximised.

Table 3.2 Distribution of fibre types in 2-year-old Thoroughbred horses in muscle biopsy samples taken at two different depths at the end of their first training season

Type	Superficial (4 cm deep)		Deep (9 cm deep)	
	Mean (%)	Range (%)	Mean (%)	Range (%)
I	11	0–20	24	0–35
IIA	40	32–61	47	32–61
IIB	49	33–79	30	10–55

From: Sewell *et al.* (1994).

Variations between horses of different sexes

Some studies have shown that there are differences in the proportions of muscle fibre types associated with sex differences; for example, stallions tend to have more type IIA fibres than mares, suggesting that they are more likely to have both power and stamina. It has been suggested that the fibre type differences may reflect the lifestyle of the stallion. One study of a large number of Thoroughbred stallions and mares from birth to 6 years of age showed that the difference was present from birth (Roneus *et al.* 1991). With age there was a gradual increase in the percentage of type IIA fibres, predominantly at the expense of type IIB fibres, and a small increase in type I fibres. However, the proportion

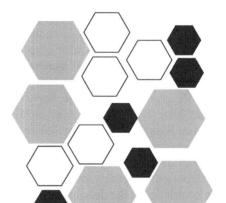

HORSE A

Frequency
%I = 33.3%
%IIA = 33.3%
%IIB = 33.3%

Relative area occupied
%I = 33.3%
%IIA = 33.3%
%IIB = 33.3%

HORSE B

Frequency
%I = 33.3%
%IIA = 33.3%
%IIB = 33.3%

Relative area occupied
%I = 15%
%IIA = 26%
%IIB = 59%

Fig. 3.10 When considering proportions of fibre types it is important to consider the relative area occupied by each fibre type. Type I = black; type IIA = white; type IIB = grey.

of type IIA fibres was always around 5% higher in the stallions at all ages. Other studies have not found any significant sex differences.

Variations between individual horses of the same breed

Even within the same breed, individual horses show differences in their muscle composition. Knowing this, attempts have been made to predict for which distance individual Thoroughbred horses are best suited, so that they can be trained accordingly. In practice this has not proved successful because there are so many other factors that contribute to the suitability of horses for certain distances and also problems with using one muscle biopsy sample to accurately reflect the total percentage of muscle fibres within all major locomotory muscles of a horse.

Variations between muscle biopsy samples

As already described, muscle fibre type distribution varies according to the depth within the muscle,

with more type II fibres being found superficially, and also according to the exact sampling site. One single sample is therefore not necessarily representative of the whole muscle. When considering proportions of muscle fibres, we should be thinking about proportion of total cross-sectional area of muscle, not simply numerical percentages. As an example (Fig. 3.10), if we have Horse A and Horse B, both with the same percentage of type IIB fibres, but in Horse B the type IIB fibres are larger, this will result in a greater cross-sectional area of type IIB fibres. So although the percentage of the different muscle fibre types are the same, Horse B will be capable of developing greater power because the relative area occupied by type IIB fibres is nearly double that of Horse A.

If we were to try and use results from muscle biopsy samples to indicate performance we would need to make sure that we took samples from the same relative area in the muscle for all horses and that the horses were at the same stage of training, because we know training can alter the proportions of fibre types to a certain extent.

KEY POINTS

- Horses have around 700 individual muscles making up around 40–50% of the total body mass.
- The three main types of muscle are smooth (involuntary), striated (skeletal or voluntary) and cardiac (heart).
- Muscles are subdivided into muscle bundles, which in turn are made up of muscle fibres; each muscle fibre is a single muscle cell.
- Muscle cells are organised into motor units. A motor unit consists of the motor nerve and the muscle fibres it activates (innervates) which are always of the same fibre type.
- For fine movements there may be only ten muscle fibres per motor nerve, but for power there may be up to 2000 muscle fibres per motor nerve.
- All muscles receive a baseline level of stimulation known as tone. If the nerve is cut and tone is absent the muscle atrophies (wastes).

- Muscle cells contain nuclei, glycogen granules, fat droplets, myoglobin, mitochondria and contractile proteins (actin and myosin). The functional unit of contraction is the sarcomere.
- Nerve impulses are transmitted into and through the muscle via the sarcolemma and the transverse tubules, leading to an influx of calcium ions from the sarcoplasmic reticulum into the cytoplasm of the muscle cell.
- ATP is required for both contraction and relaxation.
- The strength of contraction is proportional to the number of motor units activated (recruited).
- Narrow diameter nerves have a lower threshold and are stimulated (recruited) before larger diameter nerves.
- It is not possible to recruit all motor units under voluntary control.

- Isotonic contraction = same tension contraction. Tension is constant and the length of the muscle changes (shortens). Also referred to as a concentric contraction.
- Isometric contraction = same length contraction. Muscle length is constant but tension changes (increases).
- Length and tension – all voluntary muscles are always under slight tension and have an optimum length at which they will be able to develop the most tension.

- Muscle is composed of two main fibre types – I (red or endurance) and II (white or sprinting). Type II fibres can be further subdivided into IIA and IIB fibres.
- Fibres are usually recruited in the order of the size of their motor nerves, i.e. I $\rightarrow$ IIA $\rightarrow$ IIB, and their speed of contraction.
- Most muscles are made up of different proportions of type I, IIA and IIB fibres; these proportions vary with factors such as muscle location, function, depth, breed, sex and age of individuals.

Chapter 4

Connective tissue

Various types of connective tissue together with the skeletal muscles make up the musculoskeletal system. The connective tissues have very important and diverse functional roles, reflected in their structure. The most significant component of the skeletal system is bone itself. Other types of connective tissue are:

- Cartilage (found on ends of bone and has various other roles within the skeleton)
- Derma (skin)
- Tendon (attaches muscles to bone)
- Ligament (connects bones together at joints)
- Fascia (a form of internal skin, surrounding muscles and separating muscle groups).

All of these tissues contain relatively few cells and lots of extracellular material. The only way in which they are different is in the types of cells that exist within them. For example, cartilage is cartilage because it contains cartilage cells or chondrocytes; tendon is tendon because it contains tendon cells or tenocytes. The cells sit within an extracellular matrix made up of a mixture of fibres and 'ground substance'. This mixture of collagen and elastin fibres is held together by the ground substance that acts like a glue. The ground substance is actually made up of proteoglycans (compounds containing both protein and carbohydrate components), proteins, water and solutes.

Connective tissue types vary according to the proportions of elastin and collagen and the arrangement of the fibre types within them. Tendons and ligaments have fibres arranged in parallel, whilst hyaline cartilage has layers in which fibres run either parallel or perpendicular to the joint surface. Collagen is the major fibrous element of all connective tissue types and contributes to the tensile strength of the tissue. In fact, weight for weight, collagen is as strong as steel. Large quantities of elastin give a tissue rubber-like qualities and

flexibility. Ligaments in the necks of all grazing animals are high in elastin; however, there is relatively little elastin in tendons and skin. The proteoglycan element of the connective tissue confers resistance to compressive forces. Thus, the articular (hyaline) cartilage found at the ends of bones contains high quantities of proteoglycan.

Tendons and ligaments

Tendons link muscle to bone and transmit the forces generated by the contracting muscle to the bone in order to effect movement at a joint or simply to support a joint. The superficial digital flexor tendon (SDFT) supports the fetlock in the standing horse, transmits the forces of the flexor muscles to the digit and acts as a biological spring, effectively reducing the energetic cost of locomotion and no doubt contributing to the high speed of the horse. The SDFT is particularly susceptible to injury by virtue of its functional responsibility and also its position within the limb. Every time the foot hits the ground and the fetlock sinks, the tendon is required to stretch, absorbing the energy before rebounding and returning this energy to the limb. Whilst the tendon must be elastic enough to act as a spring in this way, it must not be too elastic because it would not then be able to support the fetlock joint effectively. During galloping the downward force on the fetlock is sufficient to produce maximal extension and the fetlock nearly hits the ground; at this point the tendon may be stretched by as much as 8 cm! Because it is the most superficial structure on the palmar (rear) aspect of the forelimb, the SDFT is also prone to injury caused by the hind limb striking into it when the horse is galloping or jumping.

Reflecting the importance of their role in supporting the fetlock and acting as a powerful spring,

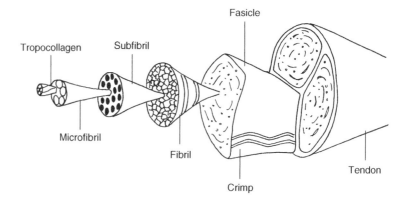

Fig. 4.1   Structure of tendon.

the flexor tendons tend to be stronger and stiffer than extensor tendons. The cross-sectional area and shape of tendons does, however, vary considerably between tendons and between individual horses. The cross-sectional area of the SDFT is approximately 140 mm² in Thoroughbreds, whereas that of the deep digital flexor tendon (DDFT) is approximately 150–190 mm². The cross-sectional area of the suspensory ligament is approximately 150–200 mm² and that of the common digital extensor tendon (CDET) just 25–30 mm².

Ninety-five percent of the collagen in tendons is type I collagen. Tendons are made of bundles of longitudinally orientated collagen microfibrils consisting of the protein tropocollagen (Fig. 4.1). The strength of tendons is increased by cross-linking between overlapping collagen molecules. Microfibrils and subfibrils are bundled into fibrils. There are two populations of fibrils based on cross-sectional area, those around 35–40 nm in diameter and those around 165–215 nm. The fibrils are surrounded by a small volume of non-collagenous matrix, including proteoglycans, glycoproteins, elastin, tenocytes, ions and water. Tendon cells (fibroblasts and tenocytes) tend to be arranged along the longitudinal axes of the fibrils. Fibroblasts are 'active' tendon cells which produce the tendon matrix.

Groups of fibrils are known as fascicles, within which the fibrils are arranged in a helical spiral. In the unloaded state, fibrils have a wavy appearance known as crimp that contributes to their elasticity. The greater the crimp angle, the more elastic the tendon. Crimp angles vary throughout the tendon cross section, i.e. central fibres seem to have less crimp than peripheral fibres, particularly in older horses; thus tendon appears to lose its elasticity with age.

The gross structure of ligament is very similar to that of tendon, with certain differences reflecting the role of ligament in providing resistance to the forces acting on joints in order to maintain the integrity of the joint. Ligaments contain less elastin than tendons whilst the cellular component of ligament seems to be greater than that of tendons, with the cells in ligaments known as desmocytes.

Bones

What do bones look like?

A typical immature long bone (Fig. 4.2) has the following regions:

- Diaphysis (or shaft)
- Epiphyses (or head; singular = epiphysis)
- Metaphyses (singular = metaphysis).

Each metaphysis contains an epiphyseal growth plate (sometimes referred to as the metaphyseal plate but they are one and the same thing). The growth plates are the only points at which a bone can grow in length. The bone itself is made up of two types of bone tissue: dense (or compact) bone found on the outside of the bone shaft and spongy (or cancellous) bone found on the inside of the shaft. The dense bone is lined by two membranes; the periosteum on its outer surface and the endosteum on its inner surface.

Spongy bone is made of the same material as dense bone but does not have the same ordered

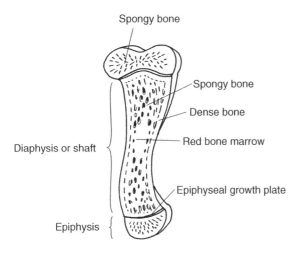

Fig. 4.2 A typical immature long bone.

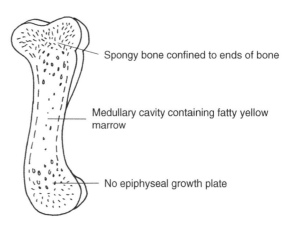

Fig. 4.3 Mature bone.

structure or the same strength. Spongy bone is so called because it is full of holes. The holes are filled with red bone marrow, responsible for producing red blood cells, white blood cells and platelets. In young animals, all bones have red bone marrow, but in adults, red blood cells are only produced in certain areas of the skeleton, namely the pelvis, ribs, sternum and by the marrow at the very ends of long bones.

The basic long bone structure mimics a cylinder, with its strength largely conferred by its particular geometrical shape. A cylinder is better at supporting weight acting down its longitudinal axis than across its transverse axis; thus long bones are orientated so as to confer the greatest possible mechanical strength for any given mass of bone. The bone is not dense throughout, because this would vastly increase its mass for relatively little increase in load-bearing ability. Notice also that the ends of the bone are slightly flared, increasing the cross-sectional area of the bone at the points where it forms joints with other bones. Again, this decreases the local stress on the bone and increases its ability to withstand the forces applied to it, as well as acting as sites for tendon and ligament attachment.

From the immature to the mature state (Fig. 4.3) bones grow not only in length but in 'girth' or cross-sectional area, and this is usually accompanied by an increase in the thickness of the cortex, i.e. the outer layer of dense bone. A medullary cavity containing fatty yellow marrow forms where once

there was spongy bone and red bone marrow. This means that spongy bone is now only found towards either end of the bone shaft. Perhaps the most significant change, and the one that clearly marks the 'coming of age' of the bone, is the disappearance of the growth plate, preventing any further longitudinal growth. This process is often referred to as the growth plates 'closing' and can be detected by radiography (X-ray).

Microanatomy of bone

The dense bone is made up of very ordered structures called Haversian systems or osteons. Each Haversian system is a series of concentric rings called lamellae. Throughout each Haversian system there is a central canal through which nerves and blood vessels run (Fig. 4.4). The central canals branch to form smaller canals called lacunae (meaning little lakes), which run throughout the Haversian system. The lacunae are joined to each other by canaliculi, which are the smallest canals. This arrangement of networks within the bone is similar to that of arteries, arterioles and capillaries within the general circulation. The extent of the network of channels throughout the bone enables very small blood vessels and nerves to reach individual bone cells.

Bone is different to other types of connective tissue in that the extracellular matrix is overlaid with inorganic salts. This unique component of bone is what makes the bone so much harder than

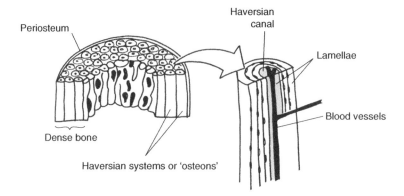

Fig. 4.4   Haversian systems.

other forms of connective tissue. The inorganic salts are in the form of hydroxyapatite that has the chemical formula $Ca_{10}(PO_4)_6(OH)_2$. Hydroxyapatite crystals contain calcium and phosphorus in a ratio of approximately $2:1$; this is the rationale for providing calcium and phosphorus in the horse's diet in the ratio $2:1$. The inorganic part of the bone gives it hardness; if it is removed by soaking the bone in dilute acid the bone becomes flexible enough to tie in a knot! If the organic part is removed the bone becomes totally brittle, so the organic part gives the bone flexibility.

Bone cells

Bone cells are responsible for the constant turnover of bone and are instrumental in the repair of bone should injury occur. There are three different types of bone cells (Fig. 4.5):

1. Osteoblasts

Osteoblasts are bone-forming cells found near both surfaces of the dense bone, lining the endosteum and periosteum. They synthesise and extrude the collagen and proteoglycans that form the extracellular bone matrix. The matrix then becomes mineralised over a period of days. As the mineralised bone surrounds the osteoblast the cell gradually reduces the rate of production of matrix until it becomes an osteocyte.

2. Osteocytes

Osteocytes are mature osteoblasts found at or near the lacunae. They play an important role in cell-to-cell signalling, sensing changes in the mechanical

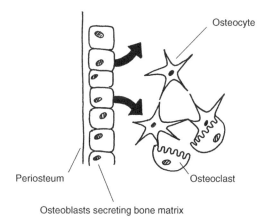

Fig. 4.5   Bone cells.

environment and signalling to osteoblasts and osteoclasts in order to modify their activity. They have long processes by which they can transfer nutrients (primarily calcium) to different regions within bone and from the matrix to extracellular fluid compartments within bone.

3. Osteoclasts

Osteoclasts digest the collagen of the bone matrix using enzymes such as collagenase, lysosomal enzymes and phosphatase. By digesting the fundamental structural support of the bone matrix, the osteoclasts tunnel their way throughout the bone, releasing calcium and phosphorus into extracellular fluid. It may seem unusual that there are cells whose sole purpose is to break down the very structure of bone, but the osteoclasts have a very important role in 'remodelling' and repairing bone as well

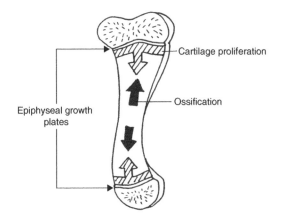

Epiphyseal growth plates

Cartilage proliferation

Ossification

Fig. 4.6 Endochondral ossification.

as providing a mineral pool within bone which acts as a ready supply of calcium should the level of free calcium in the blood fall.

Bone growth

The predominant type of bone formation normally occurring in the body is known as endochondral ossification or intracartilaginous ossification. This is the process by which growth occurs at the epiphyseal plates. Endochondral ossification involves laying down minerals on the basic cartilaginous structure found at the ends of long bones. Epiphyseal cartilage proliferates by producing chondrocytes and this results in the diaphysis being pushed away from the epiphysis (Fig. 4.6). The new cartilage is then ossified to form bone. As the bone reaches maturity, the rate of ossification overtakes the rate of proliferation and the growth plates close. Epiphyseal growth plates close at different stages in the horse's life depending on the bone in which they are found. In general, distal bones (those at the furthest ends of limbs) have growth plates that close earlier than those found proximally (closer to the body); for example, the growth plates of the cannon bone close at 9–12 months whilst those of the tibia close at around $3\frac{1}{2}$ years. Some of the last bones to mature are those of the spine. Growth plate closure seems to be related to the intensity of the impact or loading applied to the bone, because the more distal bones that are subject to relatively large impact loads tend to close earlier. Similarly, too much mechanical stress placed on an immature

bone can cause the growth plates to close prematurely. Early growth plate closure could occur for a number of reasons but overweight youngsters would be susceptible, particularly if they are also required to work. If the horse has well formed limbs and good foot balance, the growth plate should close uniformly; however, in some youngsters uneven loading of the growth plate, either due to poor conformation or injury, may lead to uneven growth plate closure and a permanent angular limb deformity (deviation of the limb in the frontal plane).

Reshaping the bone

Each bone has a template or outline for a predetermined size and shape according to the horse's genetic make-up. Bone growth occurs both at the growth plates of a bone, thereby increasing its length, and also within the shaft of the bone, leading to an increase in bone circumference. Bone growth other than that resulting in an increase in length can be called modelling. Modelling results in a net increase in bone mass otherwise known as hypertrophy. Modelling occurs on the periosteal and endosteal surfaces, bringing about increases in bone width by adding bone material to the outer surfaces of the dense bone. Firstly, the bone matrix is secreted by osteoblasts; then between 6 and 12 hours later most of the minerals are deposited. The complete mineralisation process is not completed until 10 days later. Once completely mineralised, i.e. at 60–70% mineral by mass, the bone matrix surrounds the osteoblast which then stops producing matrix and becomes an osteocyte.

Remodelling describes bone turnover. Bone is adaptable to a certain extent, and can make some adjustments to its size and shape by remodelling. Exactly like sculpting with clay, pieces of the structure can be added or removed to arrive at the desired shape. Removal of bone is carried out by osteoclasts, whilst addition of bone is carried out by osteoblasts: in this way bone material is constantly recycled. Rebuilding the bone takes longer than the initial removal stage, so if there is a high rate of remodelling in a whole bone or in a certain region of bone, the bone will literally be full of little holes until the bone material is completely reformed. As remodelling appears to leave the bone in a particularly vulnerable state, it may seem like a rather unnecessary evil; however, it is absolutely necessary for three reasons:

(1) *Bone repair*. The process of remodelling allows for 'clean-up' of damaged bone tissue in the event of various types of minor and major fractures followed by reformation of completely new bone tissue indiscernible from the original structure.

(2) *Improvement and or adaptation of poor original growth*. Bone turnover confers flexibility to the bone structure, a useful feature when the physical demands on the bone may vary enormously throughout life. The ability of the bone to adapt in response to functional demands was first recognised by Julius Wolff in the 1870s.

(3) *Calcium homeostasis*. Ninety-nine percent of the body's calcium is found within the skeleton. Calcium is a very important mineral, being involved in such diverse processes as blood clotting, muscle contraction and hormone and enzyme action. The skeleton is often called upon to relinquish some of this calcium in times of need so that these essential functions are not compromised. Remodelling means that there is a constant calcium pool within the bone

structure that can be used in times of low blood calcium.

In an animal receiving adequate nutrition in terms of mineral content, there should not be any net bone loss throughout the process of remodelling provided the bone is loaded sufficiently. There is a critical minimum amount of stress that is required if bone mass is to be maintained: any less than this critical level and there is net decrease in bone mass. This may occur if a horse is not allowed to move freely, as in prolonged periods of box rest, or if a limb is non-weight bearing. Astronauts exposed to long periods of weightlessness also experience problems of loss of bone mass. When we break a leg and it is held in a cast, bone mass (as well as muscle mass) tends to be lost. Once the limb is allowed to bear weight again bone mass is slowly regained. Following a fracture, the level of exercise should be built up cautiously because of the vulnerability of the bone structure at this stage. Whilst there is a threshold level of activity required to maintain bone mass, loading throughout a training programme can actually result in net gain of bone mass as we shall see in Chapter 8. At normal rates of remodelling, the entire calcium content of the mature skeleton can be replaced every 200 days.

KEY POINTS

- The musculoskeletal system is made up of connective tissue (bone, cartilage, ligaments and tendons) and the skeletal muscle.
- Connective tissues vary in the proportions of elastin and collagen and this determines their properties and relates to their function.
- Tendons link muscle to bone and transmit forces generated by muscles to effect movement.
- Tendons must be elastic enough to act as springs but still be able to support limbs.
- Ligaments connect bones together and help stabilise joints.
- The structure of ligaments is similar to tendons but ligaments contain less elastin.
- Bone is made up of two basic types of tissue – dense or compact bone found on the outside of the shaft and spongy or cancellous bone found on the inside of the shaft.

- Both spongy and dense bone are made of the same material, but the components are more ordered in dense bone.
- Spongy bone is so called because it contains 'holes' which accommodate red bone marrow that produces red and white blood cells and platelets.
- Bones grow in both length and girth (cross-sectional area) and maturation of bone is considered to have occurred when the growth plates have disappeared or closed.
- Bone is different to other types of connective tissue because its extracellular matrix is overlaid with an inorganic salt known as hydroxyapatite.
- Hydroxyapatite is a mixture of calcium and phosphorus in the ratio of $2:1$ and gives bone its hardness.

- Bone cells are responsible for growth, turnover and repair.
- Osteoblasts are bone-forming cells; osteocytes are responsible for nutrient exchange; osteoclasts can digest bone matrix releasing calcium and phosphorus, and are important in remodelling of bone and providing a source of calcium for other tissues and organs in times of dietary deficiency or increased use.
- The predominant type of bone formation normally occurring in the body is known as endochondral ossification or intracartilaginous ossification. This is the process by which growth occurs at the epiphyseal plates (growth plates).
- In general, distal bones have growth plates that close earlier than those found proximally.
- The growth plates of the cannon bone close at around 9–12 months of age whilst those of the tibia close at around $3\frac{1}{2}$ years. Some of the last bones to mature are those of the spine.
- Bone growth other than that resulting in an increase in length can be called modelling. Modelling results in a net increase in bone mass otherwise known as hypertrophy.
- Bone is adaptable to a certain extent and some adjustments in its size and shape can be made by remodelling.
- Remodelling may leave the bone weaker but is necessary for bone repair, improvement and or adaptation of poor original growth and calcium homeostasis.

Chapter 5

The respiratory system

Respiration, breathing, ventilation

Respiration defines the process by which ATP is produced using oxygen. Unicellular organisms are small enough to obtain all the oxygen they need by the passive process of diffusion. Diffusion of oxygen into the unicellular organism is driven by a gradient of higher oxygen concentration outside the cell to lower oxygen concentration inside the cell. The greater the gradient, the faster the rate of diffusion. Similarly, all the carbon dioxide they produce as a result of cellular oxidative mechanisms is removed by diffusion. They respire but they don't breathe. In higher animals, both the gas exchange surface and the sites of oxygen usage are too far removed from atmospheric gases for diffusion alone to be effective. Animals need a method of bringing gases from the atmosphere to the gas exchange surface, i.e. the lung, and this is achieved by breathing. Breathing is a process whereby gases are brought to the gas exchange surface and removed from it by bulk flow. Bulk flow means that all the gases move en masse. Another term for this movement of air in and out of the lungs is ventilation.

The composition of dry atmospheric air is 20.98% O_2 (oxygen), 0.04% CO_2 (carbon dioxide), 78.06% N_2 (nitrogen) and 0.92% other gases, mainly argon. The air that the horse breathes also contains a variable amount of water vapour, with the degree of saturation indicated by the relative humidity. Whether atmospheric humidity is 5% or 95%, the incoming (inspired) air is warmed (to close to body temperature) and saturated with moisture, i.e. to 100% humidity, within the nasal passages before entering the lungs. The horse will take into the lungs anything that is 'airborne' including all gases and particulate matter, desirable or otherwise (e.g. dust, moulds, viruses, pollen, etc.), found in the atmospheric air to which it is subjected. Breathing in is not selective; it is necessary to take the rough with the smooth. Atmospheric gas is breathed in and a modified version of it is breathed out. Expired air (air breathed out) is saturated with water vapour and at rest contains somewhere around 17% O_2 and 3% CO_2. From this you can see that not all the oxygen which is inspired (breathed in) is used up. If it were, mouth-to-mouth resuscitation would be useless!

An important difference between the respiratory systems of humans and horses is the way in which they most commonly respond to disease. If we have some form of respiratory disease, such as a cold (i.e. an infectious disease) or asthma (i.e. an allergic disease), one of the first obvious signs to someone else is that we cough. If we cough it's a fairly clear indication that we have some form of infection or disease and vice versa, if we are not coughing in all probability our lungs are fine. Horses are very different. Compared to us they are much less likely to cough, even when they have quite severe respiratory disease. Burrell *et al.* (1996) showed that coughing has an 84% specificity but only a 36% sensitivity for detecting the presence of respiratory disease or infection in horses. What this means, in simple terms, is that if a horse is coughing there is a very high chance that it has a respiratory tract infection or some other form of respiratory disease (high specificity), but if it is not coughing there is only a small chance that it is healthy (low sensitivity). It's very common to hear people say that their horse never has any respiratory problems despite being on straw and dusty hay, but that the horse coughs once or twice each time it's taken to be exercised: these horses probably have respiratory disease that should be investigated.

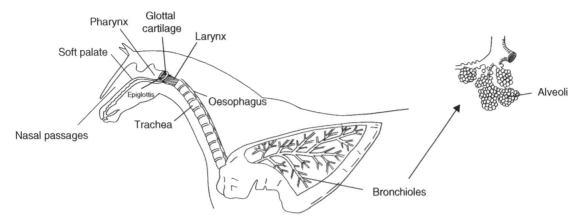

Fig. 5.1   The equine respiratory system.

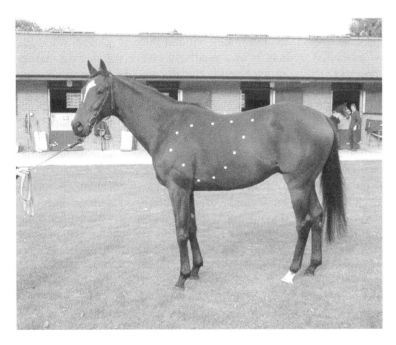

Fig. 5.2   External lung border.

Anatomy of the respiratory system

If we made a journey from the atmosphere, down through the airways, we would pass through the following structures (Fig. 5.1): nostrils, nasal passages (nares), pharynx, larynx, trachea, carina, bronchi, bronchioles, alveolar ducts and alveoli.

The respiratory system can be likened to a tree, with the trachea representing the trunk and all the airways following on from it representing the branches. We can number each generation of branching of the respiratory system, with the trachea being generation 0, the first generation of bronchi branching from the trachea as generation 1, and so on. In the horse, the division of each airway is described as being monopodial and means that each daughter airway arising from the division of a single parent airway is smaller than the parent. In man, division of airways is often described as symmetric, and daughter airways can be either the same size as the parent or smaller.

The number of airway generations from the trachea to the alveolar ducts varies greatly between different species. For example, in the respiratory tract of man, there are on average 23 divisions or generations. The number of generations in the horse is thought to be much higher and of the order of 38–43. As the airway generations of the horse have not been well described, we will use the human lung as an example. Generations 0–16 are considered to be conducting airways: no significant gas exchange occurs across their walls and their primary function is to move air down to the gas exchange surfaces; no diffusion can occur across the walls of the conducting airways because they are too thick. Generations 17–23 are considered to represent respiratory airways where gas exchange can occur by diffusion. The walls of generation 0–16 airways are lined with ciliated epithelial cells (the cilia beat to help move mucus and other unwanted material out of the airways), from generations 17 to 20 the air moves through alveolar ducts, whilst generations 20–23 consist purely of alveoli. In man, the number of alveoli ranges from around 200 million to 600 million depending on height (i.e. body size), and the mean diameter varies with lung volume but is around 0.2 mm or 200 μm at functional residual capacity (see p. 46). The total alveolar number in horses is likely to be somewhere in the order of 10^{10}–10^{11} as estimated from a lung surface area of 2500 m^2 and an average alveolar diameter of 70–180 μm, giving a mean alveolar surface area of 15 000–100 000 μm^2 based on the approximation that alveoli are spherical (they are actually polygonal). The actual surface area of the lung where gas exchange can occur is about 85 m^2 in humans and about 2500 m^2 in horses. This accounts for around 85% of the total volume of the lung. A doubles tennis court has an area 261 m^2 (2808 ft^2) and therefore the horse's gas exchange surface area is almost equivalent to ten doubles courts! In comparison to the gas exchange area, the capillary surface area of the equine lung has been estimated to cover 1700 m^2. Horse lungs also have good collateral ventilation, meaning that air can move between regions within the lung at the level of structure known as the lobule. Cattle and pigs have almost no collateral ventilation between adjacent lobules, whilst dogs and cats have a very high degree of collateral ventilation.

The total volume of air that can be contained by the lung (total lung capacity) is about 6–7 litres in man and around 40 litres in a 500 kg horse. Lung capacity is related to body size, so larger individuals will have a bigger lung capacity. The position of the horse's lung is shown in Fig. 5.2. However, lung size does not necessarily relate to lung function. Indeed, the size of the horse's chest is often falsely thought to be associated with performance, and there is no reason why a wide and deep-chested horse should have better lung function than a narrow and shallow-chested horse. If the wide-chested horse has a larger lung capacity this may not be an advantage as he will probably also have more muscle tissue that will need to be supplied with oxygen.

The airways will be at their widest when the smooth muscle around them is relaxed, when the lung is at a relatively higher volume, e.g. during exercise, and in the absence of respiratory disease. Horses affected by recurrent airway obstruction (RAO; formerly known as equine chronic obstructive pulmonary disease (COPD)), for example, will tend to have narrowed airways and therefore increased airway resistance and decreased dynamic compliance (increased lung stiffness; see p. 50) due to a combination of factors including bronchoconstriction (or bronchospasm; contraction of the smooth muscles around the airways), thickening of the walls of the airways making the internal diameter smaller, and obstruction of the airways by mucus.

The lung has two blood circulations. The pulmonary circulation brings venous blood into close contact with the gas exchange surface. However, the lung tissue itself must also have a blood supply providing oxygen and nutrients to its cells. This is called the bronchial circulation. This is similar to the heart, which also has a coronary circulation providing the heart muscle with oxygen and nutrients.

How much air goes in and out?

Ventilation can be measured to quantify the volume of air that goes in or out of the lung. The total amount of air moved either into or out of the lung each minute is known as the minute ventilation and can be calculated as follows:

Minute ventilation (litres/min) = tidal volume

(litres) × respiratory frequency (breaths/min)

Tidal volume V_T refers to the depth of the breath, and respiratory frequency (f_r) is simply the number of complete breaths taken per minute. The relationship can be expressed in symbols as follows:

$$\dot{V}_E = V_T \times f_r$$

The dot above the V indicates that minute ventilation is a rate, i.e. something per unit time (in this case litres/min). Lung volumes such as minute ventilation and tidal volume should always be stated under the same conditions. This is because volume is affected by barometric pressure, temperature and moisture content. The universal convention for lung volumes is BTPS. This stands for body temperature and pressure, saturated. The precise conditions are 37°C, 101.3 kPa (760 mmHg), and 100% relative humidity (RH) at 37°C. A similar convention is used for volumes of oxygen taken up and volumes of carbon dioxide produced (exhaled). This is known as STPD (standard temperature and pressure, dry; see Chapter 18).

At rest an average sized Thoroughbred horse (500 kg) might have a minute ventilation of somewhere around 50–60 litres/min, produced by taking breaths of 5–6 litres, ten times a minute. Not all of these 50–60 litres will come into contact with the gas exchange surface. A large proportion of the air is simply moved in and out of the conducting airways. The gas that is not exchanged but simply moved in and out of the lung is known as wasted or dead space ventilation (V_D). This gas would actually have the same oxygen (~21%) and carbon dioxide (0%) composition on expiration as when it was breathed in. In a healthy horse at rest, around 60% of the volume of a single breath constitutes dead space. This dead space is made up of two components: the first is the anatomical dead space ($V_{D\,anat}$), which refers to the proportion of a breath that fills the conducting airways and never gets in contact with a respiratory surface (i.e. alveolar–capillary membrane or respiratory bronchiole surface); the second component is the physiological dead space ($V_{D\,phys}$), which refers to air that is brought in contact with a respiratory surface but gas exchange does not occur

because the region is not currently being perfused (supplied) by blood.

What makes the air go in and out of the lung?

There are two concepts to understand before we can study more closely how gases behave:

(1) Gases move from regions of high pressure to regions of low pressure, like the gas escaping from a punctured tyre.
(2) Boyle's law: this states that the pressure of a fixed mass of gas (gas has mass the same as fluids or solids) at constant temperature is inversely proportional to its volume.

To understand Boyle's law, imagine a certain mass of gas held in a container. Any gas held within a container exerts a pressure due to collisions of the gas molecules with the container walls. If we put the same gas in a smaller container, i.e. we decrease the volume in which it is contained, it would exert a greater pressure because there would be more collisions of gas molecules with the container walls. If we put the same mass of gas in a larger container, there would be more room for the molecules, and relatively fewer collisions with the container walls, and so the pressure exerted by the gas would be lower (see Fig. 5.3).

To get atmospheric gas to move into the lung in inspiration, we must create a pressure gradient for gases to move by bulk flow. We cannot change atmospheric pressure, but the pressure inside the lung can be changed by altering the lung volume. When the volume of the lung is increased during inspiration, the pressure within the lung decreases (becomes more negative).

The lung volume is increased during inspiration by contraction of the diaphragm and expansion of the chest (see Fig. 5.4). As a result, the pressure within the alveoli is made more negative (or less positive, whichever you prefer). Air rushes in from the atmosphere because a pressure gradient has been created, and gases will move from a region of high pressure (the atmosphere) to a region of lower pressure (the lung) until the two regions have equal pressure. During normal, quiet breathing, intra-alveolar pressure (the pressure of gas within the

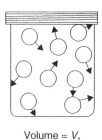
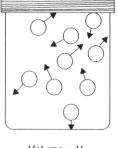
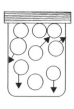

Volume = V_1

Pressure = P_1

Volume > V_1

Pressure < P_1

Volume < V_1

Pressure > P_1

Fig. 5.3 Boyle's law: the pressure of a fixed mass of gas at constant temperature is inversely proportional to its volume.

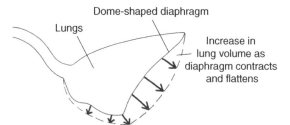

Lungs

Dome-shaped diaphragm

Increase in lung volume as diaphragm contracts and flattens

Fig. 5.4 When the volume of the lung is increased during inspiration, the pressure within the lung decreases (becomes negative).

lung) only changes by 0.1–0.2 kPa (1–2 cmH₂O) above and below atmospheric pressure.

The rate at which the air moves into the lung is given by the following equation:

$$\text{Rate of flow }(\dot{V})$$
$$= \frac{\text{Atmospheric pressure} - \text{Alveolar pressure}}{\text{Airway resistance}}$$

The flow rate of air into the lung is therefore greater if there is a large pressure difference between the atmospheric pressure and the alveolar pressure, and if there is little resistance to flow, with resistance largely being determined by the size of the airways. A more appropriate term for airway size is calibre.

Actions of the respiratory muscles

The major inspiratory muscles are the diaphragm and the external intercostals. During gentle inspiration at rest, 80% of the work of breathing is done by the diaphragm, and 20% by the external intercostals. In humans, inspiration is a purely active process, meaning that it requires energy. When we inspire, the diaphragm is contracted, and flattens, thereby increasing the volume of the thoracic cavity with a consequent increase in lung volume. At the same time, the external intercostal muscles lift the ribcage up and outwards to further increase chest (and therefore lung) volume. As the lung distends, elastin fibres within the diaphragm are stretched, which stores energy. At the end of inspiration the diaphragm and the external intercostals relax and air is squeezed out. In other words, expiration is passive; no muscular work is done to breathe out during quiet breathing at rest.

In a forced exhalation, such as when coughing or when playing a wind instrument, the internal intercostal muscles are also used to actively pull the ribs down. The abdominal muscles may also be contracted and contribute to forcing air out of the lung. Only in these instances of forced expiration do we see active expiration in humans. Horses adopt a different breathing strategy to humans. Horses have what is known as a biphasic inspiration and expiration. Fig. 5.5 shows schematically how respiratory action differs between the two species.

Both human and horse lungs have a normal, resting volume. This is known as the functional residual capacity (FRC) and is sometimes referred to as the end expiratory lung volume (EELV); it corresponds to the lung volume when the lung is at rest, neither breathing in, nor breathing out. Humans ventilate the lung by actively increasing the lung volume above FRC, and then allowing the lung passively to return to FRC. Notice in Fig. 5.5 that if the lung volume is returning to FRC, that part of the respiratory cycle is passive, and if the lung volume is

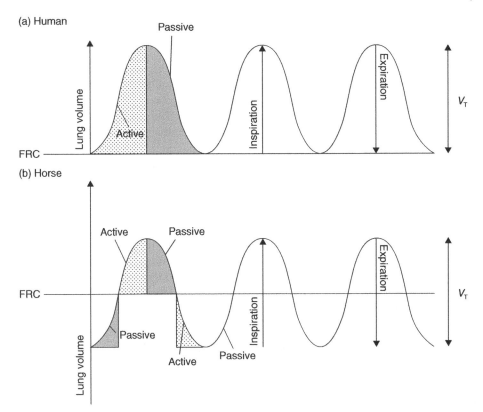

(a) Human

(b) Horse

Fig. 5.5 Breathing strategies of humans and horses.

moving away from FRC, that part of the respiratory cycle is active. We say that humans breathe from or above FRC at rest. You will see then that normal inspiration in the horse has both an active and a passive part, and normal expiration in the horse has both an active and a passive part. This is because at rest horses breathe *around FRC (i.e. both above and below)*, *not just above it*, as do humans. It is thought that it may be less expensive in energy terms for the horse to breathe like this, because it has a stiffer chest wall than humans. In other words, this strategy may help to reduce the work of breathing.

Air moves in and out of the lung as the diaphragm and ribs are moved to bring about changes in the size of the thoracic cavity, but what makes the lung move along with the chest wall?

Pleural membranes

The lung volume changes in accordance with movements of the chest wall because of the existence of pleural membranes. There are two pleural membranes:

- Visceral (nearest the lung)
- Parietal (nearest the chest wall).

The cavity between the two membranes is filled with a very thin layer of pleural fluid. Only a few millilitres of pleural fluid fill the entire area between the two membranes, known as the pleural cavity. Pleural fluid acts as a lubricant, and as an adhesive. It literally sticks the chest wall and the lung together.

At rest, i.e. at FRC, the pressure within the pleural cavity, known as intrapleural pressure or P_{pl}, averages −0.3 to −0.5 kPa (−3 to −5 cmH$_2$O); in other words, there is a negative pressure between the lung and the chest wall. Both the chest wall and the lung possess a degree of elasticity, such that they will always tend to return to FRC. If the chest wall volume is decreased below FRC, it will tend to spring back to FRC, and if the chest volume is increased, it will also tend to spring back to FRC.

Thus FRC is the absolute volume of the chest at which the tendency of the chest to spring outwards is exactly opposed by the tendency of the lung to collapse inwards. As lung volume increases during inspiration, P_{pl} becomes more negative, reflecting the tendency of the lungs to move away from the chest wall. As the lung volume decreases during expiration, P_{pl} becomes less negative, reflecting the tendency of the chest wall to expand and recoil back to FRC. Intrapleural pressure changes are not easy to measure directly. Inserting a catheter into the pleural space carries a risk of introducing air. This would result in the pleural membranes no longer being held tightly together and the area of lung where the air had entered would collapse inwards. This is what is known as a pneumothorax. An additional risk would be introducing bacteria into the pleural cavity and causing a bacterial pleuro-pneumonia. However, although pleural pressure is not usually measured directly it is quite easy to estimate, as the pressure within the mid-thoracic oesophagus closely approximates the pressure within the pleural space. This is because the oesophagus passes through the thoracic cavity in which the lungs (and heart) are contained. Therefore, although the oesophagus is not within the lung, it is subject to the same changes in pressure that occur within the thorax during breathing. In fact, the heart is also affected by changes in intrathoracic pressure associated with breathing. One example of this is respiratory sinus arrhythmia that can often be clearly seen on an electrocardiogram (ECG) after exercise. After exercise the respiratory rate and efforts are often both quite high and therefore quite large swings in intrathoracic pressure occur with breathing. These are reflected by a periodic and intermittent slowing of the heart rate in time with the breathing. Increases in intrathoracic pressure during expiration reduce the flow of venous blood back to the heart and the heart responds to this by decreasing its rate. As the horse breathes in, the intrathoracic pressure becomes negative; this restores venous return and so heart rate increases. This effect is also seen in human weightlifters and is referred to as the Valsalva manoeuvre when they try to exhale against a closed mouth, nose and glottis which causes a dramatic increase in intrathoracic pressure and a decrease in heart rate. You can demonstrate this effect with a heart rate monitor or ECG.

The oesophageal pressure is usually measured by recording the pressure changes within a condom placed over the end of a long catheter that is inserted through the nares (nostrils) and pushed down the oesophagus. The position of the tip of the catheter is estimated first by holding the catheter up against the outside of the horse and marking the length at the nares. Approximate intrapleural pressures for inspiration and expiration are given in Table 5.1. In healthy horses during normal breathing at rest, intrapleural (or oesophageal) pressure only changes by around 0.3–0.5 kPa (3–5 cmH$_2$O), and is nearly always negative (e.g. −0.1 to −0.4 kPa = −1 to −4 cmH$_2$O). During maximal exercise such as galloping, there are large swings in intrapleural pressure up to 6.9 kPa (70 cmH$_2$O) with P_{pl} on expiration becoming positive.

Ventilation–perfusion matching and mismatching

The ventilation and perfusion of the whole lung is not uniform, and gradients of ventilation and pulmonary blood flow (perfusion) exist between the apex (i.e. top) and the base of the lung, both in man and in the horse. In the horse, this was first shown by Amis *et al.* (1984) using scintigraphy. Both ventilation and perfusion are greater at the base of the lung than at the apex. The ventilation gradient occurs as a result of an intrapleural pressure gradient. Intrapleural pressure is more negative at the apex of the lung than at the base, so at FRC alveoli at the apex are stretched and at a greater volume than those at the base; consequently, these alveoli are also stiffer than those further down the lung and during inspiration they are less compliant and therefore much harder to inflate. As a result, the majority of air tends to go towards inflating alveoli further down the lung.

Historically, the perfusion gradient in relation to vertical lung height has been thought to be primarily due to the effects of gravity. Whilst this is probably true for anaesthetised horses, Hlastala *et al.* (1996) showed that in conscious, unsedated standing horses, gravity did not play a major role in determining blood flow at different vertical heights

Table 5.1 Approximate intrapleural pressures for inspiration and expiration

	kPa	cmH$_2$O
Inspiration (normal breathing)	−0.4	−4
Expiration (normal breathing)	−0.1	−1
Inspiration (maximal exercise)	−3.9	−40
Expiration (maximal exercise)	−2.9	30

in the lung. However, it is likely that although the horse cannot control where ventilation goes within the lung because this is determined by physical factors, it is able to control where perfusion does or does not go by vasodilating and vasocontricting different blood vessels. This has important physiological consequences for achieving optimal gas exchange.

For the lungs to be totally efficient, ventilation ($\dot{V}$ in l/min, measured at the nostrils) and perfusion ($\dot{Q}$ in l/min, i.e. cardiac output) in any region of the lung should be matched as closely as possible. There would be little point in sending lots of blood to a region not being ventilated. Imagine if half the pulmonary venous blood flow, i.e. the venous blood flowing from the right heart through the pulmonary artery, went to regions of the lung that were not being ventilated; if this then mixed with blood that had been through ventilated regions, instead of having an arterial oxygen tension (Pa_{O_2}) of around 13.3 kPa (100 mmHg), the result would be a much lower arterial tension. This would be because any venous blood that does not come into contact with a ventilated gas exchange surface effectively stays as venous blood. If the venous Pa_{O_2} was 5.3 kPa (40 mmHg), and half the blood stayed as venous and the other half increased to 13.3 kPa (100 mmHg), when all the blood mixed together back in the pulmonary veins and left ventricle, we would have a mean arterial Pa_{O_2} of (5.3 kPa + 13.3 kPa)/2 = 9.3 kPa ((40 mmHg + 100 mmHg)/2 = 70 mmHg). This is, in fact, what happens in many instances of respiratory disease.

Because the lung does not have mechanisms that can effectively control where airflow goes, it tries to 'match' areas of high and low ventilation with high and low perfusion by controlling the blood flow to these areas. An ideal ventilation perfusion or $\dot{V}/\dot{Q}$

ratio for the whole lung would therefore be unity (1), i.e. on a global level if minute ventilation was equal to cardiac output. In reality, the $\dot{V}/\dot{Q}$ ratios across the whole lung probably vary between 0.8 and 1.2 in healthy horses at rest, with a mean close to 1. We can also think of $\dot{V}/\dot{Q}$ ratios on a whole lung basis or on a regional basis. For example, a small region of lung may have a low $\dot{V}/\dot{Q}$ ratio but the whole lung would have a $\dot{V}/\dot{Q}$ ratio close to unity.

A $\dot{V}/\dot{Q}$ ratio of zero would equate to no ventilation despite some level of perfusion, whilst a $\dot{V}/\dot{Q}$ ratio of infinity would equate to no perfusion despite some level of ventilation. $\dot{V}/\dot{Q}$ ratios below unity may be the result of a decrease in $\dot{V}$ despite a normal $\dot{Q}$ or an increase in $\dot{Q}$ despite a normal $\dot{V}$. Similarly, ratios above unity may result from an increase in $\dot{V}$ or a decrease in $\dot{Q}$.

Since there are similar gradients of increasing ventilation and perfusion with vertical distance from the top to the bottom of the lung, the $\dot{V}/\dot{Q}$ ratio is fairly uniform from the top to the bottom of the lung during normal, quiet breathing. Thus at the top of the lung, a ratio of unity will usually be the result of a relatively low $\dot{V}$ and low $\dot{Q}$, whilst at the bottom of the lung a ratio of unity will usually be the result of a relatively high $\dot{V}$ and high $\dot{Q}$. In fact, ventilation and perfusion are better matched in horse lungs than in human lungs. It is commonly accepted that poor matching of perfusion to ventilation is the main reason for impaired gas exchange as a result of respiratory disease.

How easy is it to inflate the lungs?

In horses, during normal resting breathing, the pressure swing within the lung itself to move around 6 litres of gas in and out is only a matter of 0.3–0.5 kPa (3–5 cmH$_2$O). A balloon requires a pressure gradient of 26.5 kPa (270 cmH$_2$O) for the same increase in volume. This is around 200 times the pressure change required to inflate the lung by 6 litres. The ease or difficulty with which the lung inflates is called its compliance. Static compliance refers to the ease or difficulty with which the lung can be inflated either when it has been removed from the body or during anaesthesia when the animal's respiratory muscles have been paralysed and it is being artificially ventilated. Dynamic compliance refers to the same ease or difficulty of inflation during normal breathing when the animal is conscious, sedated or anaesthetised (but not paralysed). The easier the lungs are to inflate, the greater the compliance and the greater the increase in lung volume for any given change in intrapleural pressure (P_{pl}). Compliance can be related to the pressure gradient that has to be created in order to increase the lung volume by the following equation:

$$\text{Compliance } (C) = \frac{\text{Change in lung volume (litres)}}{\text{Change in } P_{pl} \text{ (cmH}_2\text{O or kPa)}}$$

$$\text{or} \quad \frac{\Delta V}{\Delta P_{pl}} \quad (\text{where } \Delta \text{ means 'change in'})$$

Thus units of compliance are usually either l/cmH$_2$O or litres/kilopascal (l/kPa).

Compliance values for a healthy horse at rest would be around 0.1–0.2 l/kPa (1–2 litres/cmH$_2$O). Human lung compliance at rest is around 0.02 l/kPa (0.2 litres/cmH$_2$O), so the horse's lungs are more compliant than human lungs during normal resting breathing. Lung compliance is not the same under all circumstances. For example, at very low lung volumes compliance is low, meaning that it requires more energy to inflate a collapsed area of lung than to continue to ventilate a region of lung that already has air in it. At very high lung volumes the lung tends to become stiffer as the constituent elastin fibres approach their maximum length; thus, at high lung volumes compliance is also reduced. The lungs in a horse with moderate to severe RAO are often less compliant than those of healthy horses, and compliance may be as low as 0.001 l/kPa (0.1 l/cmH$_2$O) in such cases. The lungs of the RAO horse would therefore require ten times the change

in pressure as those of a healthy horse to move the same volume of air.

Compliance varies according to the elasticity of the lung. Normal lungs are very elastic. At high lung volumes, at the peak of inspiration, the recoil of the lung tissue tends to return the lungs to their original volume. In a person suffering from emphysema, a disease often caused by smoking, the lungs have lost their elasticity, and these people find it extremely difficult to exhale. For emphysema sufferers, expiration during normal breathing at rest is no longer a purely passive process. Similarly, horses with RAO may also have to work harder to exhale, giving rise to the characteristic 'heave' line found in those badly affected, due to over-development of the abdominal muscles used in expiration. 'Heaves' is a common term for RAO that is used mainly in North America. In the UK, the term 'broken winded' is probably the most common lay term.

The term RAO has been adopted to avoid confusion when discussing human and equine COPD which are entirely different conditions. The human form of COPD is caused primarily by smoking, whereas equine COPD is primarily an allergic disease commonly caused by exposure to moulds and similar in many features to human asthma.

The high compliance of the lung is also related to a substance called surfactant that helps to keep the alveoli open. Alveoli are small, fluid lined spheres. The fluid lining the alveoli is similar to extracellular fluid (fluid surrounding cells) and is therefore largely salt and water. The water molecules on the inner alveolar wall attract each other, producing a surface tension within the alveoli (see Fig. 5.6). The resultant force of these many water–water molecule attractions is directed towards the centre of the alveoli, producing a collapsing pressure which

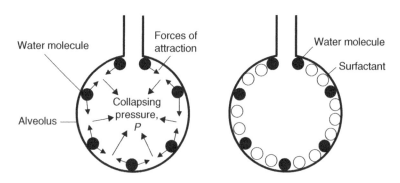

Fig. 5.6 Surface tension effects within alveoli.

depends upon, (1) the surface tension (T) and (2) the radius of the sphere, such that

$$\text{Collapsing pressure } (P) = \frac{2T}{r}$$

where T is the surface tension and r is the radius of the sphere. This is known as the law of Laplace. This tendency for the alveoli to collapse inwards at low volumes is bad news. As small, water lined spheres, they should be subject to a large collapsing pressure. Thankfully, both human and horse lungs have a mechanism that reduces the potentially large surface tension effect within alveoli, by producing a substance within the lung called surfactant. Surfactant is made primarily (90%) of phospholipids and a small amount of protein. The two main phospholipids are dipalmitoylphosphatidylcholine (or DPPC for short) and phosphatidylcholine (PC), which have a hydrophilic (water soluble) head and a hydrophobic (water insoluble) tail. Surfactant gets in between water molecules, thereby lowering surface tension effects by reducing the attraction of water molecules to each other. This decreases the tendency for the alveoli and small airways to collapse at low volumes, which increases compliance and decreases the work of breathing. Surfactant is stored in lung cells known as type II pneumocytes and is secreted into the airways. Each day around 10–15% of the surfactant lining the lungs may be lost as it is moved out of the smaller airways, into the trachea and swallowed along with mucus and other debris. Therefore surfactant is continuously secreted onto the lung surface. In man, sighing, which increases the lung volume, is a potent stimulus for surfactant release. Although horses do not 'sigh' as such, they do occasionally take almost double normal tidal volume breaths during exercise which may help to increase surfactant secretion.

Getting gases across the alveolar–capillary membrane

Air is moved from the atmosphere to the alveoli by bulk flow through the active process of ventilation. Once the air has reached the alveoli the oxygen has to get into the blood across the alveolar–capillary membrane (also sometimes called the blood–gas barrier). At the same time, carbon dioxide in the blood (formed by metabolism) must diffuse out into the alveoli so that it can be breathed out. In normal circumstances, all of the nitrogen in the air breathed in is also breathed out. During maximal exercise, in each breath there may be as little as a quarter of a second for gas exchange to take place. The key point about diffusion is that it is a passive process. It does not require energy, which may be thought of as an advantage. The disadvantage is that the animal cannot do anything to speed up the process of diffusion.

There are several factors affecting the rate at which gases diffuse across the alveolar–capillary membrane and their relationship to the rate of diffusion is described in Fick's law of diffusion which may be expressed as follows:

$$\text{Rate of diffusion, } \dot{V} = \frac{\text{Area}}{\text{Thickness}} \times \Delta P \times D$$

Let us take each of these factors in turn and discuss their impact on the rate of diffusion of oxygen and carbon dioxide.

Area

The rate of diffusion of a gas is proportional to the area available for gas exchange.

In the horse lung, the surface area available for gas exchange is approximately $2500\,\text{m}^2$. In humans who smoke, and in horses with RAO, the area available for diffusion may be decreased because there is damage to lung tissue and airways that may be blocked with mucus. In these cases, less oxygen can diffuse across the alveolar–capillary membrane, meaning that the partial pressure (also referred to as oxygen tension) of oxygen in arterial blood will be lower than normal. The partial pressure of oxygen considered normal in arterial blood of a horse at rest is $12.0\,\text{kPa}$ ($90\,\text{mmHg}$) or above (up to about $14.7\,\text{kPa}$ ($110\,\text{mmHg}$)). A horse with moderate to severe RAO would normally have a resting arterial partial pressure of oxygen less than $11.3\,\text{kPa}$ ($85\,\text{mmHg}$). This condition of low arterial oxygen tension is known as arterial hypoxaemia. When this occurs, the body attempts to compensate for the fact that there is less oxygen arriving in the bloodstream by producing more red blood cells so that their number in the circulation is increased (polycythaemia). Respiratory rate and heart rate may also be slightly increased above normal to compensate for the decrease in Pa_{O_2}.

In the normal, healthy lung, the surface area available for diffusion does not limit the rate of diffusion of gases. Consider the situation in the normal, healthy horse, where the total surface area available for diffusion is $2500\,m^2$ and the volume of air brought into the lung with each breath during rest is about 6 litres. About one half of this will actually find its way to a respiratory exchange surface, so 3 litres of air is presented to a gas exchange surface of $2500\,m^2$ – no problem!

Thickness

The rate of diffusion of a gas is inversely proportional to the thickness of the exchange surface.

The thicker the surface across which diffusion takes place, the slower the rate of diffusion. The thickness of the alveolar-capillary membrane may be increased if there is a lot of mucus within the lung, if there is pulmonary oedema (leakage of interstitial fluid into the alveoli or airways) or if blood is present in the airways as a result of exercise-induced pulmonary haemorrhage (EIPH). In the normal healthy horse lung, the thickness of the alveolar-capillary membrane is no more than $0.5\,\mu m$ (or $0.0005\,mm$), and does not significantly limit the rate of diffusion. To illustrate how thin the blood–gas barrier is, a horse red blood cell is around $5\,\mu m$ in length, ten times the size of the barrier that holds the cells on the blood side of the blood–gas barrier. Both the horse and man have a particularly thin blood–gas barrier or alveolar-capillary membrane that is around 0.2–$0.5\,\mu m$ at its thinnest part. This is approximately 200 times thinner than a human hair. A thin blood–gas barrier enhances diffusion and may partly explain the horse's high capacity to use oxygen during exercise, but it has also been suggested that this is why the horse is prone to EIPH.

Diffusion constant

The rate of diffusion of a gas is proportional to the diffusion constant, D.

Each individual gas has a diffusion constant; the higher the diffusion constant, the greater the rate of diffusion. D is a value describing both the solubility of the gas in the medium lining the gas exchange surface (remember, the lungs are kept moist) and the size of the gas molecule.

$$D \propto \frac{Solubility}{Molecular\ weight}$$

The molecular weight of O_2 is 32 and that of CO_2 is 44.

On the basis of their molecular weights, CO_2 should diffuse more slowly than O_2 because it is a bigger molecule. However, CO_2 is around 22 times more soluble than O_2, and so the diffusion constant for CO_2 is actually greater than that for O_2. The solubility coefficient for oxygen in blood at 37°C is $0.023\,ml\ O_2$ (STPD)/100 ml blood/kPa ($0.0031\,ml\ O_2$ (STPD)/100 ml blood/mmHg), whilst the solubility coefficient for carbon dioxide in blood at 37°C is $0.519\,ml\ CO_2$ (STPD)/100 ml blood/kPa ($0.0692\,ml$ CO_2 (STPD)/100 ml blood/mmHg) ($0.519/0.023$ or $0.0692/0.0031 = 22.3$). STPD means standard temperature (0°C) and pressure ($101.3\,kPa = 760\,mmHg$), dry (0% relative humidity, i.e. saturated vapour pressure, SVP = $0\,kPa$ ($0\,mmHg$)). This is an accepted convention for expressing gas volumes. Remember that the volume of a gas is dependent on pressure, temperature and moisture (SVP). The STPD convention is also used for expressing oxygen uptake and carbon dioxide production (see Chapter 18).

Looking back at Fick's law, and if all other factors are equal, CO_2 *should* diffuse across the membrane faster than O_2. We shall see whether or not this is the case in a moment.

Pressure gradient

The greater the pressure gradient between the gas within the alveoli and pulmonary arterial blood, the greater the rate of diffusion.

In this case, gases will be moving from a gas to a fluid, so we need to use a measure that will allow us to express their concentration regardless of whether they are in a gas mixture or in a fluid. For this we talk about the gas in terms of its partial pressure.

The partial pressure of a gas in a gas mixture or in a solution is that proportion of the total gas pressure which corresponds to the percentage by volume of the particular gas.

This may sound rather complicated but is really

Table 5.2 Partial pressures of oxygen and carbon dioxide within the atmosphere, and on either side of the alveolar-capillary membrane

	Atmosphere		Alveoli		Pulmonary artery	
	kPa	mmHg	kPa	mmHg	kPa	mmHg
O_2	21.3	160	13.3	100	5.3	40
CO_2	0.04	0.3	5.3	40	6.1	46

quite simple in practice. The following example shows how partial pressures are calculated:

Atmospheric pressure = 101.3 kPa (760 mmHg)
Percentage O_2 by volume = approximately 21%
Partial pressure of O_2 = 101.3 × (21/100)
= 21.3 kPa or (760 × (21/100) = 160 mmHg)

This would be the case for dry air. If the air has moisture in it we have to account for this before working out the oxygen partial pressure. As an example, the pressure exerted by moisture in air that is fully saturated at 37°C is 6.3 kPa (47 mmHg) and is known as the saturated water vapour pressure. To calculate the partial pressure of oxygen in saturated (100% RH) inspired air at body temperature (37°C) and at an atmospheric pressure of 101.3 kPa (760 mmHg): 101.3 kPa − 6.3 kPa = 95 kPa × (21/100) = 20.0 kPa (760 mmHg − 47 mmHg = 713 mmHg × (21/100) = 150 mmHg).

In Table 5.2, there is quite a difference between the partial pressure of oxygen in atmospheric air and alveolar air. At first sight this may seem surprising. However, the air in the alveoli at any one time is actually a mixture of inspired gas and dead-space gas, and so we can expect that the partial pressure of oxygen would be lower than atmospheric, because the incoming air is to some extent 'diluted' by the dead-space gas. From Table 5.2, we can work out the pressure gradients for gas diffusion:

For O_2: 13.3 kPa − 5.3 kPa = 8.0 kPa
(100 mmHg − 40 mmHg = 60 mmHg)

For CO_2: 6.1 kPa − 5.3 kPa = 0.8 kPa
(46 mmHg − 40 mmHg = 6 mmHg).

Earlier, we predicted that CO_2 would diffuse faster than O_2 if all other things were equal, but in fact they are not: the driving pressure for the diffu-

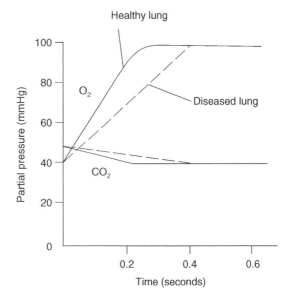

Fig. 5.7 Diffusion of gases across gas exchange surface with time.

sion of O_2 across the alveolar-capillary membrane is greater than that for CO_2. In reality, both gases diffuse at a similar rate. It takes no more than about 0.5 s for the diffusion of gases to occur and an equilibrium to be reached across the blood-gas barrier.

During normal quiet breathing in horses, the respiratory cycle lasts about 6 s and there is more than enough time for diffusion to occur. However, if for some reason the rate of diffusion is compromised, for example due to disease or the horse is asked to exercise, the diffusion of gases may not reach an equilibrium in the short time that they are in contact with the gas exchange surface (Fig. 5.7).

It seems that the lung is built with a substantial safety margin. In the normal lung, there is more than enough time for diffusion to occur. Sometimes it is only possible to diagnose respiratory disorders when the horse is exercised maximally on a treadmill, as only then will the system be challenged sufficiently for any limitation to gas exchange become apparent.

The same goes for the human lung, which unfortunately lays it open to abuse, as smokers may not realise that their lung function is reduced until they try and perform any strenuous exercise or they are further compromised by disease, by which time it may be too late!

KEY POINTS

- Respiration is the process whereby ATP is regenerated from ADP using oxygen.
- Unicellular (single celled) organisms respire but don't breathe.
- Breathing is the process of actively moving gases from the atmosphere to a gas exchange surface.
- Inspired air is conditioned by being warmed to body temperature and humidified in the upper airways.
- Cough is a good indicator of respiratory disease in horses but when cough is absent it is not a good marker of health.
- The total surface area available for gas exchange in the horse's lung is equivalent to around ten doubles tennis courts.
- Total lung volume in a 500 kg horse is around 40 litres.
- The lung has two separate blood circulations, the pulmonary and bronchial circulations.
- Minute ventilation is the tidal volume multiplied by the respiratory rate and is around 50–60 litres/min in a 500 kg horse at rest.
- When the diaphragm flattens and or the respiratory muscles make the chest wider, the pressure inside the airways and alveoli becomes more negative than outside the horse and air moves into the lung.
- Gas which is moved in and out of the respiratory system without ever taking part in gas exchange is referred to as dead space ventilation and consists of anatomical and physiological dead space.
- The horse has active phases (requiring muscular effort) to both inspiration and expiration, unlike humans.
- The relaxed or resting volume of the respiratory system is called the functional residual capacity (FRC) or end expiratory lung volume (EELV).
- At rest, horses breathe around their FRC, whilst humans breathe from FRC.

- The outside of the lung is covered by the visceral pleura and is held close to the parietal pleura, which lines the inside of the chest. The two pleural surfaces are not physically joined but are held together by a small volume of pleural fluid. During gentle breathing at rest the pressure changes in the pleural cavity (the space between the pleural surfaces) between 0.3 and 0.5 kPa (3 and 5 cmH$_2$O).
- Oesophageal pressure is a good approximation to pleural pressure and easier to measure.
- The level of ventilation and perfusion both increase from the top to the bottom of the lung.
- The lung tries to match the level of perfusion in any one region to the level of ventilation. This is known as $\dot{V}/\dot{Q}$ matching and may be disturbed in disease ($\dot{V}/\dot{Q}$ mismatch).
- The lungs are very compliant and it only takes a change in pressure of 0.3–0.5 kPa (3–5 cmH$_2$O) to move 6 litres of gas in and out. A balloon would require around 26.5 kPa (270 cmH$_2$O) for the same change in volume.
- The inner surface of the airways and alveoli is lined with surfactant which protects the lung and reduces the tendency of the smaller airways and alveoli to collapse at low lung volumes.
- Surfactant consists of around 90% phospholipid.
- Ventilation (moving air into and out of the lungs) is an active process requiring energy. Exchange of gases across the blood–gas barrier occurs by the passive process of diffusion.
- The rate of diffusion of a gas is governed by the area available for gas exchange, the thickness of the blood–gas barrier, the molecular weight of the gas molecule and the difference in the pressure of the gas (diffusion occurs from areas of high to lower pressure).
- The horse has a large lung capacity even accounting for its size and this is an important factor in high intensity exercise.

Chapter 6

The cardiovascular system

The cardiovascular system consists of the heart (cardio) and the blood vessels (vascular) that circulate blood around the body. The blood vessels form two main circuits known as the systemic and pulmonary circulations. The systemic circulation refers to the blood vessels that supply the whole body, i.e. those vessels going from the left hand side of the heart, to all organs and tissues, and then back to the right hand side of the heart (Fig. 6.1). The arterial blood that flows away from the heart in the systemic circulation is under high pressure (mean pressure around 13.3 kPa (100 mmHg) at rest in the horse) and has a long distance to travel, with a large amount of blood having to be moved against gravity. The systemic circulation carries gases, nutrients, waste products, hormones and heat around the body.

The pulmonary arterial circulation consists of all the blood vessels flowing out of the right hand side of the heart, to the lungs. The vessels taking blood from the lungs to the left hand side of the heart comprise the pulmonary venous circulation. The blood flowing within this loop is under lower pressure (mean pressure approximately 2.0–3.3 kPa (15–25 mmHg) at rest in the horse) than that within the systemic circulation. The primary purpose of the pulmonary circulation is to bring venous blood into close contact with the respiratory surface to increase the amount of oxygen and unload carbon dioxide so that it can be exhaled. The lung tissue itself also requires nutrients and oxygen and this is supplied by the bronchial arterial circulation. This arises from the main arterial outflow from the left side of the heart (the aorta). The heart (which is a muscle) also has its own special circulation known as the coronary circulation. This is a network of arteries and veins running over the heart. In man, if these vessels (most often the coronary arteries) become blocked by fatty deposits, a heart attack may occur. In a coronary heart attack, the blood supply to a region of the heart fails, and with no blood and oxygen supply that region of the heart is damaged. Heart attacks are fairly rare in horses. However, this should not surprise us: horses are vegetarian, they don't eat high fat diets (especially not saturated fats), they don't drink excessively, don't smoke and they take plenty of exercise.

Types of blood vessel

Arteries

Arteries are the most substantial of the blood vessels. They have thick, muscular walls, which you would expect of vessels that carry fluid under high pressure (Fig. 6.2). There are no valves in arteries, because being under high pressure, there is no risk of significant backflow. All arteries carry blood away from the heart and, as such, carry oxygenated blood; the exception to this rule is the pulmonary artery which carries venous blood on its way to be reoxygenated. Blood with high oxygen content is bright red, and so arterial blood coming from a wound is easily recognisable, both due to its colour and the fact that it spurts out of the wound with the same frequency as the pulse rate.

Arteries are lined with elastin, which helps to modulate the 'on–off' effect of the heart's contraction, so that the flow of blood downstream of the large arteries is almost continuous rather than intermittent. The muscle found within arteries is smooth muscle (also known as involuntary muscle) and is the type of muscle that is controlled by the autonomic nervous system. Smooth muscle contractions allow alterations in the cross-sectional area of the arteries and thus provide a mechanism for regulating blood flow.

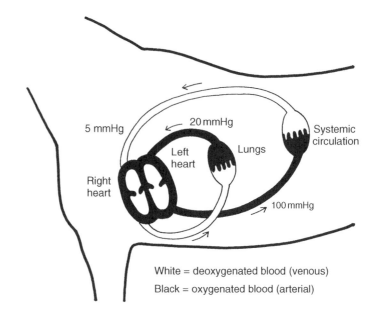

Fig. 6.1   Pulmonary and systemic circulations.

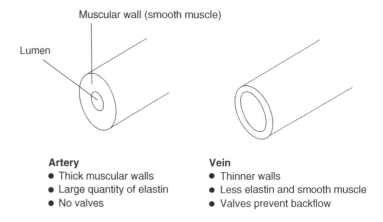

Fig. 6.2   Blood vessels.

Artery
- Thick muscular walls
- Large quantity of elastin
- No valves

Vein
- Thinner walls
- Less elastin and smooth muscle
- Valves prevent backflow

Veins

Veins are thinner walled vessels which carry blood back to the heart; they have less elastin and smooth muscle than arteries. The blood flowing through them is described as 'deoxygenated' and is darker in colour than arterial blood. There is less oxygen in venous blood than arterial blood, because much of the oxygen has been unloaded at the tissues, but it is never completely devoid of oxygen. Thus the term 'deoxygenated' is perhaps misleading. Veins carry blood under lower pressure than arteries, so there are valves to prevent backflow. In people suffering from varicose veins, the valves are incompetent and so pooling of blood occurs in the lower limbs and the pressure of blood returning to the heart is low. Even in normal individuals, about 70% of the total circulating volume of blood is found in the venous circulation. As in arteries, the cross-sectional area of veins can be altered by the autonomic nervous system to regulate blood flow and pressure (Fig. 6.3).

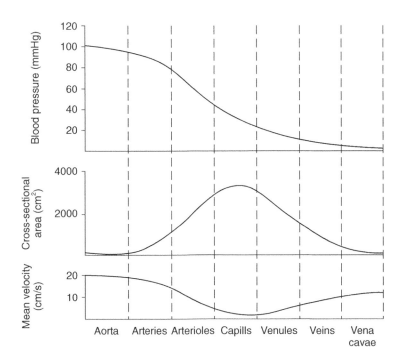

Fig. 6.3 Graph of pressure, flow velocity and cross-sectional area of circulation.

Capillaries

Capillaries are simple walled structures. At any time only about 5% of the total volume of blood in the circulation is found within capillaries. The average capillary pressure is approximately 2.7 kPa (20 mmHg), being lower at the venous end than the arterial end. The walls of capillaries are only one cell thick; this is thin enough to allow diffusion of nutrients and gases between capillaries and tissues. Blood flows very slowly through capillaries, which allows time for the exchange of gases and nutrients between the capillary blood and surrounding cells by diffusion. The same laws that govern diffusion in the lung also operate at the level of the capillaries. It takes about 1–2 seconds for blood to flow from the arterial end to the venous end of a normal sized capillary. During exercise the blood flow through certain tissues, e.g. the lungs, is faster, which can present problems in that the blood has travelled through the capillary and out to the venous circulation before complete exchange of oxygen has taken place. In tissues that are relatively inactive during exercise, e.g. the gastrointestinal tract, the arterioles (small arteries) supplying the capillary network are constricted and so blood flow through that tissue is reduced. In this way, blood is directed to areas of the body that require it the most – primarily the muscles.

The heart as a pump

The heart is a muscular pump made up of four chambers: two atria and two ventricles. The atria are smaller and less muscular than the ventricles, and their function is to assist with filling of the ventricles. The heart is made up of a special type of smooth or involuntary muscle, which is known as cardiac muscle or myocardium. The flow of blood through the heart is shown in Fig. 6.4.

The left ventricle is larger than the right ventricle and its walls are more muscular because it must pump against the 'back' pressure of the arterial circulation. For this reason the left ventricle is often referred to as a 'pressure' pump whilst the right ventricle is referred to as a 'volume' pump. If the heart is to be an effective pump, blood must be prevented from flowing back into the venous

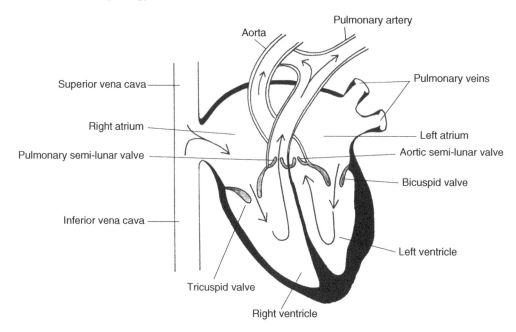

Fig. 6.4   The heart and the flow of blood through it.

circulation when contraction takes place. For this reason, valves are found both between the atria and ventricles (atrioventricular valves), and between the ventricles and the arteries (semilunar valves) to prevent backflow of blood.

The valves are passive. Whether they are open or shut depends entirely on the relative pressures of blood on either side of them. For example, when the pressure in the atria is greater than the pressure in the ventricles, the atrioventricular valves are open. When the pressure in the atria is less than the pressure in the ventricles, the valve is closed. Similarly, when the pressure in the ventricles is greater than that within the arteries, the semilunar valves are open and vice versa.

The arterial pressures in the systemic circulation alternate between what are known as 'systolic' and 'diastolic' pressures depending on whether the heart is in contraction or relaxation. In man, when the heart is in a state of contraction, the pressure in the vessels is high at around 16.0 kPa (120 mmHg; systolic pressure) and when the heart is in a state of relaxation, the pressure in the vessels is around 10.7 kPa (80 mmHg; diastolic pressure). In medical terms this is usually referred to as a blood pressure of 120/80 (120 over 80 mmHg or 16.0/10.7 kPa). The

equivalent pressures in the horse are very similar under true resting conditions but are greatly influenced by heart rate and excitement.

Cardiac output

Cardiac output ($\dot{Q}$) is the amount of blood that flows out of the left hand side of the heart per minute. It depends directly upon two variables:

(1) Heart rate (f_c or HR) = how many times the heart beats in a minute
(2) Stroke volume (SV) = the volume of blood pumped out of the heart at each beat, such that:

$$\dot{Q} \text{ (litres/min)} = \text{HR (beats/min)} \times \text{SV (litres)}$$

The dot over the Q indicates that we are dealing with a rate (as for minute ventilation, $\dot{V}_E$). The SV, and therefore the cardiac output also, is dependent upon the amount of blood returning to the right hand (venous) side of the heart (preload), the force of contraction of the heart during each beat (myocardial contractility) and the pressure in the arterial systemic circulation (afterload).

For a person, cardiac output is between 4 and 6 litres/min, increasing up to anything between 25 and 35 litres/min during exercise in elite human athletes when demand for oxygen and hence blood flow, is increased.

For a horse, resting cardiac output is in the region of 25 litres/min (our maximum during exercise) and increases up to 300 litres/min in elite equine athletes during exercise. Despite the fact that the horse is a much larger animal and will obviously have a higher oxygen requirement due simply to its larger muscle mass, the horse is still capable of a cardiac output greater than that of a human. If we 'normalise' for body mass by simply dividing the maximum cardiac output by the body mass for each species, we see that the human maximum cardiac output is around 0.35 litres/min/kg body mass and that for the horse is 0.7 litres/min/kg body mass. Therefore the horse is capable of twice the cardiac output of the human when the values are scaled for differences in body size.

Cardiac output is increased in response to the increased demand for oxygen that occurs during exercise; however, in addition it is redistributed, so that a greater proportion of the cardiac output goes to the muscles and the heart, and a smaller proportion to the stomach, intestines, kidney and other organs. During low to moderate intensity exercise a significant amount of cardiac output is also directed to the skin to aid thermoregulation. In man, the skin blood flow is also significant during intense exercise. However, during intense exercise the horse is able to decrease the amount of blood flowing to the skin. This has the advantage of increasing blood flow and oxygen delivery to the locomotory muscles, but has the disadvantage of making the horse hotter. The body will match supply of blood flow to demand as far as possible, even during maximal exercise.

Electrical conduction through the heart

Cardiac muscle cells are shorter than skeletal muscle cells and are branched. They touch end to end, providing a direct electrical connection between adjacent cells via special regions known as intercalated discs. The electrical resistance between cardiac muscle cells is low and so electrical nerve impulses pass easily between adjacent cells. As a result, when one cell is stimulated the stimulus will spread directly to all the other connected cells.

Electrical impulses are, however, prevented from passing directly between atria and ventricles by the presence of a fibrous ring. This ring prevents electrical coupling of atrial and ventricular cells. The only point at which electrical activity can pass between the atria and the ventricles is via Purkinje tissue found in the wall between the left and right ventricles.

Because atria and ventricles are essentially electrically isolated, they are prevented from contracting simultaneously. For the heart to be an effective pump atrial contraction must occur before ventricular contraction. In this way, both the atria contract together to fill the ventricles with blood and then the ventricles contract together to pump this blood out into the pulmonary artery (right ventricle) or aorta (left ventricle). The most unusual thing about the heart muscle is its ability to contract rhythmically without a nervous supply. It is possible to take the heart out of the body, having removed all nerves which supply it, and keep it beating for several hours by simply bathing it in a solution which supplies oxygen and nutrients. In contrast, smooth muscle and skeletal muscle both require nervous stimulation in order to contract. The heart is capable of maintaining rhythmic contractions without any nervous input. This is a particular feature of cardiac muscle and it is known as inherent rhythmicity.

The unusual ability of the heart to beat without external nerve supply is due to the fact that heart muscle generates the electrical impulse responsible for the mechanical contraction 'on site'. The heartbeat is initiated in a region of specialised cardiac tissue known as the sinoatrial (SA) node, more commonly known as the pacemaker, which is found on the right hand side of the right atrium (Fig. 6.5). The electrical activity then spreads from cell to cell across the atria, with the right atrium contracting slightly before the left. The electrical signal quickly reaches another node found at the bottom of the right atrium near the septum called the atrioventricular node (AVN). Conduction of electrical activity across the AVN is slow compared with the conduction across atrial and ventricular muscle.

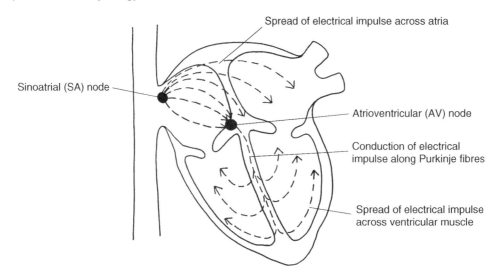

Fig. 6.5   Electrical conduction through the heart.

The slow transmission across the AVN ensures that the atria have finished contracting (and therefore finished filling the ventricles) before ventricular contraction starts. In this way there is plenty of time for blood to flow from the atria into the ventricles before ventricular contraction. There would be little point in contracting the heart muscle before the ventricles were full of blood.

In the condition known as atrial fibrillation, which is one of the more common cardiac conditions of the horse, the atria contract at a fast rate that is not related to the rate of contraction of the ventricles. In effect the atria and ventricles are out of phase. This is not an uncommon finding in racehorses and is usually associated with poor performance and an increased frequency and/or severity of exercise-induced pulmonary haemorrhage (EIPH). Because the atria are contracting more rapidly and also out of phase with the ventricles, the filling of the ventricles is reduced and therefore so is stroke volume and hence cardiac output. The reduced cardiac output is the most likely reason for the reduced performance. Many horses that develop atrial fibrillation will spontaneously convert back to normal. For this reason, if atrial fibrillation is diagnosed the horse is often left for around a week before being treated to see if it can convert back to normal function on its own. If the horse does not convert, the condition can often

be treated successfully medically using quinidine sulphate. However, quinidine is both toxic and irritant. For this reason it is administered by nasogastric tube rather than intravenously. Side effects can include low blood pressure, lethargy and colic, and in rare cases sudden death. About 75% of horses with atrial fibrillation respond to quinidine treatment, but it is not uncommon for the condition to recur in some horses.

From the AVN the electrical signal passes down specialised conducting fibres called Purkinje fibres found within the bundle of His. The fibres within the bundle of His divide and spread upwards into the left and right ventricles forming the Purkinje network. The electrical signal reaches the apex of the ventricles very quickly and then spreads upwards throughout the ventricular muscle. In effect, the blood is wrung out of the heart, with the contraction beginning at the bottom of the ventricles; blood is pushed out of the ventricles from the closed end to the open end, rather like the way toothpaste *should* be pushed out of the tube!

An ordered electrical wave which brings about the heartbeat thus takes the following route through the heart muscle (see Fig. 6.5): sinoatrial node, atrial muscle, atrioventricular node, bundle of His, Purkinje fibres, ventricular muscle.

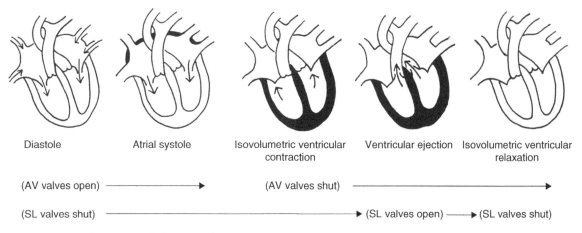

| Diastole | Atrial systole | Isovolumetric ventricular contraction | Ventricular ejection | Isovolumetric ventricular relaxation |

(AV valves open) ⟶ (AV valves shut) ⟶

(SL valves shut) ⟶ (SL valves open) ⟶ (SL valves shut)

Fig. 6.6 The cardiac cycle. Actively contracting areas are shown in black.

The cardiac cycle

Venous blood flows continuously into the right atrium from both the inferior vena cava (blood coming back from the head and neck) and superior vena cava (blood coming back from all other parts of the body) and into the left atrium from the pulmonary vein. Let us follow the cardiac cycle from the point when the heart is relaxed, i.e. in diastole.

(1) At this stage of the cardiac cycle when venous blood is flowing into both atria, the atrioventricular valves are open and blood flows straight through the atria into the ventricle. When the ventricle is about 70% full, the atria contract and propel blood into the ventricles. This phase of the cardiac cycle is called atrial systole (see Fig. 6.6).

(2) After a short pause the ventricles contract, decreasing the volume within them. As the ventricular volume is decreased, the pressure within the ventricle is increased. The pressure within the ventricles rises above that of the atrium causing the atrioventricular valves to shut, making the first heart sound, 'LUP'.

(3) The continuing increase in ventricular pressure forces open the semilunar valves. The pressure within the aorta and the pulmonary artery are both at their lowest before this, a value referred to as the diastolic blood pressure (about 10.7 kPa (80 mmHg) in the aorta at rest in a

healthy person and similar in a horse). Blood is then ejected into the systemic and pulmonary circulations. At the point at which blood is forced into the arteries it is at its highest pressure, corresponding to the systolic blood pressure (about 16.0 kPa (120 mmHg) at rest in a healthy person and, again, similar in a horse).

(4) When ventricular contraction stops, ventricular pressures drop below pulmonary arterial and aortic pressures, the semilunar valves close, and the ejection of blood from the heart stops. The closing of the semilunar valves corresponds to the second heart sound, 'DUP'.

At rest at a heart rate of 30 beats/min two-thirds to three-quarters of each cardiac cycle is spent in diastole and only one-third to a quarter in systole. To some extent the exact proportions of systole and diastole may vary slightly depending on the criteria used to define systole and diastole. For example, using echocardiography (ultrasound) and Doppler (a technique to visualise blood flow in the heart) to look at aortic flow, diastole would be defined as the period when the aortic valve is closed and there is no blood flowing out of the left ventricle.

So, for 25–33% of the cardiac cycle, the heart is actively contracting and for the remaining 66–75% of the cycle the heart muscle is relaxed and the heart is filling. When the heart rate increases, diastole tends to be shortened more than systole, so that at maximal exercise systole and diastole are approximately equal in duration. In other words, if any part of the cardiac cycle is compromised at high heart rates it is filling time (diastole) that is lost, not contraction time (systole).

The electrocardiogram (ECG)

The ECG is a measure of the sum of the electrical activity within the heart throughout the course of each heartbeat. It is measured at the skin surface and has a characteristic shape. Electrodes placed in strategic positions on the skin surface pick up the electrical activity and the exact positioning of the electrodes can affect the shape and size of the ECG recorded. The ECG represents the sum of all the electrical activity occurring in all the cardiac muscle cells in one beat. The pattern of the ECG corresponds to specific events within the cardiac cycle as outlined below (Fig. 6.7b).

The timing values for each phase of the ECG given below are for resting mature horses with a heart rate of around 30 beats/minute.

- *P wave*. This represents the electrical signal passing across the atria or the depolarisation of the atria and at rest lasts for around 0.12–0.14 seconds.
- *PQ interval* (approximately 0.35–0.55 seconds' duration). This corresponds to the passage of electrical activity through the AV node, bundle of His and Purkinje network. Because these structures are electrically isolated from the rest of the cardiac cells, the heart appears to be electrically silent at this point.
- *QRS complex* (0.10–0.15 seconds' duration). This corresponds to the electrical stimulation (or depolarisation) of the ventricles. It has a much greater amplitude than the P wave because the ventricular mass is greater than the atrial mass and thus the amount of active cells within the ventricles is greater.
- *T wave*. This corresponds to the relaxation (or repolarisation) of the ventricles, the electrical signal having passed. There is also a wave corresponding to the relaxation of the atria but this occurs at the same time as the wave of depolarisation passes through the ventricles and is swamped by it.

The duration from the start of the QRS (i.e. the Q wave) to the T wave is known as the QT interval and is around 0.6 seconds.

The ECG changes dramatically in nature from rest (Fig. 6.7a,b) to exercise (Fig. 6.7c). The most striking change is often the dramatic increase in size of the T waves. The ECG provides information to the clinician about both the quality of the heartbeat and its rhythm (Fig. 6.7d,e). ECGs are used to monitor the heart throughout anaesthesia, throughout a field or treadmill exercise test, or simply to aid in the diagnosis of a suspected heart abnormality such as atrial fibrillation.

In man, the convention for taking a standard Lead I ECG is that the negative electrode is placed on the right arm and the positive electrode on the left arm. This gives the characteristic ECG shown in physiology or medical texts, which has a positive (upward) R wave. The equivalent Lead known as a base–apex ECG in a horse is taken with the negative electrode placed on the neck or withers and the positive electrode placed on the sternum or other point below the vertical height of the heart (e.g. under the chest in the midline). However, if we compare a human and horse ECG taken in this way, the horse ECG appears to be 'upside-down'. The reason for this is that in the horse the network of Purkinje fibres is very extensive and penetrates very deeply into the myocardium. This means that when the electrical impulse spreads from the atria into the ventricles, the majority of the myocardium depolarises at the same time, with the exception of the very lowest part of the intraventricular septum (between the left and right ventricles at the base of the heart). Thus, whilst in the human ECG we see the wave of depolarisation as it spreads throughout the ventricles, in the horse the wave of electrical excitation travelling from the base to the apex (giving a positive R wave in people) is cancelled out. The only depolarisation wave that is seen is the one travelling in the opposite direction and therefore it appears negative rather than positive.

Control of blood flow

Various tissues have differing requirements for blood at different times depending on the activities of the body. There is a finite amount of blood in the body which is insufficient to supply all of the body, all of the time, especially during exercise. The horse is able to increase its blood volume from about

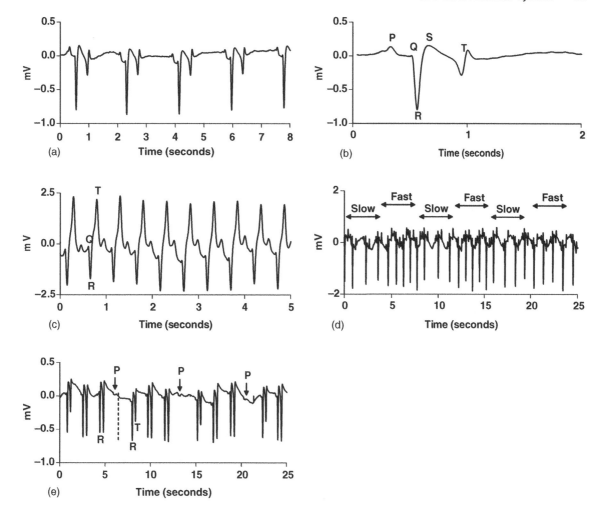

Fig. 6.7 (a) The resting electrocardiogram (ECG); (b) resting ECG showing one heart beat; (c) exercising ECG; (d) exercising ECG showing respiratory sinus arrhythmia; (e) exercising ECG showing second degree AV block.

40 litres at rest to around 50 litres during maximal exercise by a combination of releasing extra blood cells stored in the spleen and shifts and redistribution of fluids. We cannot do this. However, even with this extra volume of blood, the body must choose where it is best directed. If the requirement of skeletal muscle for oxygen is increased by exercise, the increase in blood flow to muscle can be achieved by:

(1) Diverting blood away from less active organs or organs not required during exercise, e.g. the gut.
(2) Decreasing thermoregulation by decreasing skin blood flow.

(3) Increasing cardiac output.

The ability of the circulatory system to regulate blood flow to all the tissues within the body is quite amazing; in fact, the tissues themselves play a part in regulating their own blood flow by a process known as autoregulation. When a tissue becomes active its blood vessels automatically dilate in response to the increase in activity. This occurs because active tissues release what are known as vasoactive substances into the bloodstream. Vasoactive stimuli include high levels of carbon dioxide, low levels of oxygen, high concentrations of hydrogen ions (which make the blood more acidic), high levels of potassium ions, high levels of lactate, and heat. All of these result from an increase in cellular activity, coupled with an inadequate blood supply. The resulting accumulation of metabolites leads to dilation of blood vessels and a consequent increase in blood flow. Once the metabolites have been cleared as a result of the increased blood flow, the flow is reduced by vasoconstriction to bring the vessels back to their original state. A control mechanism such as this, whereby the end result tends to switch off the initial stimulus, is called negative feedback and is the most commonly used type of physiological control. Autoregulation ensures that tissues that are working hard and using oxygen have relatively more oxygen delivered to them and is just one of the ways in which the body attempts to exactly match demand for nutrients such as oxygen, carbohydrate and fat with supply.

Another method by which blood flow is matched to demand is via nervous control. Smooth muscle in blood vessel walls is controlled by sympathetic nerves that are part of the autonomic nervous system. If the frequency of impulses within the sympathetic system increases, vasoconstriction occurs. Sympathetic nerves are generally active, constantly sending impulses that liberate the neurotransmitters noradrenaline and adrenaline, and cause the smooth muscle to contract. If the sympathetic supply is cut the vessels dilate, demonstrating that there is constant sympathetic tone. Tone means that there is a basal level of stimulation, i.e. the system is never 'fully relaxed'.

Supposing all the tissues in the body required an increase in blood supply, all the vessels would be dilated and it would not be possible to maintain the blood pressure. An analogy would be to have all the taps in your house turned on full at once. The water pressure in each would be reduced and some taps would not have any supply at all. Regulatory mechanisms are important not only to match blood supply to demand but to prioritise blood flow and to maintain blood pressure in spite of increased demand.

Control of blood pressure

Blood flows down a pressure gradient. Arterial blood pressure must be maintained or circulation

could not continue. Arterial blood pressure is a consequence of the cardiac output $\dot{Q}$ and the peripheral resistance P, i.e. the resistance of the blood vessels to flow, which is largely dependent on the degree to which the vessel is dilated. If the vessel is dilated resistance is low, and if the vessel is constricted the resistance is high. If cardiac output increases and resistance stays the same, i.e. the blood vessels stay the same size, blood pressure increases. If resistance decreases and cardiac output stays the same, blood pressure decreases. In other words, blood pressure is related proportionately to both cardiac output and resistance.

Blood pressure = cardiac output
× peripheral resistance

Potentially large swings in blood pressure are usually avoided by altering cardiac output. This is mediated by baroreceptors (special cells that act as 'pressure sensors') found within the blood vessels that are sensitive to changes in blood pressure. If the baroreceptors detect an increase in stretch of the major arteries there is an increase in frequency of nerve impulses sent to the medulla in the brain, which responds by bringing about a reduction in vasoconstriction and a reduction in heart rate via the autonomic nervous system. Small fluctuations in blood pressure are modulated purely by varying peripheral resistance at the level of the arterioles. In normal healthy individuals, blood pressure is stable over periods of hours. Fig. 6.8 shows the relationship between blood presure, heart sounds and ECG over one cardiac cycle.

The composition of blood

Blood makes up around 10% of the body mass of the horse – approximately 50 litres or 5 bucketfuls! Blood consists of plasma, red blood cells (RBCs), white blood cells (WBCs) and platelets.

Plasma

If we take a blood sample from a horse, add an anticoagulant (a substance to stop it clotting, e.g. EDTA) and place it in a test tube, after about 30 minutes it will have separated into a clear yellow fluid uppermost in the tube and a red, semiopaque

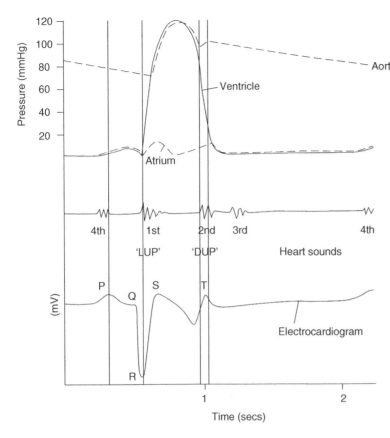

Fig. 6.8 Relationship between blood pressure, heart sounds and electrocardiogram. First and second heart sounds are most obvious, but two other heart sounds may be audible; third heart sound correlates to ventricular filling; fourth heart sound or 'atrical sound' is associated with atrial contraction and end of systole.

layer at the bottom of the tube (see Fig. 6.9). The clear yellow fluid is called plasma. It clots when exposed to air unless an anticoagulant is added. Plasma with the clotting agents removed is known as serum. This is formed by taking a blood sample and leaving it to clot in a tube. The clot can then be removed leaving the serum. Plasma is largely water (92%) and protein (6%), with the remainder being made up of substances which are dissolved and suspended within it, e.g. glucose, fats, amino acids, hormones, electrolytes, antibodies and vitamins. A very small amount of oxygen is also carried around the body dissolved in the plasma, but around 99.9% is carried bound to haemoglobin in the red blood cells.

Plasma proteins consist of albumins, globulins and fibrinogens. Albumins are often used to bind steroid hormones so that they may be transported around the body without being filtered out of the circulation and into the urine by the kidney (albumins are too large to be filtered at the kidney). Globulins form antibodies used in defence against

disease, and fibrinogen is responsible for blood clotting. Capillary walls are largely impermeable to proteins which at normal blood pressures do not pass freely between the blood vessel and surrounding tissues; consequently, they tend to exert an osmotic pull on water in surrounding tissues. The 'osmotic pull' is given by the osmolarity of a solution expressed in osmoles, with one osmole of a solute calculated as follows:

1 osmole (osm)

$$= \frac{\text{Molecular weight of a substance (in grams)}}{\text{Number of freely moving particles each molecule liberates in solution}}$$

The large molecular weight of the proteins when in solution tends to produce a high osmolarity and large osmotic potential. Osmotic potential describes the extent to which water will pass through a semipermeable membrane (in this case the capillary wall) in order to travel down a solute concentration gradient. Generally, the osmolarity is the same between the plasma and the interstitial fluid (the fluid between cells), due largely to the free movement of water between the two fluid compartments.

If all the blood in the circulation were drained out and the red blood cells separated from the plasma, the plasma volume would be around 30 litres in a 500 kg horse or around 10% of the total body water content, i.e. about 300 litres. Plasma volume does differ between breeds, with Thoroughbreds tend to have a plasma volume of around 75 ml/kg bodyweight whilst heavier breeds may have plasma volumes as low as 55 ml/kg.

Red blood cells (erythrocytes)

Red blood cells (RBCs) are biconcave discs with no nucleus, i.e. they are anucleate. This means they have more room available for storing haemoglobin, the pigment that makes the blood cells red and carries oxygen around the body. Why is haemoglobin contained in RBCs and not just free in the plasma? Even though haemoglobin is a large protein, it would still be excreted by the kidney if it was not held in the erythrocytes. Myoglobin molecules are of similar size and structure to haemoglobin, and when severe muscle damage occurs myoglobin can be found in the urine, colouring it dark brown. The same would happen to haemoglobin if it were not contained in erythrocytes.

The biconcave shape of erythrocytes maximises their surface area for gaseous exchange, and they are highly flexible to enable them to squeeze through narrow capillaries in single file. Unlike nearly all other cells in the body, RBCs do not have mitochondria. They obtain their ATP solely from anaerobic glycolysis of glucose taken up from the plasma and produce lactic acid that diffuses back out into the plasma. If a blood sample is left at room temperature after being taken, the blood

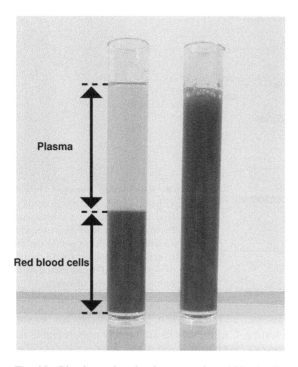

Fig. 6.9 Blood samples, showing separation of blood cells from plasma on standing. The PCV of the sample shown is 0.44 litre/litre or 44%.

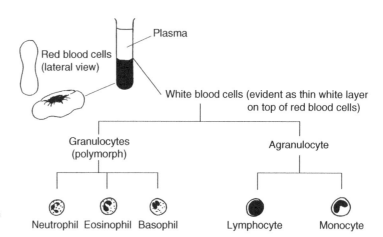

Fig. 6.10 Appearance of red and white blood cells.

glucose concentration will drop and the lactate concentration will increase as a result of RBC metabolism. RBCs have a maximum lifespan of around 3 months. New RBCs are produced in the bone marrow and old cells are removed and broken down by the spleen. The waste products of the breakdown of RBCs are further processed by the liver to produce bilirubin. Horses in training tend to have a higher rate of turnover of RBCs.

There are between 8×10^{12} and 15×10^{12} RBCs per litre of blood at rest, with the number tending to increase with training. Each cell is around $5\,\mu m$ in diameter. During exercise, the contraction of the spleen can double the number of RBCs in the horse's circulation.

White blood cells

There are far fewer white cells than red cells in whole blood. When a heparinised blood sample (a sample treated with heparin to prevent it clotting) is allowed to settle out, the white cells are seen as a thin white line between the RBCs and the plasma (Fig. 6.9, 6.10). White blood cells (WBCs) are also called leucocytes and, as shown in Table 6.1, can be divided into two main groups according to their appearance.

WBCs are responsible for defence against disease, including viral, bacterial and parasitic infection. They are also involved in allergic reactions to substances such as pollen and moulds. Their functions can broadly be separated into those which fight non-specific immune responses to infection and inflammation, and those which deal with acquired immune responses. The lymphocytes are primarily responsible for acquired immunity whilst the others take care of non-specific infections. There are approximately 3.5×10^9 lymphocytes per litre in whole blood, but the numbers increase further in response to an infection. Total WBC

count is usually around 6×10^9 to 12×10^9 cells/litre and high values often indicate infection, although low counts can be seen with viral infection.

Non-specific immunity

If the horse's skin is broken, many different species of microbes enter the body. This stimulates the surrounding tissue and ultimately stimulates basophils to release histamine and heparin into the bloodstream. Heparin increases the flow of blood into the damaged tissue, whilst histamine causes vasodilation and increases permeability of the local blood vessels. Due to the increased permeability, plasma proteins and RBCs leak into the injured site. Eventually clotting occurs with the aim of trapping the microbes in one place. Thereafter, tissue macrophages move in. If infection persists neutrophils move in to kill and phagocytose the microbes, and if further assistance is required, agranular monocytes are enlisted. During the course of these reactions the total number of WBCs circulating in the bloodstream increases.

Acquired immunity

Lymphocytes attack invading bacteria and viruses with antibodies specifically designed to deal with the particular invading organism. This is because either the body has previously been invaded by the particular organism and has a 'memory' of it or because a 'memory' has been created following vaccination. The aim of vaccination is to inject into the body deactivated viruses or bacteria that are unable to induce a true infection but which are able to induce the same type of immune response as if they were normal live or active organisms. Non-pathogenic viruses or bacteria may be produced by treatment with chemicals, by killing them (by exposure to high temperatures or UV light, for example), or by altering them genetically.

Platelets (thrombocytes)

There are somewhere in the order of 400000 platelets/ml of blood. They have a lifespan of 9–11 days. Their function is to help with clotting by forming platelet 'plugs' when blood vessels are damaged. If the skin is cut the walls of capillaries and other small blood vessels are damaged and blood leaks out (haemorrhage). Fibrinogen, which

Table 6.1 Approximate percentages of white blood cell types in the healthy horse at rest

Granulocytes	Agranulocytes
Neutrophils (~55%)	Monocytes (~5%)
Eosinophils (~4%)	Lymphocytes (~35%)
Basophils (~1%)	

is normally dissolved in plasma, is converted to fibrin in the presence of calcium. Fibrin forms a long fibrous network that traps RBCs, forming a 'clot'. The clot then shrinks and serum escapes leaving a 'scab'. Clotting is also necessary internally and not just at the skin surface. For example, worm larvae may damage blood vessel walls causing internal haemorrhage. A blood clot formed within a blood vessel can become so large that it blocks the blood vessel leading to tissue death.

Haematology and clinical biochemistry

Some vets recommend regular blood testing for horses in very hard work; for example, racehorses in training. A blood test may consist of both haematological and biochemical analyses, where haematology refers to the study of the red and white blood cells, and the biochemical analyses (often referred to as clinical biochemistry) give information relating to the chemical substances dissolved in the plasma. In the past, both haematology and clinical biochemistry testing had to be carried out manually. Smears of blood were examined under a microscope and individual biochemical tests were run in a laboratory. Machines called autoanalysers are now available to carry out automated haematology and biochemistry tests. The operator has only to load the sample, put in the reagents (chemicals needed to run the tests) and select which tests to run on each sample. The machine actually runs all the tests. Blood samples for both haematology and biochemistry are normally taken from the jugular vein. The jugular vein is chosen as it is large, superficial and easily accessible. There is virtually no difference in the haematology or biochemistry results for arterial and venous blood. Because the arteries lie deeper in the body and the blood in them is at higher pressure, it is harder to stop them from bleeding after a needle has been inserted and withdrawn, so they are usually not used for routine blood sampling. The exception is when we want to know about blood gas and acid–base status, in which case an arterial sample is essential.

The blood sample is taken using a large (at least by human medical standards!) 0.8–1.2 mm (21–18 gauge) needle. An excessive vacuum should not be used to draw the blood into the syringe because this can damage the cells (haemolysis). Blood coagulates shortly after exposure to air, so for most purposes blood samples have to be collected in tubes that contain an anticoagulant. A number of different anticoagulants are used depending on what analysis is to be carried out on the blood sample. Blood samples for both haematology and biochemistry should be handled with care. Haemolysis occurs if samples are left lying around in hot conditions, if samples are roughly handled, e.g. shaken, or if the blood sample is squirted into a sample tube from a syringe with the needle still in place. Samples for either haematology or biochemistry should be mixed with the anticoagulant in the sample tube by gentle rolling and inversion. Blood samples should not be frozen because this will also cause haemolysis. However, once RBCs have been separated from samples for biochemistry testing the plasma or serum should be stored at around 4°C, or frozen if analysis is not going to take place immediately.

Haemolysis causes several different problems, mainly interference with biochemical assays and false elevation of some measurements. For example, RBCs contain much higher concentrations of potassium than the plasma. If a sample is haemolysed, the plasma potassium concentration will be artificially high. The blood sample in the syringe is separated into tubes containing particular anticoagulants depending on what tests are going to be performed. Blood is usually collected into tubes containing the anticoagulant ethylenediaminetetraacetic acid (EDTA) for haematology, and into tubes containing lithium, sodium or ammonium heparin for plasma biochemistry. Fluoride/oxalate tubes are used for plasma glucose and lactate analysis. Fluoride/oxalate prevents clotting and also stops the RBCs metabolising glucose, which would lead to low glucose and high lactate levels.

Interpretation of blood test results is not an exact science. It is not simply a case of taking the numbers produced by the analysers and comparing them with a chart of normal ranges. Interpretation is often undertaken by a specialist haematologist, clinical biochemist or clinical pathologist. There are common patterns that may point to the likelihood of one disease or another, but interpretation may be complicated by factors such as age, breed, sex, vaccination, nutrition, time of sample collection, stage of disease and whether more than one disease process is present. The clinical pathologist provides an interpretation taking into account not only these factors, but also the clinical history and details of the clinical examination provided by the vet who sent in the sample.

There is a common misconception that blood samples can be used to indicate 'fitness'. Whilst it is true that there are changes in haematology and biochemistry readings with daily exercise and over time with training, as yet there are no reliable haematological or biochemical indicators of fitness levels. Regular blood samples are likely to be of more use in deciding when a horse is unfit to run.

Normal ranges for various haematological and biochemical parameters differ between breed types, individuals within a breed, and between ages and sexes. To be able to draw conclusions based on a blood sample from a particular horse, the results of previous tests performed on that horse should ideally be known. For a 'one-off' blood test they will only be able to state whether or not the horse lies within the normal range as defined by that laboratory. To pick up on subtle changes a horse would require regular blood testing. Any deviation from normal for that particular horse may then be more significant, provided of course that the samples were taken under similar conditions. Blood samples should ideally be collected at the same time of day, preferably before feeding and exercise. This is particularly important for haematology samples, which are often collected first thing in the morning or during late afternoon (assuming the horse was exercised in the morning and last fed at midday). Exercise increases the RBC count, the WBC count and also changes the proportions of the different white cells. Exercise also increases total plasma protein and affects concentrations of electrolytes in the plasma such as potassium, sodium and chloride. Feeding can have similar effects. Blood samples should be taken before feeding or exercise; feeding a hay meal increases plasma protein and increases haematocrit as a result of the substantial amounts of saliva produced and fluid shifts. Exercise causes increases in packed cell volume, haemoglobin concentration, plasma protein and leucocyte numbers.

Resting samples should therefore be taken before or at least 4 hours after feeding or exercise. Most training yards that use regular blood sampling do so to get early warning of infections, for example indicated by an increase in the WBC count or fibrinogen, and to pick out horses with muscle problems which are indicated by increased levels of the muscle enzymes creatine phosphokinase (CK) and aspartate amino transferase (AST).

Haematology

A haemogram (a profile of the cells within blood) may include measurements of the following parameters.

Red blood cell (RBC) count
The resting normal mean is approximately 8×10^{12} to 15×10^{12} cells/litre of blood; it may also be referred to as the erythrocyte count.

Haemoglobin
The resting normal mean is approximately 11–17g haemoglobin per dl of blood (1 decilitre = 100ml) or 110–170g/l.

MCV or mean corpuscular (red cell) volume
The resting normal mean is approximately 35–45fl (1 femtolitre = 10^{-15} litres). Human RBCs are almost twice the volume of those in horses at around 70–100fl in healthy adults.

MCH or mean red cell haemoglobin content
The resting normal mean is approximately 10–17pg (1 picogram = 10^{-12} gram).

MCHC or mean corpuscular haemoglobin concentration
The resting normal range is 30–40g/dl.

WBC or white blood cell count
The resting normal mean is approximately 6×10^9 to 12×10^9 cells/litre of blood. It is normal for an increase in WBC count (up to 30%) to be seen following short-term exercise; however, prolonged submaximal exercise is normally associated with a transient reduction in WBC count known as leucopenia. This is also accompanied by a change in the WBC profile, namely an increase in neutrophils (neutrophilia) and a decrease in lymphocytes

(lymphopenia). An increase in the neutrophil/ lymphocyte ratio in this manner is typical of the reaction associated with stress and has been suggested by some to indicate overtraining in some horses. Maximal exercise causes splenic contraction and the release of lymphocytes as well as red blood cells into the circulation. The exercise-induced increase in lymphocytes lasts a few hours following cessation of exercise.

PCV or packed cell volume

This is sometimes referred to as the haematocrit (HCT). The difference between the two is that the PCV is usually obtained by spinning down a small sample of blood in a thin glass capillary tube at high speed so that the RBCs are all packed at the bottom of the tube. This technique is normally called a microhaematocrit method. The proportions of RBCs to total volume are then measured using a special reader. The proportion of RBCs in 1 litre of blood is then expressed as litre/litre (e.g. 0.35 l/l). An HCT is essentially the same as a PCV but is usually a value calculated by an automated haematology analyser such as a Coulter Counter. The HCT is usually expressed as a percentage, e.g. 35%. Thus the PCV or the HCT indicate the volume of a blood sample occupied by the RBCs. At rest, the PCV is normally between 0.28 and 0.45 l/l. A PCV of less than 0.28 l/l may indicate anaemia and would then be likely to be associated with other physical signs, such as pale mucous membranes. Anaemia may actually be secondary to a bacterial or viral infection, which suppresses the production of RBCs within red bone marrow, or a heavy parasite burden. A PCV of more than 0.55 l/l at rest may be due to fluid loss as a result of heavy exercise, transport, diarrhoea, or excitement during the process of taking the blood sample itself. The harder a horse has worked, the higher will be the PCV, up to a maximum of about 0.65–0.70 l/l. The PCV increases with exercise as a result of the splenic mobilisation of RBCs resulting from exercise, with a lesser proportion of the increase occurring due to fluid loss as a result of sweating during more prolonged exercise. There is actually a linear relationship between PCV and speed of running up to the maximum PCV. Falsely high values for PCV may be recorded if a resting horse is in a state of nervousness or excitement when the blood sample is taken. It takes about 30–60 seconds for full splenic mobilisation to occur as a result of increased circulating levels of adrenaline. Provided the vet can get a blood sample within 30 seconds of arriving in the horse's stable, a resting blood sample should not be altered too much by splenic contraction. It may take 1–2 hours for RBCs to be resequestered within the spleen following full splenic contraction, although the majority are probably returned within the first 30 minutes.

Biochemistry

Typical clinical biochemistry measurements include plasma protein, electrolytes and muscle and liver enzymes.

Plasma proteins

Plasma proteins are made up of albumins, globulins and fibrinogen. Normal values for total plasma protein are approximately 6.0–7.0 g/dl or 60–70 g/l of plasma. The majority of the total plasma protein is made up of albumin and globulin, with a smaller amount of fibrinogen. The normal range for albumin in the laboratory at the Animal Health Trust is 32–40 g/l and the normal range for total globulin is 22–40 g/l.

In healthy horses at rest the albumin/globulin ratio is around 0.7:1 to 1:1. When the horse is dehydrated, total plasma protein, i.e. both albumin and globulin, increases as a result of the concurrent water losses. In severe dehydration, plasma protein may reach 12 g/dl (120 g/l). Globulin can be divided up to show five different subtypes (alpha 1 and alpha 2, beta 1 and beta 2, and gamma) using electrophoresis. The different globulin types have slightly different functions, but in general, an elevation in total globulin can be due to dehydration, inflammation, infection or parasite burden, e.g. worms, or stimulation of the immune system, whilst albumin levels increase with dehydration but may decrease as a result of disease. Therefore an increase in total protein with a decrease in the ratio of albumin to globulin would tend to point towards disease or inflammation rather than simply dehydration. Increases in fibrinogen are often indicative of inflammatory conditions, which may be either infectious or non-infectious in origin.

Plasma electrolytes

These include potassium, sodium, chloride, calcium, magnesium, phosphorus, iron and bicarbonate ions, all of which are dissolved in plasma. As plasma volume is only around 10% of the total body water stores, unless a horse is very ill or has a very serious electrolyte disturbance, plasma electrolyte concentrations are not usually a good indicator of electrolyte imbalance or deficiency throughout the whole body. Losses of potassium, sodium, chloride and calcium ions occur as a result of fluid losses due to prolonged or very heavy sweating or diarrhoea. Horses on high grain diets with little fibre may be potassium deficient, but hay usually contains high levels of potassium. Low plasma concentrations of calcium and phosphorus ions are uncommon because plasma calcium and phosphorus are strictly controlled within narrow ranges by parathyroid hormone, the active form of vitamin D and calcitonin, even if the body stores are extremely low. Bicarbonate reflects the acid–base status of the horse, with high levels of bicarbonate associated with alkalosis (increased arterial blood pH) and low levels associated with acidosis (decreased arterial blood pH). Alkalosis is most usually encountered in endurance horses as a result of both hyperventilation as a response to increased body temperature and electrolyte losses, whilst acidosis is more frequently associated with increased lactic acid production by muscle during short duration, intense exercise such as flat or jump racing.

Enzymes

Lactate dehydrogenase (LDH), creatine phosphokinase (CK) and aspartate amino transferase (AST) are all enzymes present in skeletal and heart muscle. These enzymes are large proteins that normally remain within the cells unless the cell membranes become more 'leaky' or are damaged. Levels of these enzymes in plasma (correctly termed activity) usually increase slightly following exercise, but abnormally high activities may indicate muscle damage or tying-up (rhabdomyolysis).

Gamma-glutamyl transferase (GGT), alkaline phosphatase (AP) and sorbitol dehydrogenase (SD) are all found in high levels in the liver; thus elevated levels of these enzymes in a sample may indicate liver damage. GGT activity may also increase as a result of obstructive diseases of the large colon. GGT activity can increase throughout a training programme and abnormally high activities may be associated with subclinical disease or injury or poor performance in some horses.

KEY POINTS

- The cardiovascular system consists of the heart (cardio), the blood and the blood vessels (vascular).
- The main circulatory systems are the systemic and pulmonary circulations.
- The systemic circulation essentially supplies all of the organs and tissues of the body. All venous blood flow passes through the pulmonary circulation which serves to bring the venous blood to the gas exchange surface.
- The heart and lungs have their own special circulations known as the coronary and bronchial circulations, respectively.
- Arteries are thick walled muscular blood vessels lined with elastin that carry blood at high pressure and generally lie deeper in the body than veins which are thin walled, carry blood at low pressure and have valves to prevent backflow.
- Arteries divide into progressively smaller vessels (arterioles) and then into capillaries where gas

- exchange with surrounding tissues actually takes place.
- The left side of the heart supplies the systemic circulation and the right side of the heart pumps blood through the pulmonary circulation.
- The pressures in the chambers of the left heart and in the arterial system are high; the left ventricle is muscular and is often referred to as a pressure pump. The pressures in the right heart and pulmonary circulation are lower; the right ventricle is thinner walled and often referred to as a volume pump.
- Heart valves are passive and only open and close in response to differences in pressure on each side of them.
- The peak blood pressure during a heart cycle is the systolic pressure and the lowest pressure is the diastolic pressure.
- The cardiac output is the stroke volume (volume pumped out of the left ventricle with each beat)

multiplied by the heart rate and is around 25 litres/min at rest in the horse.

- The left and right atria contract together to fill the ventricles and then the ventricles contract synchronously.
- The heart beat is generated by the sinoatrial (SA) node which is a specialised tissue in the wall of the right atrium also known as the pacemaker.
- The electrical activity generated in the SA node spreads through the wall of the right atrium to the left atrium and also to the atrioventricular (AV) node and down into the ventricles via the bundle of His.
- At rest at a heart rate of 30 beats/min, around two-thirds to three-quarters of each cardiac cycle is taken up by diastole (filling) and only one-quarter to one-third by systole (emptying).
- The ECG corresponds to the sum of all the electrical activity in the cardiac muscle in one beat.
- The appearance of the ECG changes dramatically from rest to exercise.
- The proportion of cardiac output flowing to different regions changes with factors such as exercise, disease, digestion and thermoregulation.
- Tissues and organs are able to control their own blood flow to some extent by the process of autoregulation.
- Blood pressure is a function of both cardiac output and arterial resistance.
- Blood makes up around 10% of the body mass of a 500 kg horse and consists primarily of RBCs, WBCs and plasma.
- RBCs are unusual in that they do not have a nucleus or mitochondria.
- Haematology and clinical biochemistry describe the fields of science and/or medicine involved in analysis of blood.

Part II
Exercise and Training Responses

Chapter 7
Muscular responses

The muscular response to exercise

The metabolic changes seen within horse muscles are generally more extreme than those of even elite human athletes; this is yet another example of the superior athletic ability of the horse. Horses have very high maximal oxygen uptake, very high levels of the enzymes in muscle associated with energy generation and metabolism, and they are able both to produce and tolerate high levels of muscle lactate.

Oxygen uptake

Oxygen uptake increases from around 5 ml/min/kg (STPD) (see Chapter 5 for an explanation of this convention) at rest to around 160 ml/min/kg (STPD) during high intensity exercise in an average Thoroughbred racehorse. The increase in oxygen utilisation is almost completely accounted for by increased usage by mitochondria within locomotory muscles, although non-locomotory muscles such as the diaphragm and intercostal muscles also increase their oxygen utilisation. In order to be delivered to the muscle from the blood, and ultimately to the mitochondria, oxygen must dissociate from haemoglobin; the tendency for haemoglobin to 'unload' its oxygen is increased in conditions associated with hard working muscle, i.e. increased muscular content of carbon dioxide and potassium, low pH and high temperature. These conditions exist both within the muscle and its local blood supply. The increased tendency for oxygen to be downloaded in these conditions is known as the Bohr shift (see Fig. 7.1), after the scientist who discovered the phenomenon. The haemoglobin then replaces the downloaded oxygen with either hydrogen ions or carbon dioxide ions. By soaking up the hydrogen ions, haemoglobin acts as a buffer and reduces the amount by which the acidity in muscle and blood will increase. The Bohr shift results in harder working tissues preferentially being supplied with oxygen and, like the mechanism of local vasodilation, is another example of a mechanism for matching oxygen supply to demand.

Blood flow

The increases in muscle blood flow during exercise are quite incredible. At rest, the muscles take only 15% of the cardiac output or about 4 litres/min. During exercise, muscles may demand up to 80% of the total cardiac output, i.e. 200 litres/min, a 40-fold increase from resting levels!

Temperature

As muscle activity (strength and frequency of contractions) increases, there is a progressive increase in muscle temperature, up to around 46°C. An increase in temperature of about 1°C actually increases the activity of enzymes within the muscle, so muscle literally needs to 'warm-up' for optimal function. Overheating of the muscles, however, may be associated with weakness, fatigue and tissue damage.

Use of fuel stores

During low intensity exercise, initially type I and type IIA fibres are recruited, with the type IIB fibres generally only recruited at higher speeds or at lower speeds when the glycogen stores of types I and IIA are depleted (see Fig. 7.2). Following exercise, repletion of glycogen stores occurs in the opposite order to recruitment, i.e. the fibres recruited last are restored first.

Low to moderate intensity exercise involves mainly the use of free fatty acids and the aerobic metabolism of glycogen to supply fuel. The body's stores of free fatty acids are large and are unlikely ever to be depleted. Fatigue during prolonged low to moderate intensity exercise (or following 3–5 repeated maximum sprint intervals) will occur due to depletion of glycogen stores rather than depletion of fat stores.

In high intensity exercise where all muscle fibres are recruited, glycogen usage and therefore depletion is greatest in type IIB fibres and least in type I fibres. During maximal exercise muscle glycogen will be responsible for the majority of ATP production. The duration of exercise will determine the balance between aerobic and anaerobic metabo-

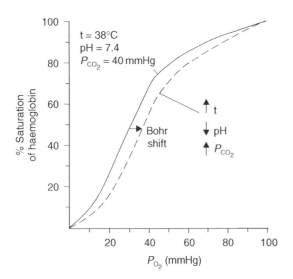

Fig. 7.1 Oxyhaemoglobin dissociation curve.

lism of glycogen. In events lasting less than 30 seconds the majority of energy will be derived from anaerobic metabolism of phosphocreatine and glycogen through glycolysis to lactate. As the duration of exercise increases, aerobic metabolism of glycogen through glycolysis occurs; pyruvate then enters the mitochondria and is metabolised through the TCA cycle to provide a greater amount of energy per molecule of glycogen. Interestingly, whilst muscles can take up glucose from the blood to use as an energy source during low to moderate intensity exercise, during high intensity exercise, although glucose can still be taken up from the blood, it is blocked from entering the glycolytic pathway if glycogen breakdown is rapid. Remember that 95% of the body's glucose stored as glycogen is actually within the muscles, whilst only 5% is in the liver and the liver has to supply all the other tissues and organs via the circulation.

In chapter 2 we described glycogen breakdown by glycogen phosphorylase resulting in the formation of only glucose-1-phosphate; however, whilst glucose-1-phosphate is the major product of glycogenolysis, because of its structure, glycogen breakdown also results in a small amount of free glucose.

Lactate kinetics

During exercise at speeds greater than about 8–10 m/s (500–600 m/min) anaerobic energy pathways will be recruited, resulting in the production of lactic acid within the muscle. The speed at which this occurs varies with factors such as breed, type of training, level of fitness, muscle fibre type, health

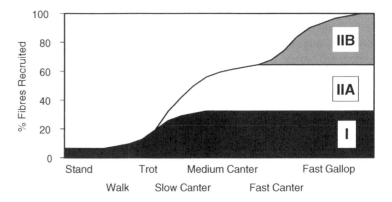

Fig. 7.2 Relationship between muscle fibre type recruitment and speed of running.

and ground conditions, and the range could be any-where from 5 to 15 m/s (300 to 900 m/min). When lactic acid is produced it dissociates into lactate ions and hydrogen ions. As lactate accumulates within the muscle (from ~24 mmol/kg dry muscle at rest up to values as high as 240 mmol/kg dry muscle) it diffuses from areas of high concentration to areas of lower concentration: this is referred to as diffusion down a concentration gradient. The lactate may initially diffuse into adjacent muscle fibres which are not producing lactate (or which have a lower lactate concentration), or into the blood via the capillaries surrounding each muscle fibre. The onset of blood lactate accumulation (OBLA) is commonly considered to occur at the speed at which the horse's blood lactate concentration reaches 4 mmol/l (see Fig. 7.3). Further increases in speed above this point lead to more rapid increases in blood lactate up to as high as 20–35 mmol/l.

OBLA is often now more frequently referred to as V_{LA4} – the velocity at which blood lactate reaches 4 mmol/l. Another term widely used to refer to the intensity at which blood lactate starts to increase more rapidly in blood is the 'anaerobic threshold'. Whilst the use of this term in scientific circles is understood, it can be confusing because, taken literally, it suggests that there has been a sudden change to using anaerobic pathways. This is definitely not the case. As explained in Chapter 2, with increasing speed from a slow start (i.e. excluding the more complicated issue of rapid acceleration), anaerobic energy generation with lactate produc-tion is gradually called upon more and more, as more and more muscle fibres, especially type IIB fibres, are recruited.

V_{LA4} or OBLA can be determined either on a treadmill or in the field (see Chapter 18). Although lactate production in muscles stops as soon as exercise intensity drops, e.g. when pulling up after a race, the peak in blood lactate following short duration (e.g. 3–5 minutes) moderate to intense exercise is often not seen until 5–10 minutes or so after exercise has finished. This is because at the end of exercise a gradient in lactate still exists between muscle and blood, with the lactate concentration in the muscle still being greater than in the blood. If exercise has been of sufficient intensity to increase blood lactate concentration above 10–12 mmol/l, the peak blood lactate level will generally occur after the end of exercise: the higher the concentration, the later (up to around 10 minutes) the peak concentration will generally be. Below 10 mmol/l, the blood lactate concentration will generally start to fall as soon as exercise ends. Therefore the time after exercise at which you take a sample for lactate is important.

The rate of lactate removal from the blood depends on the level of activity undertaken during the recovery period following an exercise bout (see Fig. 7.4). For example, lactate is removed from the blood 40% faster at trot compared with walk and 60% faster at walk compared to standing. This means that at trot, lactate is cleared twice as fast from the blood as when standing. Horses that have

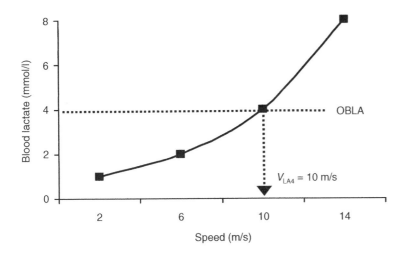

Fig. 7.3 Onset of blood lactate accumulation.

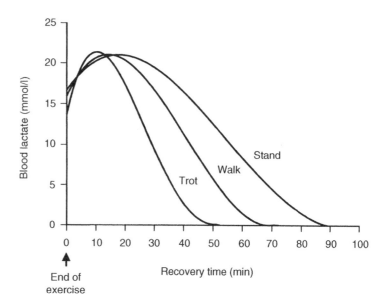

Fig. 7.4 The rate of lactate removal from blood depends upon the level of activity undertaken during the recovery period.

exercised at high intensity, for example after the steeplechase phase of a three-day event speed and endurance test, should slow down gradually, coming down from gallop, into canter, through trot and finally into walk. This form of 'warm-down' maximises the rate of lactate clearance from muscle and blood. Lactic acid production is associated with increases in muscle acidity, varying in onset and severity between fibres. Muscle pH drops in type IIB fibres first, as they have the highest glycolytic (and lowest aerobic) capacity and produce lactate at the fastest rate.

Lactic acid produced and accumulated in muscle during exercise is often described as a 'waste product' or 'metabolic by-product' and is treated as something to be avoided during exercise. This is extremely misleading. If muscle could not produce any lactic acid, exercise would be limited to low and moderate intensities only; lactic acid production is essential for acceleration, speed and explosive efforts. There is a genetic defect in man called the McArdle's syndrome in which the enzyme glycogen phosphorylase is absent so that lactic acid cannot be produced during exercise; people affected in this way are unable to accelerate rapidly or sprint.

Following high intensity exercise to the point of fatigue, we or our horse may experience acute muscle soreness during or immediately after exer-

cise. In this case soreness is related both to the production of lactic acid and the effects of the hydrogen ions (rather than the lactate) and to tissue oedema (an increased fluid uptake into the interstitial spaces between the muscle cells). The sensation normally disappears shortly after exercise and may be aided by proper warm-down exercise. Warming down keeps the muscle blood flow elevated and helps to remove hydrogen ions and resolve the oedema. This would be particularly important where a second bout of exercise is to be undertaken; for example, during the speed and endurance phase of a three-day event, or in show-jumping competitions where multiple rounds are jumped, or in a polo match where horses are ridden in one chukka, rested and then ridden in a second.

The muscle soreness and stiffness that occurs much later following an exercise bout (usually within 24–48 hours) is referred to in human sports medicine as delayed onset muscle soreness (DOMS). This is a result of structural damage to muscle fibres with the release of intracellular contents, including CK and AST, and subsequent inflammation. This has been shown not to have anything to do with lactic acid. In fact, in one human study, blood lactate levels were higher at the end of exercise in the athletes that did not subsequently experience DOMS (Schwane *et al.* 1983). In the horse, as in man, a similar scenario with a horse being fine at the end of exercise and stiff the next day is more likely to be explained by insufficient fitness or over-exertion (even in a very fit animal). These two forms of 'stiffness' associated with exercise are distinct from exertional rhabdomyolysis (tying-up). Remember that classic tying-up can occur within minutes of starting exercise, in some cases even as the horse is walking out of the stable.

Muscle buffering

The buffering capacity of muscle refers to its ability to both soak up and remove hydrogen ions from its constituent cells, thereby either avoiding a change in muscle pH or minimising the decrease in muscle pH. A high buffering capacity delays fatigue occurring due to hydrogen ion accumulation within the cells. The buffering capacity of muscle can be calculated in a number of different ways, including by calculating the slope of the decrease in muscle pH as lactate increases, from levels measured in muscle biopsy samples taken during exercise or by acid titration, e.g. using hydrochloric acid (HCl), of homogenised muscle samples obtained by biopsy. The precise conditions under which measurements are made are extremely important, and whether the muscle is wet or dry can make a significant difference to the results. However, if horse and human muscle are compared under the same conditions, it is evident that the muscle buffering capacity of the horse is around 60% greater than that of man.

Potassium loss

Different intensities and durations of exercise can result in changes in plasma electrolyte concentrations, primarily of sodium, potassium and chloride. With intense exercise, plasma potassium increases from about 4 mmol/l up to 10 mmol/l and above. During exercise there is a large efflux of potassium ions from muscle (where they are in a very high concentration compared with the plasma). Combined with this, the sodium–potassium pump in the muscle membranes, which would normally pump potassium back into the cells, is impaired when hydrogen ion concentrations rise, thus resulting in the net loss of potassium from the muscle cells and an increase in plasma potassium. Interestingly, the concentrations of potassium in plasma that occur

during high intensity exercise in the horse would produce dramatic disturbances to the normal resting heart rhythm, i.e. induce dysrhythmia, if produced at rest by infusion of a solution of potassium; such high concentrations of potassium in the blood at rest could even cause the heart to stop, but have no ill effects during exercise when adrenaline is released.

Following completion of exercise, plasma potassium concentrations return to those before exercise after a few minutes. If samples of blood are taken 1–2 hours after the end of exercise, the plasma potassium concentration may well be below that before exercise. This is a normal response and is thought to be due to the muscle taking up a little more potassium than was actually lost during exercise. However, within a few more hours the system balances itself out and the plasma concentration usually returns to normal. The one possible exception might be during prolonged exercise such as endurance where a significant proportion of the body's potassium store has been lost in sweat. Increases in plasma potassium are highly correlated with lactate concentrations.

The muscular response to training

The adaptations that take place within individual muscle fibres as a result of training depend upon the age of the horse, its previous level and type of training, its genetic make-up, and indeed the intensity and type of work to which it is subjected. All the training in the world will not transform the naturally lean human athlete into a Mr Universe; an individual's genetic make-up will limit their capacity to respond to any given training programme. This point must be borne in mind when studying the scientific literature on the subject of skeletal muscle adaptations to exercise. The same training programme could potentially bring about different training responses depending on the breed or type of horse and its natural predisposition to endurance or power sports. Many of the changes that will be described are more pronounced when a horse is trained for the first time. The mature horse may need to be exposed to a greater training load for adaptations to continue. With a few exceptions, most of the training programmes that are used for horses increase aerobic capacity.

Here is a run-down of the top ten ways in which muscle function can be improved in response to training.

Increased capillarisation

Training induces an increase in the capillary supply to muscle fibres. This may be due to increases in the number of capillaries or a relative improvement due to decreases in the size of fibres with training without a change in actual capillary numbers (see Fig. 7.5). Improvements in capillary supply improve delivery of oxygen to muscle and hence the availability of oxygen to the muscles for oxidative phosphorylation. It is more relevant to talk of capillary density than capillary number, because it is the capillary supply per unit volume of muscle fibre, i.e. capillary density, that it is important. Studies of training in man have shown that in general terms the capillary supply to muscle is improved by aerobic training but decreased by heavy resistance training. Training programmes in horses are primarily aerobic. This is consistent with the decrease in fibre size seen in many studies. However, muscle capillary supply in horses has been reported either not to change or to increase; in the studies in which an increase was observed it is difficult to separate out a possible ageing effect.

Increased transit time

As capillary density increases, the network of capillaries through which blood traverses the muscle is increased. This means that the blood flow through the muscle is slower and the transit time is longer, giving more time in which equilibrium can occur between the oxygenated blood and the working muscle. As a result of the greater opportunity for gas exchange to occur, more oxygen can be unloaded at the muscle and more lactate buffered by haemoglobin.

Increased arterial–venous difference

The increased capillary density and the increased transit time lead to more oxygen being unloaded at the muscle and a greater extraction of oxygen from the bloodstream. In addition, venous blood returning to the lungs will have a lower oxygen content, improving the gradient for the diffusion of oxygen from the alveoli across the blood–gas barrier and into the pulmonary capillaries. The increase in oxygen uptake at the muscle therefore has knock-on effects for oxygen diffusion across the alveolar–capillary membrane within the lung.

Increased oxidative capacity

In the early stages of training a previously untrained horse, such as a 2-year-old racehorse, the first 3–4 months of training may make some fibres stain as type IIA which before training stained as type IIB. This has been established by looking at muscle biopsies of horses before and after training. The type IIB fibres do not actually turn into type IIA fibres but stain and function more like a type

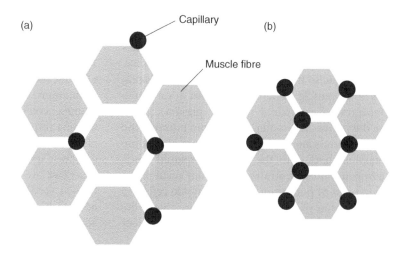

Fig. 7.5 Improvement in capillary density occurs following training. (a) Before training; (b) after training.

IIA fibre. That is they become more reliant on the aerobic metabolism of fat and glycogen than the anaerobic metabolism of glycogen to lactate. The absolute number of muscle fibres is not thought to change (an increase in fibre number would be referred to as hyperplasia), but the properties of the existing fibres do appear to respond to training. The type IIB fibres do not disappear completely, but their number may be significantly reduced.

The decrease in type IIB fibres and the increase in type IIA fibres increases the overall capacity of the muscle to use oxygen to break down fuel aerobically. This has benefits for horses competing in almost all primarily 'aerobic' disciplines, because it aids in delaying the onset of lactate production as an increased number of fibres have a greater capacity to use aerobic pathways. The downside to maximising aerobic capacity is that the horse may lose a little at the very top end, i.e. have a slightly lower maximum speed over a short distance.

As the horse matures to around the age of 4 years, the percentage of type I fibres within the muscle as a whole seems to increase by around 5%. At the same time the percentage of type IIA fibres also increases, mainly at the expense of a similar decrease in the percentage of type IIB fibres. It is still unclear whether this is simply an effect of ageing, an effect of training, or a combination of both. This contributes to the natural improvement in stamina (endurance) from youth to maturity. For example, at Olympic level, elite athletes may initially compete in the 200 and 400 metres, and after 8 years may be running in the 400 and 800 or even 1600 metres, although still at Olympic level. It is not yet clear how much of this change is due to the training that mature horses or athletes have received, or simply part of maturation (ageing).

Overall muscle mass seems to increase with training, but such increases may be difficult to distinguish from increases in muscle mass due to growth in young horses. The majority of fibres are likely to decrease in diameter, because the general trend is for fibres to become more aerobic and this is associated with a better capillary supply. Therefore, as well as each fibre being in physical contact with more capillaries, the decrease in fibre diameter also means that the distance for diffusion of oxygen from the capillary to mitochondria is reduced. Nevertheless, training programmes often appear to induce increases in muscle mass. Whether

this is due to hypertrophy (increase in the size of individual muscle fibres) increased muscle tone, or to increases in actual numbers of fibres (hyperplasia), remains to be demonstrated in horses. Both effects would potentially increase the power output of an individual muscle because power output is proportional to muscle cross-sectional area. Hypertrophy seems unlikely based on most biopsy studies in horses, and hyperplasia has only been infrequently demonstrated in cats following very heavy resistance training and in human weightlifters. As resistance training would not feature in any conventional training programme, hyperplasia would seem an unlikely explanation for increases in muscle mass in horses.

Increased activity of aerobic enzymes

The activity of aerobic enzymes such as citrate synthase (CS) and 3-hydroxyacyl-CoA dehydrogenase (HAD) improve with training. CS is responsible for the production of citrate at the start of the TCA cycle and HAD is involved in the beta-oxidation of fatty acids before their entry into the TCA cycle. Both these enzymes are found within the mitochondria. In research studies, the activity of enzymes within these pathways is used as an indication of mitochondrial density and to monitor changes in aerobic capacity. The first few months of a training programme can lead to a doubling of these enzymes compared with the levels before training. The changes in skeletal muscle enzymes such as CS and HAD seem to be maintained for up to 16 weeks following cessation of training, suggesting that the horse will maintain its improvement in aerobic capacity, e.g. as estimated by changes in $\dot{V}_{O_2max}$, even after a rest period. This is in contrast to human athletes who appear to lose fitness much more rapidly following cessation of training. Thus the implications of a horse missing 1 or 2 weeks' training through a minor injury such as a bruised sole are less than for a human athlete.

Increased capacity to use fat as a fuel

Training increases the mobilisation of FFA from adipose tissue. Trained horses and humans are more likely to utilise fat as an aerobic fuel source than carbohydrate. This has a glycogen sparing effect and thus delays the onset of fatigue due to glycogen depletion. However, fat can only be used as a major source of fuel when the exercise intensity is low to moderate. Fast cantering and galloping will stimulate rapid glycogen breakdown, and some of the intermediate products in glycolysis are able to block the metabolism of FFA. This probably occurs around a heart rate of 160 beats/min.

Increased myoglobin content of muscle

With training there is an increase in the amount of myoglobin found within muscle, the major increase being seen in type I muscle fibres. Myoglobin is a pigment similar to haemoglobin, but it only unloads its oxygen at very low partial pressures of oxygen (around 0.13–0.27 kPa (1–2 mmHg)), such as those found in hard working muscle fibres. Even in a horse working maximally, the pressure of oxygen in the arterial blood would only fall from around 13.3 kPa (100 mmHg) at rest to around 9.3 kPa (70 mmHg). Whereas haemoglobin should only be found within red blood cells, myoglobin should only be found within muscle cells and not in the bloodstream. Increased myoglobin content in muscle leads to an increased oxygen storage capacity. This helps to buffer fluctuations in oxygen supply and demand both temporally and spatially within the muscle fibres, particularly at the onset of exercise and with the intracellular movement of oxygen. Horses that have experienced a severe bout of tying-up (setfast or exertional rhabdomyolysis) may have very dark urine. This condition, known as myoglobinuria, is caused by severe damage to the muscle fibres which results in myoglobin leaking out into the plasma and being excreted by the kidneys into the urine.

Increased glycogen content

Training results in a greater glycogen storage capacity of muscle, increasing the fuel store available for both anaerobic and aerobic energy production. By being able to store more glycogen, glycogen depletion (a potential cause of fatigue in horses working both aerobically and anaerobically) is reduced or delayed. The glycogen content of horse muscle is approximately 300–500 mmol/kg dry muscle before training and may increase to as much as 800 mmol/kg dry muscle after training. The increase is likely to be the most in horses with lots of large type IIB fibres, i.e. in horses with the characteristics of a sprinter. The normal storage capacity of the horse is similar to that for humans. However, by exercise and dietary manipulation, human athletes can increase their muscle glycogen content to around 1000 mmol/kg dry muscle. When the term glycogen depletion is used in relation to exercise, this can imply total depletion in endurance events or only partial depletion, e.g. 50% reduction, following high-speed exercise.

Increases in anaerobic muscle enzymes

Following specific high intensity training, some studies have demonstrated increases in enzymes associated with glycolytic capacity, such as phosphofructokinase (PFK), lactate dehydrogenase (LDH) and glycogen phosphorylase (PHOS). Other studies have shown either no difference or a decrease in such enzyme activity, especially with lower intensity aerobic training. Interestingly, a study by Sinha et al. (1991) on previously trained Thoroughbreds showed that after 6 weeks of training at 40% $\dot{V}_{O_2max}$ muscle LDH activity was decreased. However, in a second group exercised for the same time at 80% $\dot{V}_{O_2max}$ LDH was either the same or increased, and this was accompanied by an increase in muscle hydrogen ion buffering capacity. Thus an increased capacity to generate lactic acid was accompanied by an adaptation to buffer lactic acid. There was no change or difference between the groups in the muscle markers of aerobic capacity, CS and HAD activities. Thus the clear implication is that aerobic energy pathways can be trained by using either a low or medium intensity, but for anaerobic pathways only the higher intensity produced a training stimulus.

Improved motor skill

When any new motor skill (movement skill) is learnt, it requires a degree of conscious effort. Once learnt it is almost as if the instructions for performing that movement are 'hardwired' into the brain and the animal performs them effortlessly. Along with increased skill comes increased efficiency. A horse which is trained in gymnastic jumping will be able to co-ordinate its muscles in such a way as to expend less energy than the unskilled horse. The skilled horse is less likely to fatigue than the unskilled horse and is thus less likely to make unco-ordinated muscle movements that result in a fall or in musculoskeletal injury (Fig. 7.6). Horses that become fatigued are far more likely to stumble or strike into themselves. In many ways training for improved motor skill is similar to training for fitness. It is important that the right stimulus is applied at the right frequency. It is not particularly effective trying to train a horse to jump by having one jump schooling session once a week for 4 weeks. It would be much better to have a light jump schooling session morning and afternoon on two consecutive days, i.e. shorter sessions, but with less time in between. There are many examples of how horses learn better this way. Even acclimatising horses to a treadmill can be likened to a skill. The horse may well be very fit and eminently able to walk, trot, canter and gallop with a rider on grass and all weather surfaces, but on the treadmill the horse has to learn a new motor skill, that of running on a moving belt. We know that horses learn quicker and better if we train them with four or five short tread-mill acclimatisation runs, within a period of 2–3 days, rather than one session a day or every other day for 7–10 days. If they only see the treadmill once a week for 4 weeks there is strong evidence that they don't acclimatise to it at all. And it's not just horses; the same principle applies to riders.

How long does it all take?

In a 12 week training study using previously trained Thoroughbreds and, 3 weeks of low intensity, long distance training (trotting) had no effect on activi-ties of enzyme markers of aerobic (CS, HAD) or anaerobic (LDH) capacity (Lovell & Rose 1991). However, the second phase, which involved contin-ued low intensity long distance work supplemented with moderate intensity interval training, increased CS, HAD and to a lesser extent LDH, but without changes in fibre type percentages. From 6 to 12 weeks, further increases in training intensity up to three gallops at maximal heart rate, three times a week, produced a significant increase in the relative numbers of type IIA fibres and a trend to a decrease in the percentage of types IIB and I fibres. Whilst CS and HAD did not change any further from weeks 6 to 12, LDH increased from both 6 to 9 and 9 to 12 weeks. Some training program-mes have shown changes in response to training in as little as 10–14 days. These have included de-creased glycogen usage and lactate production and increases in percentage of type IIA fibres and hydrogen ion buffering capacity.

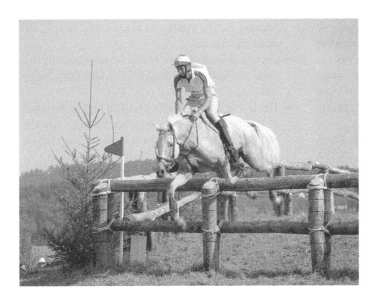

Fig. 7.6 Uncoordinated muscle movements due to fatigue may lead to a fall.

The difficulty in interpreting the results of many training studies is that the type of change, its magnitude and time-course are all likely to be affected by factors such as age, previous training history, length of lay-off if previously trained, initial individual muscle fibre composition, breed and the precise training programme. These factors should all be considered when reviewing the scientific literature relating to training studies.

How long does it all last?

Detraining describes the period following either complete cessation of a training programme or a marked decrease in training intensity. From detraining studies performed on horses, we have learnt that the reversal of training-induced adaptations in muscle due to relative inactivity is far slower in the horse than in other athletic species, such as man. Following complete cessation of training, responses of the muscles to exercise are maintained for at least several weeks. Changes in enzyme activities and glycogen content may take up to 3 months to reverse if no exercise at all is undertaken. However, in one study where horses were walked for 20 minutes a day, 7 days a week and exercise tested every fourth week to determine the time-course and nature of detraining effects, the only significant change after 16 weeks of detraining was that lactate concentrations were doubled during exercise, although exercise capacity was unchanged (Butler *et al.* 1991).

KEY POINTS

- Oxygen uptake by the muscles can increase 30-fold from rest to exercase.
- The horse's high maximal oxygen uptake is a result of both a high capacity for oxygen delivery and a high density of mitochondria (the site of oxygen consumption) in the muscles. The horse is able to increase its oxygen uptake by a factor of 40 times above resting flow at maximal exercise.
- The temperature of the muscles may increase to around 46°C during intense exercise. Reversible changes in the structure of proteins may occur at 44°C; however, the risk of permanent structural damage increases with both increasing temperature and the duration of temperature elevation.
- With increasing exercise intensity muscle fibres are usually recruited (used) in the order I > IIA > IIB.
- Horses can produce muscle lactate concentrations as high as 240 mmol/kg/dry muscle or 35 mmol/l in blood. These values are both higher than those seen in human athletes.
- The processes occurring in muscle and the reliance on anaerobic glycolysis with the production of lactic acid can be followed by measuring the appearance of lactic acid in blood or plasma.
- The speed at which blood lactate reaches a concentration of 4 mmol/l is referred to as the onset of blood lactate accumulation (OBLA) or V_{LA4} (velocity at a blood lactate concentration of 4 mmol/l).
- After intense exercise, blood lactate concentration may not peak until 5–10 minutes afterwards because lactate continues to leave the muscle and enter the blood.
- Lactate removal from blood occurs faster at trot than at walk and faster at walk than when standing.
- The horse does not only produce higher amounts of lactate than human athletes, but also has the ability to tolerate it. Muscle buffering capacity is higher in horses than in man.
- Plasma potassium concentrations may increase from 4 mmol/l to 10 mmol/l during intense exercise as a result of efflux of potassium from muscle.
- Training may result in changes in muscle capillary supply, oxygen extraction, oxidative capacity, oxidative and anaerobic enzyme activities, the use of fat and or carbohydrate (glycogen) as

fuels, muscle glycogen content, myoglobin content and motor skills.

- Reponses may be detected in muscle after as little as 10–14 days of training.

- Horses detrain much more slowly than human athletes. Little change in measurable fitness may occur after 3–4 months of reduced exercise intensity and volume.

Chapter 8

Skeletal responses

Mechanical properties of bone

When we buy horses destined for a competition career we try and select individuals with 'good' conformation. In terms of limb conformation we assess the basic morphometry of the bones of the limbs and their alignment. For example, when viewing the forelimb head on, an imaginary line drawn through the middle of the forearm should bisect the limb and hoof capsule. Limb deviations either medio-laterally or axially can produce abnormal loads and increase the likelihood of degenerative joint changes.

When selling horses or advertising stallions at stud, the amount of 'bone' a horse has, i.e. its cannon bone circumference, is often quoted as an indication of the weight (load) one should expect the horse (or progeny) to be able to carry. Such measurements are all the more useful if we consider bone circumference (in centimetres) per kilogram of body mass. After all, the horse with 17 cm of bone carrying 450 kg of its own body mass is better off than a horse with 17 cm of bone carrying 600 kg. There is a compromise between a high mass of bone (increasing energy required for locomotion) and provision of adequate bone mass to avoid fracture. In animals that have been selectively bred over many years for economy of locomotion and speed, i.e. with minimal distal limb mass, there is a high risk of fracture incidence, as seen in young Thoroughbreds trained for flat racing.

As well as the basic morphometry (size and shape) of the bone, the internal composition of the bone is important in determining its ability to withstand certain types of loading. The internal composition of bones within individual horses and between horses varies in terms of the proportion of cortical to cancellous bone, the mineral density of the bone, the porosity of the bone, the thickness of the cortical bone and the ability of the bone to withstand both tensile (stretching) and compressive forces. There are a range of methods that have been used over the last 20 years or so for measuring various aspects of bone quality and that have been applied in training studies.

The 'quality' of the bone does contribute to strength, but would be secondary to the actual bone morphometry. The quality of the bone refers to its ability to withstand an applied mechanical stress, and is governed by both the mineral and organic composition. The response of bone to an applied stress can be shown by plotting a graph of the applied stress (load) against the strain that is seen in the bone itself (see Fig. 8.1). Strain is measured as a change in length (extension or compression) and is expressed relative to the original length of the bone.

$$\text{Strain} = \frac{\text{Change in length } (l)}{\text{Original length } (l_0)}$$

Strain can be measured using strain gauges glued to the bone surface. The applied mechanical stress leads to an alteration in the electrical resistance of the strain gauge which then produces a voltage output proportional to the strain occurring on the bone surface. The sort of strain seen in bone *in vivo* (i.e. in the live horse) is very small, and is expressed as microstrain (μe, i.e. strain $\times 10^{-6}$). Note that there are two regions to the stress–strain curve:

(1) *An elastic zone*: within this zone bone immediately returns to its original shape once the stress is removed.
(2) *A plastic zone*: within this zone the stress is great enough to cause some deformation of the bone tissue.

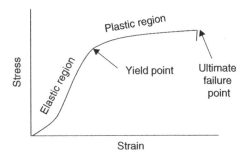

Fig. 8.1 Stress/strain curve for bone.

Bone tissue tends to have a relatively large elastic zone so it copes well with loads up to a certain magnitude. As it has a large elastic zone it is described as a pseudoductile material. A material with a relatively small elastic zone is known as a brittle material. When the rate of loading is increased, bone can actually change from having a pseudoductile behaviour to a brittle behaviour. Thus, it is not just the magnitude of the applied stress that is important, but the rate at which it is applied. The loading rate is equivalent to the number of times each limb strikes the ground, and the stress applied to the bone is the concussive force received by that limb. The estimated rates of loading which would cause a change from pseudoductile to brittle behaviour can occur in galloping horses.

The techniques currently available to study bone responses *in vivo* include the following:

(1) *Ultrasound velocity measurement.* Ultrasound velocity gives an indication of bone strength because the greater the velocity (speed) of the ultrasound through the bone, the greater the bone density.

(2) *Single photon absorptiometry.* This is a method that allows bone mineral content to be assessed. The number of photons absorbed is proportional to the bone mineral content. It can be used when combined with ultrasound measurement to give estimates of bone mineral density. Dual energy X-ray absorptiometry (DEXA) has superseded this, but at the time of writing had not been used for any *in vivo* equine training studies.

(3) *Radiography.* Radiographs have always been used to assess the maturity of the bone by studying growth plate closure. Radiography has been used to assess the thickness of the dorsal cortex of the third metacarpal (cannon) bone. Quantitative radiography has been used to estimate mineral density.

(4) *Scintigraphy.* Scintigraphy is a more recent method of imaging used as a means of identifying bone turnover and blood flow, bone deposition and pathology. Horses are injected with a substance known as a radiolabel that acts as a radioactive physiological marker. A commonly used radiolabel is ^{99m}Tc-methylenediphosphate (MDP), which is taken up into the bone matrix within 1–3 hours and can be imaged using a gamma camera. Scintigraphy will indicate where the areas of high blood flow and/or bony changes are, but the vet may need to use other diagnostic techniques to give a definitive diagnosis. Scintigraphy is expensive and only tends to be used within larger equine veterinary hospitals and research centres.

(5) *Bone markers.* Current research is aimed at finding blood markers of bone metabolism to be able to monitor the changes in bone during training and perhaps identify those at risk of fracture before this occurs, thereby reducing wastage. Recently, research has been directed towards the use of blood-borne markers of bone formation and resorption. Possible 'biomarkers', as they are called, include bone alkaline phosphatase (AP, an enzyme thought to reflect osteoblast activity), carboxy-terminal propeptide of type I collagen, hydroxyproline (Hp) produced during collagen formation, and osteocalcin which is released into the bloodstream during bone formation.

The influence of exercise on modelling and remodelling

Basic bone growth and remodelling

Throughout life there is a balance between bone formation and resorption. In the growth years formation exceeds resorption and skeletal mass increases (hypertrophy). Hypertrophy of the skeleton is maximal over the first year of life. In the mature horse hypertrophy is less, but there is still a high rate of remodelling (turnover of bone). In fact, the greatest rate of remodelling occurs in horses between 2 and 3 years of age. Remodelled bone has a lower mineral density than mature bone for several months following formation. As a result of remodelling, 50% of the horse's primary skeletal structure is replaced by the time it is 3 years old.

Bone responds to applied loads

Bone responds to imposed conditions according to Wolff's law. As described in Chapter 4, bone needs a certain amount of loading simply to maintain its mass. Applied stress below a certain magnitude leads to net bone loss and stress above a certain magnitude leads to hypertrophy of the bone and an increase in bone mass.

Applied stress is needed to both maintain bone mass and model it to maximise its ability to withstand everyday (and competitive) demands without injury. The sort of response made by the bone depends not only on the magnitude of the load and the frequency with which it is applied, but also on the previous level of conditioning. Unfortunately, exactly what constitutes a 'good' stress and a 'bad' stress is still largely guesswork. We can use heart rate monitors to obtain an idea of how hard the heart is working, but there is no easy way to know how hard the skeleton is working.

Bucked shins

A common manifestation of overloading of young racehorses in flat race training is 'bucked shins'. Bucked or 'sore' shins occur because the bone cells are unable to synthesise matrix fast enough to reduce the local tissue strains. Microdamage to the cortex of the third metacarpal bone (cannon bone) is then followed by remodelling which can result in increased porosity and the formation of secondary osteons which are weaker than primary bone.

This is a painful condition when first formed. In the early stages a bucked shin will be inflamed, and if the warning signs of inflammation are not

heeded, damage to the bone structure itself (micro-cracking) occurs. In time, the dorsal aspect of the cannon bone becomes thickened as a response to the strain applied and appears to bow slightly. Bucked shins are so common in 2- and 3-year-old racehorses that some trainers would almost consider them to be unavoidable. A bucked shin is thought to be nature's way of quickly laying down more bone in an attempt to increase the cross-sectional area of the bone and thus increase the area across which loads are applied; unfortunately, the rapidly modelled bone is made up of secondary osteons giving lower quality bone material than the primary osteons.

At the first signs of bucked shins horses should have the frequency of their high strain loading decreased, but not removed entirely. The high strain loading ensures that the stimulus for re-modelling is there, but the reduction in frequency ensures that the bone is given a little more time to adapt (Fig. 8.2).

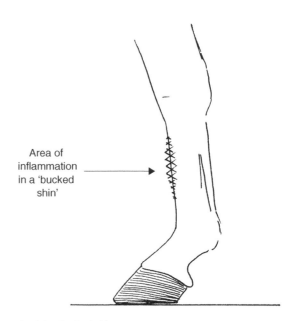

Area of inflammation in a 'bucked shin' →

Fig. 8.2   Bucked shin.

The responses of bone to training

Several studies have been carried out over the past few years in an attempt to assess the response of the skeleton to various training programmes. Most of the skeleton responds to loading by a process known as adaptive hypertrophy, i.e. increased bone mass, in accordance with Wolff's law by increasing bone mass and altering the distribution of existing bone to provide more bone where high strains occur, such as the dorsomedial aspect of the cannon bone. The dense bone of the dorsomedial aspect of the cannon bone is often thicker than the rest of the dense bone in trained horses. However, this is a positive adaptive response to training as opposed to bucked shins which are a sign of overload.

The stimulus for adaptive hypertrophy seems to be relatively short periods of high intensity work. Firth *et al.* (1999) studied two groups of Thoroughbreds, one group trained for just 4 months and one group trained for 18 months. In both groups, horses were either trained at low or high intensities. All the high intensity trained horses responded by showing increased hypertrophy at a particular site on the dorsal aspect of the radial and third metacarpal bones, whereas the low intensity trained group did not show hypertrophy of these areas.

A further response of equine distal limb bones to applied loading is microcracking. Reilly *et al.* (1997) carried out a 19 week training programme on a group of Thoroughbreds which were approximately 19 months old at the start. The horses in one group were given walking exercise only for 40 minutes per day, whilst those in the other group walked for 40 minutes per day, trotted for 20 minutes per day and carried out progressively more intense exercise on a treadmill. At the end of the training programme, samples of bone taken from the cortex of the third metacarpal bone within the mid-diaphysis region showed that the higher intensity exercise group had a greater degree of microcracking and an increase in impact strength. Microcracking is often seen following high intensity exercise and actually decreases the risk of macrocracks appearing within the bone structure, provided the loading is applied in a progressive manner over a suitable period of time. Too much loading too soon can lead to bucked shins as described above.

Work done on astronauts has shown that only 10 minutes of bone loading per day led to a training response in bone (Goodship *et al.* 1998). It seems that short periods of high impact loading will bring about an increase in bone mass, and just 10 minutes' trotting on a firm surface per day may be sufficient to bring about positive adaptations in bone, particularly in the early stages of a training programme.

Training bone in practical terms

The ability of bone to adapt to the range of stresses placed upon it may well decrease with age. The entire response of bone to an incremental increase in stress can take months to complete. The key is thus to *start early but proceed with caution*. Care should be taken to gradually expose the skeleton of the young horse to progressively increasing loads, just as the muscles are exposed to increasing demands of work. For bone to respond positively, it should be progressively loaded over a sufficient period of time. Fatigue occurs usually because loading is imposed over quite a short period of time, leading to microdamage.

One of the best ways to ensure that growing skeletons receive enough 'good' stress is to allow youngsters plenty of turn out, preferably with companions of a similar age who will engage in play together. It is vital that young horses are not allowed to carry too much load in terms of body condition (i.e. excess fat!) as this will place unnecessary strain on immature bones and joints.

You should *work at gaits that simulate the sport* for which the horse is intended. During a training programme the horse should be exposed to the kinds of surfaces and terrain seen in competition. If the horse will be required to work across country it needs to do more than work in an all-weather arena or on a nice flat gallop. As the principal strain directions are dependent upon gait, the horse should be worked at speeds that simulate the competition, so that strains are applied in the appropriate manner for a desirable training response. Short bursts of high-speed exercise or 'breeze work' are likely to be more beneficial to a racehorse, for instance, than longer, slower canters. *The more demanding the sport, the smaller the increments in training load.* Generally, you should step up the training load (stress) no more than once every 2 weeks when the horse is first trained. Just 10 minutes of high impact loading, 3 or 4 days per week is all that is thought to be necessary. Trotting fast for long periods on the road will do no more to improve bone quality than a short period of trot on the same surface.

Responses of cartilage to training

Hyaline cartilage forms the ends of the bones (the articular surfaces) of the limbs in the adult horse. The role of the hyaline cartilage is to provide shock absorption at the joint surface. Underneath the soft hyaline cartilage is a layer of calcified cartilage that separates the stiff subchondral bone from the articular surface. Having materials of very different stiffness adjacent to each other is thought to increase the risk of damage due to shear forces between the two surfaces. The calcified layer provides an interface of intermediate stiffness between the soft hyaline cartilage and the stiff subchondral bone, which is thought to reduce the magnitude of shear forces acting between the hyaline cartilage and the subchondral bone.

Carpal osteoarthritis as a result of overload is frequently seen in 2- and 3-year-old flat racehorses. The lesions are usually found at dorsal sites within the middle carpal joint. Young *et al.* (1991) demonstrated an increase in third carpal subchondral bone stiffness in response to training, whilst a study by Murray *et al.* (1998) showed that hyaline cartilage can lose stiffness with strenuous exercise at sites of clinical lesions. Therefore, strenuous exercise might be thought to increase the risk of shear forces occurring between the hyaline cartilage and the subchondral bone. More recently, a study by Murray *et al.* (1999) looked at changes in the articular cartilage of equine carpal bones. This study used two groups of horses; one group underwent 19 weeks' progressive high intensity exercise on a treadmill, whilst the other group underwent walking only. Samples were taken from eight different sites within the carpus. The group trained with high

intensity exercise had significantly thicker total cartilage and a thicker calcified layer than the low intensity trained group, but there was no difference in the thickness of the hyaline cartilage layer. The thickening of the calcified layer is thought to be a mechanism to protect the hyaline cartilage from the high impact loads. Both groups had thicker dorsal than palmar calcified layers, thought to reflect the fact that dorsal aspects of the carpal bones are subjected to high intermittent loads rather than the more constant loads experienced by palmar regions.

An appropriate amount of training introduced in a progressive manner seems to lead to an increase in thickness of the articular cartilage within the carpal joints of young flat racehorses, together with hypertrophy of the underlying subchondral bone at the same time as an increased rate of remodelling within the carpal bones themselves. These are all positive adaptive responses to the applied training load, thought to reduce the likelihood of carpal fracture (common in 2- and 3-year-old flat racehorses). However, strenuous training can eventually lead to the deterioration of articular cartilage (Murray *et al.* 1999).

The cartilage of young horses seems to be more likely to be able to adapt to imposed mechanical loads than the cartilage of adult horses. The current thinking is that cartilage may be able to respond to applied loads much earlier than it would actually be exposed in a progressive programme of exercise under a rider, and research is now aimed at inducing early adaptation of tissues so that they will be able to withstand the rigours of a competitive career.

Responses of tendons to training

Research into the response of tendons and ligaments to training is important because of the high incidence of tendon injuries in horses. Increased knowledge of the response of tendon to both exercise and training may help trainers to devise regimes that minimise the risk of tendon injury. Rehabilitation following a tendon injury is a protracted process requiring careful management of the horse's exercise over a period of months; even then, tendons never seem to be 100% recovered, with a high likelihood of recurrent injury because the damaged tissue is replaced by a connective tissue scar rather than normal tendinous tissue.

In their role as energy saving springs in locomotion, tendons are expected to achieve maximum elastic storage; this requires that tendons be stretched to their maximum. For a tendon, injury is an occupational hazard. Functional tensile strains in equine superficial flexor tendons have been recorded *in vivo* using small implanted strain gauges; such studies suggest that tensile strains of approximately 3% occur at the walk, 6–8% at the trot and up to 12–16.6% at the gallop (Stephens *et al.* 1989). The values for gallop are quite alarming when compared with another study that showed complete rupture of tendons *in vitro* (removed from the horse post mortem) occurring as a result of strains of between 12 and 19.7% (Wilson 1991). Knowing the strain we impose on the tendons at a gallop, it is no wonder that tendon injuries are so common in competition horses, and indeed amazing that there are not far more! Despite the fact that tendon injury contributes so highly to the loss of horses from competitive careers, we still do not know a great deal about the best way to train tendons in such a way as to minimise the risk of injury. However, even with the right preparation, tendon injury may occur as a result of a single badly coordinated step, either as a result of fatigue or difficult going.

Loading during stance leads to stretching and relaxation of the superficial digital flexor tendon (SDFT). Not all the energy used during stretching is returned during relaxation and the energy lost is given off as heat. During exercise core tendon temperatures can reach 46°C. A few years ago it was suggested that it was this heating of the central core that caused damage to the tendon but whilst temperatures such as these would be sufficient to kill other fibroblasts, tendon fibroblasts seem to be thermotolerant. However, we still don't know if this heating has detrimental effects on other aspects of the tendon structure, for example on the tendon matrix rather than simply the tendon cells.

We often hear people talk about 'hardening' tendons, citing this as a desirable response to road-work as part of a training programme. However, this does not appear to be based on any scientific evidence. If 'hardness' corresponds to an ability to withstand strain then it may be associated with cross-sectional area. As cross-sectional area (XSA) is related to tensile strength, an increase in XSA of the SDFT would lead to an increase in stiffness, thereby reducing its strain (increasing its hardness) but also reducing its elasticity and therefore its energy storage capacity. In other words, if the tendon did become 'harder' with training, it would presumably be less elastic and would not function so well as an elastic 'spring', thereby actually raising the cost of locomotion, which has to be an undesirable training effect.

Studies investigating the changes on tendon cross-sectional area with training have brought conflicting results. Gillis *et al.* (1993) found that the cross-sectional area of the SDFT increased as a result of 4 month race training in Thoroughbreds, but more recently, a study by Birch *et al.* (1999) found no increase in SDFT cross-sectional area in Thoroughbred horses trained on a treadmill at either low speed (walking) or high speed (up to 15 m/s). Birch *et al.* (1999) suggested that the increases seen by Gillis *et al.* (1993) may even have been due to early pathological changes in the tendon, as an increase in cross-sectional area of a tendon is one of the first signs of injury.

Whilst training does not seem to have a specific effect on the cross-sectional area of tendons, it does increase up to maturity, which appears to be around 2 years old for the SDFT and 3 years old for the deep digital flexor tendon (DDFT) (Birch *et al.* 1999). The fact that the DDFT is not fully mature during race training of 2-year-olds may not be such a problem as one might expect, because the DDFT is subject to lower peak strains than the SDFT. Another change which occurs in tendons as horses get older is the reduction in the level of crimp seen in the central core of the SDFT with resultant loss of elasticity in this region.

Recently, tendons have been shown to contain a protein called cartilage oligometric matrix protein (COMP), previously thought to exist only in cartilage. COMP plays a role in structural integrity of tendon and ligament, borne out by the fact that mutations in this protein result in lax tendons and ligaments in humans. COMP appears to be concentrated in the metacarpal region of the SDFT, being synthesised in response to a need to resist loading. It accumulates with increasing age up to 2 years old and then declines rapidly. Inappropriate or excessive exercise may damage developing tendon, resulting in reduced synthesis or increased loss of COMP (Smith *et al.* 1999). A study by Cherdchutham *et al.* (1999) was conducted using Dutch warmblood foals which were assigned to one of three exercise groups just 1 week after birth. The first group were box rested, the second group were stable kept but subjected to short sprint training of 3 minutes per day, whilst the third group were pasture kept and were seen to carry out an average of 3.5 minutes of galloping exercise per day in addition to lots of walking and trotting. After 5 months, the pasture-kept group had the highest levels of COMP. Further training up to 11 months in which all foals were housed in a barn with paddock access showed that the biochemical parameters of the previously box-kept and pasture-kept foals became similar, suggesting that the pasture exercise from age 5–11 months enabled the box-kept foals to catch up in their tendon development. However, the training group continued to have a decreased production of polysulphated glycosaminoglycans (PSGAGs), thereby increasing the risk of tendonitis in these foals. The pasture-kept exercise pattern was therefore thought to be best for the development of normal tendon in foals.

At the present time, scientists do not have all the answers regarding the best methods of inducing connective tissue responses to training, and it appears that training responses would be dependent upon breed, type of work undertaken and possibly the age at which training commences. There may also be a continuum between a desirable physiological response that increases the ability of the tissue to withstand loading and undesirable pathological change. Continued research in this area is important because musculoskeletal injury is a major cause of wastage and poor performance in competition horses. We may even find that the sort of training programme that brings about optimal adaptation in bone is not optimal for tendon or cartilage. For these reasons, it may be some time before we understand how to bring all the connective tissue types to a point of satisfactory adaptation in all types of sport horses.

KEY POINTS

- Bone strength is related to bone mass, density, shape and internal composition.
- Application of stress (loading) leads to strain, whereby strain = change in length/original length; therefore the greater the change in length, the greater the strain.
- Bone shows elastic behaviour over a wide range of applied stresses. A material with a large elastic zone is said to be pseudoductile. With elastic behaviour, when the stress is removed the bone will return to its original shape.
- At certain levels of applied stress, bone will show inelastic behaviour and when the stress is removed it will not return to its original form, i.e. it will have been deformed.

- Both the magnitude of the applied stress and the rate of application are important in determining how the bone will respond.
- The optimum way to train bone may be to expose it to short (10 minute) periods of high impact loading three or four times per week. In the early stages of a training programme this may be done by conducting short periods of trotting on roads; in the later stages it may be more appropriate to gallop on grass or on an all-weather surface.
- Carpal bones increase in bone mass in response to training and this may lead to some loss of shock absorption capacity of the articular cartilage if high loads are applied too soon in the horse's training programme.

- The articular cartilage of young flat racehorses in training responds by increasing the thickness of the calcified cartilage layer.
- The cross-sectional area of tendons increases up to maturity (2 years old for the SDFT) but does not appear to increase further with training.

- There are significant changes in the biochemical composition of the tendon matrix with training, and these changes can be both positively and negatively influenced by the sort of exercise to which the tendon is exposed at a very early age, i.e. less than 12 months.

Chapter 9

Respiratory responses

The oxygen pathway and $\dot{V}_{O_2 max}$

For a single oxygen molecule, the journey from the atmosphere surrounding the horse's nostril to a mitochondrion within a muscle cell is like going four times round the world. Considering that the oxygen molecule has to traverse several different media on its way (air, blood–gas barrier, blood, circulation, cell membranes), and the speed with which this occurs makes it even more remarkable. For sufficient oxygen to arrive at working muscle a particular chain of events must occur:

(1) The bulk flow of air from the atmosphere to the alveoli, otherwise known as ventilation.
(2) The diffusion of oxygen across the alveolar–capillary membrane or blood–gas barrier and into the red blood cells (RBCs).
(3) The transport of oxygen by the RBCs to the capillaries within the working muscles.
(4) The diffusion of oxygen from the RBCs into the muscle cells and ultimately into the mitochondria.

Maximal oxygen uptake ($\dot{V}_{O_2 max}$) refers to the maximal rate at which oxygen can be used by active tissue during exercise. It is measured in ml O_2/min/kg (expressed at STPD), i.e. the amount of oxygen that the horse takes up in a given time per kilogram (kg) of body mass. The overall oxygen delivery pathway from atmosphere to mitochondria is only as good as its slowest component, so if any one of the links in the ventilation chain (1–4 above) are compromised due to disease, poor training, or even by genetically determined factors such as a small heart, $\dot{V}_{O_2 max}$ will be lowered and the horse's performance in largely aerobic events may be impaired.

Some horses are naturally capable of a higher $\dot{V}_{O_2 max}$ than others, and these horses would be expected to be better athletes. In absolute terms, a bigger horse will use up more oxygen than a smaller horse as it has a greater muscle mass, but this is not an advantage as it also has a proportionately greater mass of bone, intestines, etc. However, if we express oxygen uptake in terms uptake per kg of bodyweight we can make useful comparisons between horses of different sizes. For example, two horses could both have a $\dot{V}_{O_2 max}$ of 70 litres/min. However, if the body mass of one is 400 kg and of the other is 600 kg, when we correct for this by dividing by mass we end up with values of 175 ml/min/kg and 117 ml/min/kg, respectively. Thus, the smaller horse has around a 50% higher $\dot{V}_{O_2 max}$ on a 'kg for kg' basis. $\dot{V}_{O_2 max}$ is one of the best physiological indicators of athletic ability when trying to distinguish between breeds and species, and poor, moderate and elite performers. However, it does have limitations and it is unlikely to distinguish between elite performers.

Ventilation

As speed of running increases, ventilation increases almost linearly. Thoroughbreds are capable of increasing their ventilation from about 50–60 litres/min at rest to over 1800 litres/min at full gallop. The amount of air a horse moves in and out each minute during a race would fill a normal sized bath in around 6 seconds. In order to move 1800 litres of air each minute in and out of the lung, the air flows at rates of up to 50 litres/second through each nostril. To get an idea of the suction necessary to create a flow of 50 litres/second, put your hand over the end of a vacuum cleaner hose! This is effectively what is happening at the nostril during peak inspiration. When the flow rates are measured during exercise in scientific studies, the maximum flow rates (known as peak flow rates) are given as the sum for both nostrils, i.e. 40 litres/second for the left nostril and 40 litres/second for the right nostril equals a peak flow of 80 litres/second. Peak inspiratory flow rates (the fastest speed for air moving into the horse) are usually around 70–80 litres/second, with peak expired flow rates around 80–90 litres/second (see Fig. 9.1). These values are often lower in horses with wind problems affecting either the upper or lower airway.

Ventilation (or more correctly respiratory minute ventilation) can be increased by increasing respiratory frequency, tidal volume or both (see Fig. 9.2). The combination of respiratory frequency (rate of breathing in breaths/min) and tidal volume (depth of breathing in litres) selected to produce any given ventilation is determined to a certain extent by the gait of the horse. During walk and trot the horse increases ventilation largely by increasing respiratory frequency, with only small increases in tidal volume. During canter and gallop the respiratory frequency is tied in to the stride frequency one for one, and so any increases in ventilation are brought about largely by increases in tidal volume, with only small increases in respiratory frequency.

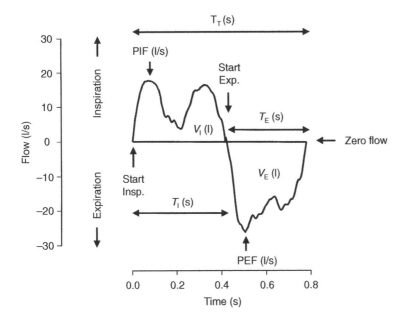

Fig. 9.1 Flow rates during inspiration and expiration. Key: PIF, peak inspiratory flow; PEF, peak expiratory flow; V_I, volume inspired; V_E, volume expired; T_I, time of inspiration; T_E, time of expiration; T_T, total breath time ($T_I + T_E$).

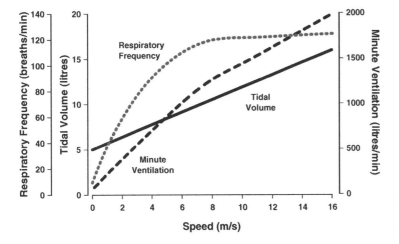

Fig. 9.2 Relationships between respiratory frequency, tidal volume, minute ventilation and speed of running.

Stride frequency is higher on the flat than on an incline and during inclined running horses adopt a lower stride frequency but must then increase tidal volume to achieve the required level of ventilation. Increases in tidal volume as a result of exercise stretch the lung and bring about an increase in the secretion of surfactant, thus helping the lung to become more compliant during exercise.

Respiratory–locomotory coupling

Respiratory–locomotory coupling describes any pattern of breathing where there is a fixed ratio between respiratory frequency and stride frequency. Normal healthy horses exhibit respiratory–locomotory coupling during fast canter and gallop with a ratio of stride to breathing of 1:1 for around 99.9% of the time. The exceptions are occasional breaths when swallowing occurs, during acceleration, and sometimes when changing leads. Think of your own breathing patterns: when running you may find that you exhale after every three strides for example, or when cycling after every pedal turn; this is respiratory–locomotory coupling, but in these examples the ratios of breathing to stride would be 1:3 and 1:1, respectively. Most people who run regularly will couple at least some of the time as it seems to have psychological benefits helping you to

concentrate on maintaining slow, deep breathing, even when you are struggling and would otherwise be inclined to breathe in a quick, shallow pattern. The difference between coupling in humans and horses is that humans can choose to breathe in time with their stride whilst horses don't appear to have any choice once working at a fast canter and gallop. The other major difference between the two athletes is that the horse's body is orientated in the horizontal plane and the human athlete is orientated in the vertical plane whilst running.

Piston–pendulum mechanical theory to explain the relationship between respiration and stride

This theory proposes that the respiratory muscles of the horse, unlike those of the human, are aided to a very large extent by the mechanics of the gait. The diaphragm and rib cage are subject to what is known as a 'piston–pendulum' effect within the horse's body as it gallops (see Fig. 9.3), an effect that actually contributes to reducing the total work (amount of energy) of breathing, reducing the effort required by the respiratory muscles.

The piston
As the forelegs hit the ground in gallop they exert a braking effect on the rest of the horse. As well as

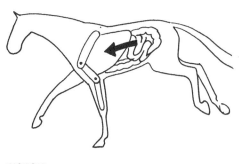

PISTON

During stance phase of forelimbs, the abdominal contents press on the diaphragm, aiding expiration.

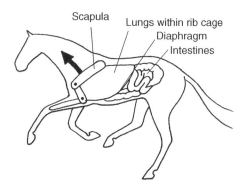

PENDULUM

Forward movement of scapula draws the rib cage forwards and outwards, expanding the thoracic cavity and aiding inspiration.

Fig. 9.3 The piston–pendulum mechanical theory.

the decelerative effect of the forelimb action, the trunk of the horse is often orientated downwards as the forelimbs land. As a result, during the stance phase of the forelimbs, the abdominal contents tend to move forwards and press onto the diaphragm, aiding expiration. At the same time, the scapula is pressed into the front of the chest which will also have the effect of compressing the rib cage. This of course can't happen in people as we run upright, but also remember that, unlike us, the horse does not have a collar bone and so to some extent the scapula is more mobile.

The pendulum

As the forelegs and forehand are raised, the scapula is brought forward by the cervical portion of the *serratus ventralis* muscle. The *serratus ventralis* muscle is connected to the ribs and therefore as the scapula is brought forward so are the ribs. This lifts the rib cage forward and outwards, thus expanding the thoracic cavity and aiding inspiration. The relationship between the respiratory and stride cycles is shown in Fig. 9.4.

Neuromuscular theory to explain the relationship between respiration and stride

On the basis of studies of respiratory muscle activity in horses during exercise, Ainsworth *et al.* (1997) proposed that rather than respiratory timing being 'passive' and driven primarily by locomotory forces, each breath is generated by the respiratory system itself and can therefore be independent of stride. This was concluded on the basis of simultaneous measurements of respiratory muscle electrical activity by electromyography (EMG), oesophageal pressure and limb movements. They concluded that although locomotory forces may contribute to airflow, this is of minimal importance and that locomotory forces do not primarily control breathing during exercise. This is supported by the observation that horses with either upper or lower airway obstruction can switch from 1:1 to 1:2 respiratory–locomotory coupling, i.e. one breath over two strides. For horses that are mildly affected, this may only represent one breath over two strides (1:2 coupling) every 20–30 breaths, with all other breaths still being 1:1. In horses with severe obstruction the coupling may switch from 1:1 into continuous 1:2 breathing.

Alveolar ventilation ($\dot{V}_A$)

Not all the air brought into the body with each breath makes it down to the alveoli. A certain proportion of each breath is 'wasted' and is referred to as dead space. This is wasted ventilation in the sense that energy was expended to bring it into the lung but that it never reached an area where gas exchange could occur. Remember that the lung has conducting airways where no gas exchange occurs and respiratory airways where gas exchange can occur. One could think of this in terms of a Tube train journey. You can go up and down the escalators all day, but until you get down to the platform you won't stand a chance of getting on a train.

Dead space ventilation (V_D) is therefore the proportion of the tidal volume that does not reach a respiratory surface for one reason or another. It can thus be thought of as 'wasted ventilation' and whatever is left, the 'useful' ventilation is known as alveolar ventilation.

$$\text{Alveolar ventilation, } \dot{V}_A = \dot{V}_E - \dot{V}_D$$

The wasted ventilation is correctly termed the physiological dead space ($V_{D\ phys}$) and is made up of anatomical dead space ($V_{D\ anat}$) and the alveolar dead space ($V_{D\ alv}$). In a normal, healthy individual, anatomical dead space ($V_{D\ anat}$) comprises the nostrils, the nasopharynx, the trachea and the larger bronchi, and should account for most of the wasted ventilation at rest – around 50–60% of the resting tidal volume. Thus the 'useful' alveolar ventilation is only 40–50% of total ventilation. As the horse exercises, anatomical dead space is not changed significantly. The upper airways, e.g. the larynx, may be dilated, but effectively the dimensions of most structures remain unchanged and this does not cause a significant increase in dead space volume with exercise. Alveolar dead space ($V_{D\ alv}$) corresponds to that proportion of the tidal volume that is wasted due to the ventilation of alveoli that are not being perfused with blood. $V_{D\ alv}$ is actually reduced during exercise because blood flow to the lung is increased and capillaries that were

(a)

Canter

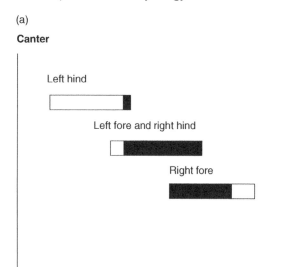

Gallop

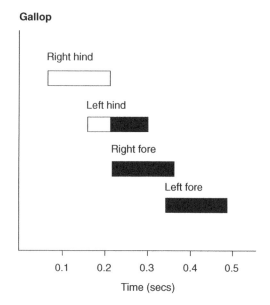

Bars represent stance duration of limbs.

☐ = Inspiration

■ = Expiration

(b)

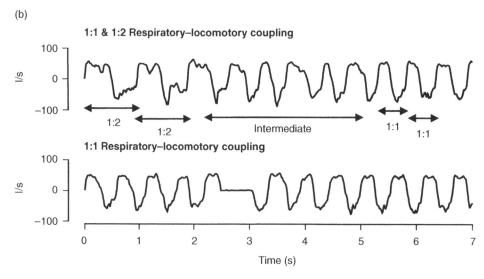

Fig. 9.4 (a) Diagram representing the relationship between the timing of events of the respiratory cycle and the timing of events in the cycle of limb movement when a normal horse is cantering and galloping (adapted from Attenburrow 1982). (b) In the top panel the horse is initially taking one breath over two strides. There is a transition period (intermediate) when the horse is either breathing 1:2 or 1:1, before settling into a regular 1:1 pattern. The bottom panel shows a horse with 1:1 respiratory–locomotory coupling. This is only broken briefly at around 2.5 seconds when the horse swallows and no airflow occurs.

previously non-functional or only receiving a very small blood flow become highly perfused.

During exercise tidal volume is increased; in fact it can be increased 3–4 times above resting levels. This causes a decrease in the dead space to tidal volume ratio ($V_D : V_T$), and an increase in alveolar ventilation (V_{alv}). For example, if anatomical dead space at rest is 2 litres and tidal volume is 4 litres, the ratio is 0.5 or 50%. At a tidal volume of 16 litres, if anatomical dead space remains at 2 litres, the ratio is only 0.13 or 13%. So a greater proportion of the breath reaches the regions of the lung actually involved in gas exchange. Thus as the horse exercises and increases its tidal volume, the percentage of each breath that is wasted is proportionally less. The V_D/V_T ratio therefore decreases during exercise due to a combination of increased tidal volume, the fact that anatomical dead space remains unchanged, and increased lung perfusion.

Is respiratory–locomotory coupling over-rated?

At first sight, respiratory–locomotory coupling would seem to be a 'good thing'. Surely it must be if it saves energy. The problem comes when the horse is pushed to maximal speeds. In order to increase speed most horses will increase stride frequency and then increase stride length. At top speeds stride frequency will also reach a maximum. In this situation, increasing respiratory frequency in order to increase ventilation is simply not an option, and the only way the horse can get more air into its lungs (given the same stride duration) is to increase the *rate* of airflow. This requires greater swings in intrapleural (alveolar) pressure. In other words, it requires more work to be done by the respiratory muscles. For any given level of ventilation, slower, deeper breathing is more effective in terms of alveolar ventilation and oxygen uptake than quick, shallow breathing. For example, a minute ventilation of 1000 litres/min can be achieved by a combination of a respiratory frequency of 100 breaths/min and a tidal volume of 10 litres or a frequency of 200 breaths/min and a tidal volume of 5 litres. However, the latter would be less effective for reasons described above.

A horse with a long stride will take fewer strides to cover a given distance at any given speed. Horses with longer strides may therefore have the edge over the short striding competition as they are less likely to reach maximal stride frequency, and hence maximal respiratory frequency, when running at any given speed. Assuming respiratory–locomotory coupling is 1:1, a horse with a long stride should be capable of a larger tidal volume than a horse with a short stride. As a rule, National Hunt horses who require more stamina than speed are taller and longer striding than their flat racing counterparts.

There are some notable exceptions to the typical 1:1 coupling ratio. Respiratory–locomotory coupling with a ratio of 1:2, i.e. one breath to two strides, is seen in Standardbred trotters at racing speed, horses with RAO, in horses with upper airway obstruction, e.g. moderate to severe laryngeal hemiplegia ('roarers' or 'whistlers'), and healthy horses cantering at slower speeds. For example, a horse may breathe 1:2 with stride when in a very steady hack canter, but should switch to 1:1 breathing when cantering at one-star level cross-country speed. Healthy horses galloping at high speeds but breathing an inspired mixture of 21% O_2 and 6% CO_2 (normally, inspired CO_2 is effectively 0%) have also been shown to adopt a 1:2 respiratory–locomotory pattern leading to speculation that arterial CO_2 partial pressure may be involved in the control of respiration and gait linkage. It is interesting that horses suffering from RAO, with a compromised airflow and gas exchange resulting from the disease often adopt a 1:2 pattern of breathing, allowing more time for inspiration and expiration. Presumably the normal coupling mechanism is over-ridden in conditions where a 1:1 pattern is no longer cost-effective, where airway resistance is dramatically increased or when the elimination of CO_2 becomes compromised. Another advantage in switching from 1:1 to 1:2 breathing is that an increase in tidal volume would further decrease the anatomical dead space as a fraction of the tidal volume.

Pulmonary resistance

Pulmonary resistance is a measure of how difficult it is to move air through the airways. High resistance is associated with low flow rates or high effort, and low resistance is associated with high flow rates or less effort, both for any given pressure difference. The pressure difference is that between the nostrils (essentially zero) and the alveoli. Total pulmonary resistance, the sum of the resistances of all the airways within the lung is known as R_{total}. The most important determinant of airway resistance is simply the radius of the airway (calibre). Think of the airways like hosepipes. The thicker the hosepipe, the greater the flow rate through it. There are various other major factors affecting R_{total}, and their relationship with R_{total} is given by the general equation for gases flowing in tubes:

$$R = \frac{8\eta l}{\pi r^4}$$

where η is the viscosity of the gas mixture flowing through the airway, l is the length of the airway and r is the radius of the airway.

If the radius of the airway is halved, it can be seen that the resistance will be increased 16-fold, as R is inversely proportional to the radius to the power 4. Normally, η and l are constants as neither the viscosity of the gas nor the length of the airway will change throughout the course of breathing. If a horse is given a less dense gas mixture to breathe, for instance a heliox mixture (79% helium and 21% oxygen as opposed to 79% nitrogen and 21% oxygen in air), the viscosity of the gas breathed is decreased, resistance is decreased, and the work of breathing is decreased. Interestingly, this also results in a significant increase in maximal oxygen uptake. During normal quiet breathing, 50% of the total pulmonary resistance is due to the nasal passages, 30% to the remaining upper airways and 20% to the intrathoracic airways (the airways con-

tained within the chest or rib cage) (see Fig. 9.5). It would therefore appear that the large upper airways present a greater resistance to moving air in and out than the smaller airways within the lung. This is not surprising if we consider which combination of hosepipes would get the garden watered quicker, one hundred 1 cm diameter hosepipes or one 10 cm one? Although the nasal passages have a larger radius than, say, the alveolar ducts, if we were to transect the lung and lay all the alveolar ducts from that section side by side we would find that the sum of the alveolar ducts presented a greater total area of airway than the two nasal passages. Resistance decreases as airway generation number (division number) increases because the *total cross-sectional area* (the sum of the areas of all airways at each level or generation in the lung) of airways increases.

The equation for R_{total} assumes that airflow is laminar, i.e. that air flows through the airway in a nice orderly fashion. Unfortunately, at the sort of flow rates that the horse produces during exercise, and partly because of the shape of the airways, flow is not usually laminar, but turbulent. Turbulent flow makes less forward progress than laminar flow, effectively increasing the resistance to airflow (see Fig. 9.6). During exercise, flow rates of air increase, and increases in turbulence and resistance are inevitable. An increase in airway resistance is therefore an unavoidable consequence of exercise. In humans as in horses, a large proportion of the total airway resistance is due to the nasal passages.

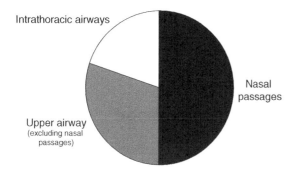

Fig. 9.5 Partitioning of total pulmonary resistance in the horse at rest.

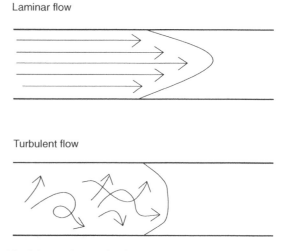

Fig. 9.6 Laminar and turbulent flow.

Humans can switch to mouth breathing in an effort to bypass this airflow bottleneck, but horses cannot as they are obligate nasal breathers. However, they still have a range of physiological tactics which they employ to offset the inevitable increase in R_{total} with exercise. They can:

- Dilate the nares
- Abduct the larynx
- Open up the lower airways (bronchodilate).

Despite these adaptations, R_{total} continues to increase during exercise to levels above that experienced at rest when the airflow was lower. During heavy exercise such as galloping, there is a two-fold increase in R_{total} despite all the above adaptations. A large component of the increase in resistance to airflow during exercise is due to an increase in inertia or inertance. Inertia is a property of matter that during motion causes it to resist change in either direction or velocity, i.e. speed. As an aircraft accelerates down the runway during take-off, you can feel yourself being pressed back against the seat as your body's inertia is overcome. Similarly, on landing as the plane touches down and there is a dramatic deceleration, you would continue in motion if it were not for the safety belts resisting your inertia. Large ships also demonstrate the property of inertia. They are hard to get going, but once going, take a long time to stop. As airflow increases its inertia is raised and it becomes harder to slow down, stop and reverse the flow; the ease or difficulty in decelerating, stopping and accelerating air in the airways is therefore referred to as inertance.

The mechanisms the horse uses to try and reduce resistance have not gone unnoticed. Various devices to dilate the nares have been used. Currently the most popular of these is a version of the human nasal dilator strip that has been produced for horses which aims to prevent the soft tissue in the nasal notch becoming sucked inwards during inspiration (p. 110).

The struggle to breathe

At certain points in the respiratory cycle, pressures on the outside of an airway are considerably greater than those on the inside, the airway becomes compressed and partial collapse can occur. This is like the drinking carton that collapses when you get to the bottom of the drink, when the pressure difference between the outside and the inside is high enough to collapse the walls of the carton. Similar, although slightly less dramatic, effects occur in the airways of all horses during maximal exercise. Different parts of the pulmonary system are affected at different stages of the respiratory cycle. During inspiration the nares, the pharynx, the trachea and the bronchii can become collapsed because their internal pressure is negative. During expiration when air is being expelled from the alveoli, the pressure across the walls of the smaller lower airways (especially those which do not have cartilage) may be enough to compress some of them. During maximal exercise at a time when we could really do without an increase in airway resistance, airways start collapsing on us, a phenomenon known as dynamic partial collapse. Dynamic partial collapse is quite normal and is something that happens to normal, healthy horses.

Dynamic partial collapse has a bearing on the apportioning or partitioning of total airway resistance, depending upon whether the horse is inspiring or expiring. During inspiration at exercise, the extrathoracic airways (airways outside the chest) are now seen to account for more than 90% of R_{total}. During expiration at exercise, the intrathoracic airways account for more than 50% of the total airway resistance (see Fig. 9.7). The dynamics of airway resistance help us to understand why some respiratory problems cause obstruction of the airways on inspiration and some on expiration. As the upper airways present their greatest proportion of R_{total} during inspiration, upper airway disorders such as left laryngeal hemiplegia ('roaring') affect inspiration more so than expiration. Lower airway disorders such as RAO are usually most apparent during expiration because this is when the contribution of the lower airways to resistance is the greatest. One possible exception is dorsal displacement of the soft palate which is a common finding in racehorses and is often suspected on the basis of frequent swallowing and is sometimes associated with a 'gurgling' noise and poor performance. Although this is an upper airway obstruction, because of the nature of the obstruction this condition affects both inspiration and expiration, although the latter usually to a greater extent.

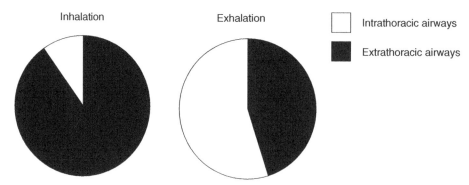

Fig. 9.7   Partitioning of the total pulmonary resistance in the horse at exercise.

It has been suggested that tracheas that are circular rather than ellipsoidal will be less prone to dynamic collapse. Extension of the trachea by encouraging or allowing the horse to stretch its head and neck may reduce turbulence and also stiffen the trachea so that it is less vulnerable to dynamic compression. Conversely, preventing a horse from extending its head and neck while working hard will increase resistance to airflow in the upper airway (particularly at the larynx) and the horse's ventilation will be compromised. In the final stages of intense exercise, such as a flat race, horses are often seen to extend their head and neck and this is most probably in an attempt to increase ventilation. Many horses that 'make a noise' during exercise are more likely to do so if their head and neck are flexed than if they are allowed to extend them. Dynamic collapse of the trachea can often be seen in horses severely affected by RAO during resting endoscopy.

After exercise the adaptations made by the horse to decrease R_{total} outweigh the physical factors which tended to increase R_{total} during the exercise, with the net result that R_{total} immediately post-exercise is actually lower than pre-exercise values. The problem of airway resistance may be compounded both at rest and during exercise by the inhalation of irritants which lead to increased mucus secretion, mucus plugging (obstruction of airways) and bronchoconstriction (constriction of the smooth muscle surrounding the airways). We can reduce these effects by keeping our equine athletes in a very low dust environment. Paying attention to little details such as mucking out the stable

whilst the horse is outside can make all the difference. Normally, debris and particulate matter are removed from the lung by the mucocilliary tract, but clearance may be compromised if the horse's head is fixed in an upright position for long periods of time such as during long journeys in horseboxes. Viral infections such as influenza also kill off large numbers of the ciliated cells lining the trachea and larger airways, so the ability to clear debris from the lung after influenza may be decreased and predispose the animal to secondary bacterial infections. Research into equine respiratory disease is pointing the way more and more towards feeding all horses, rather than just horses with RAO, minimal dust forage and keeping them on a rubber floor.

The work of breathing

Breathing in and out is most definitely an active process. It requires energy so that the respiratory muscles can perform mechanical work, the work of breathing. As ventilation increases, the work of breathing increases (see Fig. 9.8). This means that the oxygen consumed by the respiratory muscles must also increase in line with the speed of running. However, ventilation cannot increase indefinitely. It is likely that there is a critical point where any extra oxygen taken up as a result of increased ventilation would be used entirely by the respiratory muscles. In this situation, there is little point in continuing to increase ventilation. Just as it would be false economy to spend £10 on petrol to travel to a shop where your purchase would be £5 cheaper, it

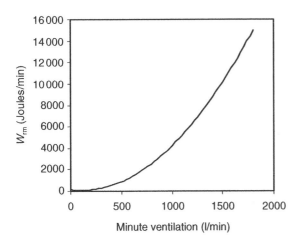

Fig. 9.8 Relationship between work of breathing and ventilation based on data of Art *et al.* (1990a).

is false economy for the respiratory muscles to continue increasing ventilation in line with speed of running indefinitely. In horses, exercise capacity may well be limited by increases in the work of breathing.

Exercise-induced arterial hypoxaemia

In chapter 5 we discussed the superb design of the lung with regard to maximising oxygen diffusion across the alveolar–capillary membrane. At rest and during moderate exercise there would seem to be no problems in getting adequate quantities of oxygen across from the alveoli into the bloodstream because the partial pressure of oxygen in the arteries is maintained at close to 13.3 kPa (100 mmHg). The fact that arterial oxygen partial pressure is stable at approximately 12.0–13.3 kPa (90–100 mmHg) throughout low and moderate levels of exercise, reflects the ability of the respiratory and cardiovascular systems to successfully match oxygen supply to demand. In fact, in going from rest to walk and trot, the partial pressure of oxygen in blood may actually increase slightly.

During high intensity exercise, however, normal, fit and healthy horses exhibit a drop in the partial pressure of arterial oxygen from around 13.3 kPa

(100 mmHg) to as little as 9.3 kPa (70 mmHg) (arterial hypoxaemia; hypo = below), which is usually also accompanied by an increase in the partial pressure of carbon dioxide from around 6.0 kPa (45 mmHg) at rest to 8.0–9.3 kPa (60–70 mmHg) during intense exercise (hypercapnia) (Table 9.1). The development of hypercapnia is taken to indicate that the horse hypoventilates during intense exercise. The horse literally does not ventilate enough for the level of work, most probably due to the constraints of respiratory–locomotory coupling.

Normally, a drop in arterial oxygen pressure increases the drive to breathe, stimulating a compensatory increase in ventilation to counteract the apparent hypoventilation (inadequate ventilation resulting in an increase in arterial carbon dioxide partial pressure). The horse is unusual in that it tolerates an arterial hypoxaemia and hypercapnia at maximal exercise without making any compensatory increases in ventilation. Human athletes normally manage to maintain their blood gas levels right up to maximal exercise levels, with arterial hypoxaemia only ever seen in elite human athletes working at very high exercise intensities. Several theories have been put forward to explain why horses experience exercise-induced arterial hypoxaemia. The most likely explanation is that arterial hypoxaemia occurs as a result of a combination of three factors:

(1) At high exercise intensities some of the pulmonary blood flow 'shunts' across from the pulmonary arterial circulation to the pulmonary venous circulation by-passing the gas exchange surface, i.e. a small proportion of the pulmonary venous blood never gets to meet fresh inhaled gas at the alveoli and mixes on the other side of the lung with blood that has been reoxygenated, thus lowering the average arterial oxygen pressure.

(2) Improvements in pulmonary perfusion and high flow rates of blood through the pulmonary circulation due to improvements in cardiac output as a result of training may actually reduce transit times across the gas exchange surface. In other words, the flow rate of blood through the pulmonary circulation becomes so fast that there is no longer enough time for adequate oxygen uptake.

(3) Finally, because of the very high pulmonary vascular pressures during exercise, some plasma is squeezed from the capillaries, leading to a transient thickening of the alveolar–capillary membrane during exercise. As one of the factors determining the rate of diffusion is diffusion distance, this will increase the time it takes oxygen to diffuse from the alveolar space into the capillaries.

In some instances the arterial hypoxaemia becomes worse in trained horses, especially in those with a large cardiovascular capacity: perhaps this is because training allows them to work at levels at which the hypoxaemia occurs, or because the blood flow improves to such an extent that pulmonary transit times are decreased, i.e. the blood flows faster through the pulmonary capillaries. The consequences of arterial hypoxaemia may well be less for the horse than the human athlete because the horse possesses the ability to increase the number of circulating RBCs from a store in the spleen. Humans are not able to do this. However, what this means for the horse, is that even though the partial pressure of oxygen in arterial blood falls with intense exercise, the amount of oxygen carried (known as the oxygen content of the blood and which is proportional to the number of RBCs) actually increases by around 30% between rest and moderate intensity exercise (50–60% $\dot{V}_{O_2max}$). With increasing intensity up to 100% $\dot{V}_{O_2max}$ or higher, the oxygen content of arterial blood falls, but still remains higher than at rest.

Table 9.1 Typical values for respiratory variables in horses

	Rest	Maximal exercise
Respiratory rate, f_R (breaths/min)	10–15	120–150
Tidal volume, V_T (l BTPS)	3–6	14–20
Minute ventilation, $\dot{V}_E$ (l/min BTPS)	40–60	1500–2000
Peak inspiratory flow, PIF (l/s)	3	80
Peak expiratory flow, PEF (l/s)	3	100
Oxygen uptake, $\dot{V}_{O_2}$ (ml/min/kg, STPD)	5	130–200
Carbon dioxide production, $\dot{V}_{CO_2}$ (ml/min/kg, STPD)	4	140–220
Arterial blood Pa_{O_2} (mmHg @37°C)	90–110	70
Arterial blood Pa_{CO_2} (mmHg @37°C)	45	70
Arterial blood pH (37°C)	7.4	7.1

Respiratory response to training

Maximal oxygen uptake has been shown in a number of different studies to increase by up to 30% in the first few weeks of training. More commonly the increase would be expected to be around 15–20%. The improvements in aerobic capacity have everything to do with adaptations at the level of the muscle and the cardiovascular system, and very little, if anything, to do with any respiratory adaptations. Surprisingly, there is almost no improvement in ventilatory capacity as a result of training. Respiratory muscle strength may increase by about 10%, but this does not contribute much to the improvement in $\dot{V}_{O_2max}$. Many people assume that there must be large improvements to the function of the pulmonary system, as their horses do not 'blow' so much when they are fit. The extent to which a horse 'blows' after exercise is related to how much it has called upon anaerobic energy pathways and body temperature. The unfit horse will rely more on anaerobic energy supply, will get hotter and thermoregulate less well than when fit. Rather than suddenly being able to take in more oxygen, the fit horse has simply become a more efficient aerobic machine, better at delivering and utilising the oxygen that is brought in. The improvement in oxygen utilisation manifests itself in a horse which can trot up the hill without blowing, where previously it could not. The fact that the lungs do not respond to training should send a clear message. If you damage your horse's lungs by keeping it in a dusty environment and on hay and straw full of moulds, any damage done cannot be overcome by training the lungs to compensate. After lameness, respiratory problems are the most common reason for horses performing below expectations.

Exercise-induced pulmonary haemorrhage (EIPH)

EIPH deserves special mention as it is probably the most common 'abnormality' affecting the horse during exercise. EIPH refers to bleeding (haemorrhage) from blood vessels within the lung (pulmonary) which occurs during exercise (exercise-induced). Lay terms include 'bleeding' and 'bursting blood vessels'. Whilst it has been documented for over 300 years that a small percentage of racehorses show blood at the nostrils after racing, e.g. Bleeding Childers, it was not until the introduction of fibreoptic endoscopes only as recently as the 1970s that it became clear that blood observed at the nostrils during or following strenuous exercise nearly always originated from the lungs, rather than from the upper airway.

With the more widespread use of endoscopy in veterinary practice and veterinary research, it is now clear that anywhere between 40 and 75% of Thoroughbred horses will have some blood in their trachea after racing. The degree of haemorrhage varies considerably between individual horses, with horses showing visible blood at the nostrils (epistaxis) often being referred to as 'bleeders' (see Fig. 9.9). The prevalence of epistaxis following racing was reported to be between 0.25 and 2.5% in a study published by Cook (1974).

There are a number of published endoscopic surveys of the incidence of post-race haemorrhage assessed by endoscopy undertaken by different groups of researchers and in different countries around the world. The reason for the relatively wide range of reported incidence is not clear, but it may be related to the time at which post-race endoscopy was carried out. As the site of haemorrhage is almost always in the caudal lung, it will take some time for blood to move cranially and ventrally along the airways, i.e. forward and downwards from the back of the lung towards the front and middle of the lung, into the trachea. Similarly, if too long a period of time is left between the end of exercise and endoscopic examination, the blood may have been cleared up the trachea and swallowed. The time now chosen by most researchers for endoscopy to assess the presence of blood in the trachea after exercise is around 30–40 minutes post-exercise (see Fig. 9.10).

Whilst blood is not always seen in the trachea following intense exercise, Whitwell and Greet (1984) suggested that more than 90% of Thoroughbreds in training that are galloped experience some degree of haemorrhage on a frequent basis. This was based on the analysis of a large number of tracheal washes from horses in training. Nearly all horses that were galloping had haemosiderophages present in tracheal washes. A haemosiderophage is a macrophage containing haemosiderin from broken down erythrocytes that it has removed from the airways. Thus, the presence of haemosiderophages indicates that haemorrhage has previously occurred. After blood is instilled into the lung it takes around 7 days for haemosiderophages to appear in tracheal washes and they can be found for at least 3 weeks. Thus, the presence of haemosiderophages is evidence that the horse has experienced EIPH at some time recently. On the basis of post mortem examinations of the lungs of racehorses in Hong Kong, Mason *et al.* (1983) reported that 94% of retired racehorses had evidence of previous EIPH, whilst the figure was 100% for horses destroyed during training.

Rather than simply record the presence or absence of blood in the trachea, many researchers have adopted scoring systems to grade the amount of blood seen in the trachea. The scoring system used at the Animal Health Trust is as follows:

- *Grade 0.* No blood visible
- *Grade 1.* Flecks of blood

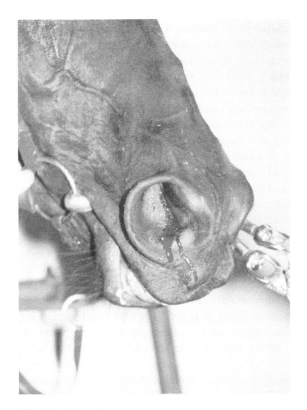

Fig. 9.9   Epistaxis.

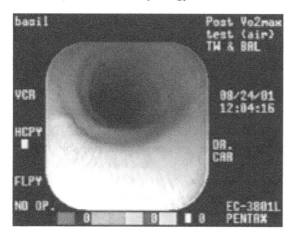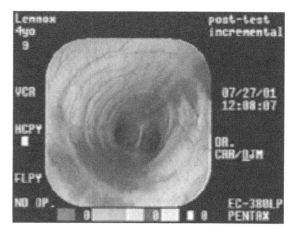

Fig. 9.10 Blood in trachea as evidence of EIPH. Image on left shows a grade 1 haemorrhage, the image on the right shows a grade 3 haemorrhage. The carina can be seen in the centre of the right-hand image.

- *Grade 2.* More than flecks, but less than a continuous stream
- *Grade 3.* Continuous stream less than half the tracheal width
- *Grade 4.* Continuous stream more than half the tracheal width
- *Grade 5.* Airways awash with blood.

With increasing age it has been found that not only the number of horses with blood in the trachea post-racing is increased, but also that the higher grades of bleeding (3 and above) are more common in the older horses.

A more refined and sensitive approach to quantifying EIPH after exercise has been the use of RBC counts in bronchoalveolar lavage (BAL) samples. In this approach the horse is first sedated. For tracheal wash alone, sedation is rarely used except in the case of very difficult horses. After the endoscope has been passed into the trachea a tracheal wash is often taken and the presence of any blood scored. The endoscope is then advanced to the carina (the point of the first division of the trachea into two) and passed into the left or right lung along the left or right mainstem bronchus. Unless a horse has airway inflammation or increased airway reactivity, it is unlikely to cough more than once or twice as the endoscope is passed down the trachea. However, almost all horses will cough as the endoscope is passed into the bronchi.

For this reason, once in the bronchi, body temperature local anaesthetic (usually 10–30 ml of a 2% solution of xylocaine or similar local anaesthetic) is infused down the biopsy channel of the endoscope as it is advanced. The solution is infused at body temperature because cold solutions may induce cough. The endoscope is advanced until it reaches an airway generation that is smaller than itself, at which point it is wedged so that there is a good seal between the outside of the endoscope and the airway wall. Around 100–200 ml of warm (37°C) sterile 0.9% saline is then infused into the lung segment beyond the point at which the endoscope is wedged, via the biopsy channel. In this case the fluid is warm because this helps the epithelial lining fluid (the fluid lining the airways and alveoli) to dissolve into the saline and also to reduce the risk of coughing. Coughing is particularly undesirable at this stage of the procedure as it can lead to the seal between the endoscope and the airway being broken and saline rushing back past the tip of the endoscope which cannot then be sampled.

Immediately the full volume of saline has been instilled it is recovered by hand-suction on the syringe, or sometimes by a suction pump. A common practice is to instil 100 ml (from two 50 ml syringes), recover as much as possible and then to instil a further 100 ml and recover it. The two recovered aliquots are then pooled together. A good sample is considered to have been collected if more than 60% of the volume instilled has been recovered. Not all the saline instilled will ever be recovered, but up to 80% is possible. The saline that remains in the lung does not do any harm and will be absorbed by the lung into the lymphatic system.

If a post-exercise BAL is performed, the number of RBCs can be counted using a haemocytometer and the RBC count expressed per volume of BAL fluid. At rest, RBC counts are almost always under 10 cells/µl of BAL, unless haemorrhage has been caused by the BAL procedure itself. It is unusual for the BAL procedure to induce haemorrhage, but this can occur if the horse does not co-operate, if the endoscope is moved in and out of the airways, or if the horse coughs frequently. Counting RBCs in BAL post-exercise is a more sensitive test for detecting EIPH than scoring for the presence of blood in the trachea. For example, after moderate to high intensity treadmill exercise, e.g. 2 minutes at 12m/s (720m/min) on a 3° incline, most horses would not show blood in the trachea but BAL RBC count may range from 300 to 3000 RBCs/µl BAL. The appearance of small volumes of blood in BAL can be quite dramatic. The technique of counting erythrocytes in BAL is now becoming used more widely than simple endoscopic scoring by groups involved in EIPH research.

Whilst originally thought to be a Thoroughbred 'problem', it is now clear that any breed or type of horse or pony undertaking strenuous exercise may experience some degree of EIPH. The condition has been observed in Thoroughbreds following flat racing and steeplechasing, in Standardbreds following racing (trotting or pacing) and in horses used for polo, showjumping, cross-country and barrel racing. EIPH has also been shown to occur in racing greyhounds, camels and humans after intense exercise.

It had been almost universally accepted that EIPH in horses was a consequence of intense exercise, such as racing. However, a post mortem study of the lungs of young racehorses in Japan (Oikawa 1999) suggested that EIPH may occur at speeds as low as 7–9m/s (420–540m/min, i.e. slow canter).

The bleeding that occurs as a result of intense exercise in horses is not randomly or uniformly distributed throughout the whole lung, but almost always affects the dorsocaudal (uppermost and rearmost) part of the lung, effectively the area of lung under the back of the saddle. In a young 2-year-old horse in training or young riding horse (around 4–5 years old), with strenuous work (fast canter and gallop and possibly jumping), the very tips of the lung will tend to be affected first. As the horse ages and the volume and intensity of exercise over time both increase, a larger amount of lung is affected and the bleeding tends to become worse (see Fig. 9.11). It may be that continual bouts of EIPH cause structural changes in the lung as a result of the repair process and this may explain the trend for more frequent and severe bleeding with age. For example, in an endoscopic study of the prevalence of EIPH in Thoroughbreds racing on the flat, Roberts *et al.* (1993) reported that 40% of 2 year olds, 65% of 3 year olds and 82% of horses

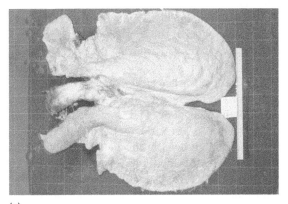
(a)

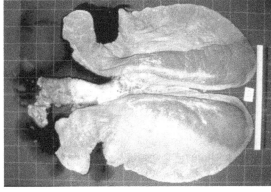
(b)

Fig. 9.11 (a) Normal, healthy lungs and (b) lungs damaged by exercise-induced pulmonary haemorrhage (areas of dark staining).

aged 4 years or over had blood in the trachea following racing.

Many trainers and veterinary surgeons in practice believe that EIPH affects performance. In a survey carried out in the UK, 26% of flat trainers and 54% of National Hunt trainers thought that bleeding affected racing performance. However, most surveys carried out in racing have not found an association between EIPH and performance. For example, Roberts (1998) found that in the UK, the incidence of EIPH was not different between horses performing to expectations and poorly performing horses. In fact, only one major study has demonstrated that severe bleeding was less common in placed horses compared with unplaced horses (Mason *et al.* 1983). However, in a treadmill study where 200 ml of autologous blood (i.e. the horse's own blood drawn from a vein) was instilled into the right and left lungs, gas exchange was impaired during intense exercise and exercise tolerance was reduced. This amount of blood instilled (400 ml) was described as giving the appearance of a grade 2–3 haemorrhage as scored on the amount of blood in the trachea after exercise.

The process of blood entering the airways can have both immediate and long-term potential effects. There is evidence that EIPH may cause permanent alterations in the blood supply to the affected parts of the lungs. Fortunately, EIPH usually only affects a relatively small amount of the total lung. During exercise, blood that enters the airways will inactivate lung surfactant and interfere with gas exchange either by increasing the distance that oxygen and carbon dioxide have to diffuse by forming a thicker layer over the blood–gas barrier or by even blocking small airways so that the alveoli beyond them cannot be ventilated at all. Thus ventilation and gas exchange could be impaired. In the longer term, as the damaged tissue is repaired it is likely that there will be some fibrosis and stiffening of the lung tissue. There may even be loss of tissue structure. Thus, the area damaged may not return to full function. Instillation of blood into the airways experimentally has also been shown to cause airway inflammation which may itself cause further damage because neutrophils produce elastases and reactive oxygen species which weaken cell membranes, possibly making haemorrhage more likely to occur during the next bout of exer-

cise. Inflammation is the process that occurs when body tissues are damaged. For example, in the case of a cut in the skin, the inflammatory response results in increased blood flow to the area, with redness, swelling, heat and pain. Finally, blood is a good medium for bacterial growth and many practitioners believe in giving antibiotic cover to a horse that has been known to have experienced a moderate to severe episode of EIPH.

Despite the fact that it is now 25 years since it was generally accepted that horses bleed in their lungs after intense exercise, the cause is still not known. A large number of factors have been proposed to be the cause of EIPH in the horse and these include:

- Mechanical stress in the lung during exercise as a result of compression by the diaphragm and movement of abdominal contents
- Asphyxia and hypoxic pulmonary vasoconstriction
- Airway inflammation and chronic lung disease
- Parasite infestation and pathogens in the blood
- Airway obstruction
- Defects in coagulation
- Uneven distribution of mechanical stress within the lung during exercise
- Compression of the chest and lung by the shoulder and generation of compression waves leading to shear stress (tearing of tissue at the microscopic level).

The most popular theory is that the bleeding occurs because of very high stresses due to high transmural pressure across the walls of the tiny capillaries in the horse's lung during exercise leading to pulmonary capillary stress failure. This is the theory proposed by the group led by the eminent respiratory physiologist John West based at the University of California. The basis for this theory is that the blood is only separated from the air spaces within the lung by a very thin membrane, the blood–gas barrier (or alveolar–capillary membrane) which facilitates uptake of oxygen by the blood. During exercise horses develop tremendously high pressures in the pulmonary blood vessels and it is hypothesised that this could be sufficient to rupture the vessel walls. Although the pressure of the pulmonary blood vessels is high, it only varies by perhaps 5.4 kPa (40 mmHg) from diastole to systole during each cardiac cycle. Thus the pressure pushing out from inside the blood vessel is relatively constant. However, the transmural pressure (the pressure across the blood vessel wall) varies throughout each respiratory cycle because the pressures in the airways change from positive on expiration to negative during inspiration and will be at their greatest during early inspiration.

Treatment of EIPH at present is problematic because the condition is still not well understood. 'Treatments' used or still being used include snake venom, antioxidants, anticoagulants, aspirin, blood removal, β_2-agonists, hormones, diuretics, water deprivation and nasal dilator strips. The range of treatments being applied is a reflection of the fact that no single treatment appears to have high efficacy.

The high pulmonary vascular pressures during exercise are the basis behind the use during racing of the drug frusemide (also known as furosemide in the USA and most commonly as Lasix). Frusemide is almost certainly the most widely used 'treatment' for EIPH. Frusemide is a diuretic which causes increased urine output and effectively dehydrates the horse, equivalent to a loss in body mass of perhaps 2–5%. The loss of fluid reduces the circulating plasma volume and therefore the blood volume. As a result, the blood pressure and most importantly, the pulmonary artery pressure, is lower both at rest and during exercise. Thus, the vascular component of transmural pressure during exercise should be reduced.

Whilst in the USA the use of frusemide is permitted during both training and racing, in the UK its use is restricted to during training, mainly for horses experiencing severe EIPH. Frusemide has been used as a treatment for EIPH for many years on the basis that the most commonly accepted explanation for EIPH is pulmonary capillary stress failure due to high pulmonary capillary transmural pressures. Because frusemide reduces pulmonary vascular pressures, it reduces transmural pressure. The efficacy of frusemide in reducing pulmonary vascular pressures during exercise has been extensively demonstrated; however, evidence for its efficacy in preventing EIPH has been lacking. For example, Manohar and colleagues reported in 1997

that whilst frusemide at 1 and 1.5 mg/kg significantly reduced pulmonary capillary pressure during intense treadmill exercise (14.2 m/s, 3.5% incline), the incidence of EIPH (although only scored as positive or negative and not graded) was the same in control and both frusemide treatment sessions. Similarly, a number of studies conducted at racetracks in the USA have shown that around half the horses treated still continue to show EIPH, but it is generally accepted that the severity is usually less after treatment. Reviews of some of the current research and of the efficacy of treatments for EIPH have recently been published (Marlin 2001, 2002).

Of course, it is possible that rather than complete prevention of EIPH as a result of frusemide treatment we should perhaps instead be looking for a reduction in severity either based on endoscopic grading or BAL RBC counts. Lester *et al.* (1999) demonstrated a reduction in peak mean pulmonary artery pressure (PAP) during maximal exercise in the field and a significant decrease in BAL RBC count, compared with control, as a result of administration of 250 mg frusemide intravenously (i.v.) 30 minutes before exercise. Interestingly, administration of 250 mg frusemide i.v. in the same horses 240 minutes before exercise (the normal time for regulated use in racing in the USA) failed to decrease peak mean PAP or BAL RBC count following exercise compared with the control session. The reduction in BAL RBC count following treatment with frusemide has also been recently replicated by both Kindig *et al.* (2001a) and Geor *et al.* (2001). These studies both demonstrated reductions in BAL RBC counts (of 90% and 80%, respectively) following high intensity treadmill exercise. However, it has also recently been found that inhaled nitric oxide (NO), which also reduces mean PAP, paradoxically, increases the severity of EIPH as measured by RBC counts in BAL (Kindig *et al.* 2001b).

Two recent studies have also demonstrated that a nasal dilator strip (Fig. 9.12) has similar efficacy to frusemide in decreasing the severity of EIPH as assessed by RBC counts in BAL. The principle behind the use of nasal dilators is that these reduce airway resistance, which reduces airway pressure changes within the lung and, in turn, these decrease the stress on pulmonary capillaries by decreasing

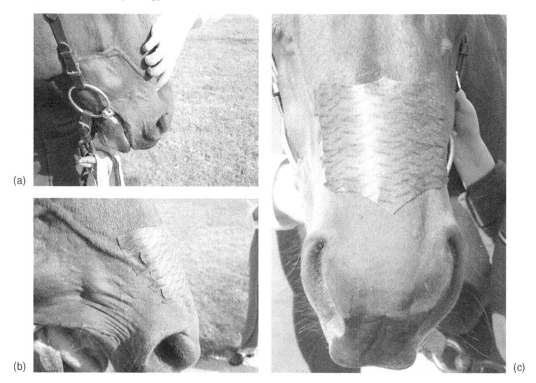

Fig. 9.12 The equine nasal dilator strip is designed to prevent or reduce the inward collapse of the skin overlying the nasal notch during inspiration (a). It contains three horizontal supporting 'springs', compared to the human versions which contain only a single support. The correct placement of the strip is critical to its effective functioning (b, c).

pulmonary capillary transmural pressure. Kindig *et al.* (2001a) reported a reduction of 44% in BAL RBC counts when horses wore a dilator strip, whilst Geor *et al.* (2001) reported a reduction of 74%. There may even be a small advantage of combining frusemide and nasal dilator strips because this reduced BAL RBC counts by 87% (Geor *et al.* 2001). At the time of writing, nasal dilator strips and frusemide are permitted during racing in most states in the USA but neither are permitted for use during racing in the UK. However, both may be used during training.

High blood pressure theories of EIPH cannot at the present time entirely explain why the bleeding occurs in the upper and rear part of the lung. For example, it has been demonstrated using the microsphere technique that blood flow to the dorsal-caudal lung increases during exercise in the horse (Bernard *et al.* 1996). However, increased flow does not necessarily equate to increased pressure. If you turn a garden hose on and keep your

finger pressed over the end, the flow is low, but the pressure is high. If you remove your finger, the flow is greatly increased but the pressure is low. Perhaps one reason for the popularity of frusemide is that it has been shown to improve performance because a treated horse will be carrying around 20–30 kg less body mass due to increased urine output before the race. For this reason frusemide is likely to be given to non-bleeders as well as bleeders in the USA where its use is permitted.

A theory has recently been proposed that EIPH results from the compression of the chest by the forelimbs during fast cantering, galloping and jumping. When the front legs are loaded during galloping, the scapula is pushed back and into the rib-cage. This is particularly so in the horse because it does not have a collar bone to stabilise the scapula. When the foot is planted on the ground, the force is transmitted to the chest and to the lung and from the compression of the lung a 'wave' of pressure passes through it. Because of the shape of the lung this 'wave' becomes amplified and most intense in the rear and upper part of the lung. The damage caused by the wave is known as shear stress. Shear stress occurs at the microscopic level and results from different parts of the tissue (in this case lung), moving at different speeds and in different directions as the pressure wave passes through it. The principle of how the damage would be caused is similar to that experienced in the lungs of people in car accidents where they are hit hard in the front of the chest by the steering wheel. In this situation, the damage and bleeding that occurs in the lung is not usually at the front of the lung where the chest has been hit, but at the back. The same is true in brain haemorrhage experienced by boxers. This usually occurs at the back of the skull, i.e. on the opposite side to where they were hit. A similar situation could exist between the back and top part of the lung and the chest wall.

At present, without knowing the true cause of EIPH, it is extremely difficult to make recommen-dations on management to prevent, reduce or treat the condition. Many suspect that airway inflamma-tion, following infection or as a result of poor stable hygiene (allowing contamination with moulds, dust and ammonia), may accentuate EIPH. Others believe that upper airway conditions such as laryn-geal hemiplegia ('roaring') may worsen bleeding. In reality, there are many factors which could poten-tially affect the strength of the blood–gas barrier and the contribution may well vary between indi-viduals. For example, most horses may experience EIPH during intense exercise due to high trans-mural pressures, whilst some individuals may bleed more severely due to exacerbation by factors such as airway inflammation and upper airway obstruc-tion. Only once we have a clear understanding of the causes of EIPH and access to techniques to accurately quantify and localise the bleeding within the lung will it be possible to improve our manage-ment of this condition.

KEY POINTS

- Ventilation increases approximately linearly with the speed of running or with workload.
- The increase in ventilation from rest to maximal exercise may be as much as 30-fold.
- Peak expired flow rates are around 10% higher than peak inspired flow rates.
- During canter and gallop healthy horses take one breath with each stride.
- Two theories have been proposed to explain res-piratory–locomotory coupling in the horse, the piston–pendulum theory and the neuromuscular theory.
- Normal 1:1 respiratory:locomotory coupling is disturbed occasionally in normal horses when swallowing or changing leads, and more fre-quently in horses with either upper or lower airway disease or dysfunction.
- Physiological dead space ventilation describes the proportion of ventilation that does not reach a gas exchange surface.
- Physiological dead space consists of anatomical dead space (conducting airways) and alveolar dead space (alveoli that are ventilated but not perfused).
- The majority of resistance to airflow during inhalation during exercise is caused by the upper airways. During expiration during exercise the lower airways are responsible for just over half of the total resistance to airflow.
- To try and minimise airway resistance during exercise, horses dilate the nares, abduct the larynx and bronchodilate the airways (cate-cholamines are potent bronchodilators).
- Dynamic partial collapse of the airways may occur during expiration during intense exercise when the pressure around the airways is very high. This can affect both large, e.g. trachea, and small intrathoracic airways.
- The work of breathing becomes proportionally greater as the level of ventilation increases.
- During intense exercise horses experience both arterial hypoxaemia (decreased oxygen tension) and hypercapnia (increased carbon dioxide tension).

- Development of arterial hypercapnia is considered to be a sign of inadequate ventilation (hypoventilation).
- Arterial hypoxaemia is thought to occur due to a combination of shunting of blood in the lung (blood that by-passes the gas exchange surface), reduced capillary transit time (blood moves along the capillary segments much more quickly due to the high cardiac output and does not have time to fully equilibrate with oxygen on the 'air' side of the blood–gas barrier) and possibly due to thickening of the blood–gas barrier due to oedema as a result of high pulmonary vascular pressures.
- The equine respiratory system *does not* respond to training.

Chapter 10

Cardiovascular responses

We have already learnt about the intricacies of the cardiovascular system at rest, hopefully demonstrating that the cardiovascular system is slightly more sophisticated than your average mechanical pump and circulation system. It can monitor and control the concentration of transported substances within strict limits, it can self-regulate the flow and pressure of the blood within its vessels, it can grow and adapt to cope with demand, and can repair itself when minor damage occurs. The cardiovascular system is a marvellous, adaptable piece of biological engineering, and with all this you usually get a lifetime guarantee.

The heart in exercise and performance

It has long been thought that a large heart corresponds to athletic ability in horses. For example, when Eclipse died a post mortem was performed and it was recorded that his heart was larger than normal for his size. Another example is that of the legendary racehorse Phar Lap, believed by many to have been the greatest racehorse ever. In a period of 4 years Phar Lap won 37 out of 51 races; in 1930 he won four races in 1 week and over 1930 to 1931 he won 14 consecutive races. When he died his heart was a staggering 6.3 kg and today is still kept in the Institute of Anatomy in Canberra University.

For many years now, stud owners and potential purchasers in the USA in particular have been scanning horses' hearts before sales using ultrasound. One of the factors contributing to the natural athletic ability of the Thoroughbred is that they tend to have large hearts. Thoroughbred horses have hearts weighing about 4–5 kg, corresponding to about 0.9% of body mass, compared with 0.76% body mass in an Arab and only 0.62%

body mass in heavier draft breeds (Kline & Foreman 1991).

Exercise physiologists are always looking for methods that would allow them to identify particularly talented individuals. To this end, attempts have been made to assess heart size in young racehorses. One method of assessing heart size was devised by Steel in 1963. He put forward the hypothesis that the size of the heart could be estimated from the resting electrocardiogram (ECG) of the horse. There is a characteristic wave on a typical ECG, known as the QRS interval, that corresponds to ventricular contraction. Steel's method was based on the hypothesis that the bigger the ventricles, the longer the QRS interval should be as the longer it would take the electrical wave to pass though the heart. The duration of the QRS in milliseconds was described as the 'heart score', which corresponded to heart size. An equation to relate heart mass to heart score was devised by measuring the heart score and then weighing hearts post mortem. For example, a heart score of 100 (equivalent to a QRS duration of 100 ms or 0.1 s) would be equivalent to a heart mass of 3 kg. Although the heart score may approximate heart size (the accuracy to which it does this is still being debated), it cannot provide any information about the stroke volume. For example, two horses of the same body mass could both have large hearts as estimated from the heart score. However, if one horse has a very muscular, thick walled left ventricle and the other has a thin walled ventricle, then the latter will have a larger stroke volume and therefore a potentially larger maximum cardiac output. Heart score measured in several studies, other than that by Steel (1963), has not been shown to be a reliable indicator of performance. This is probably because there are many more factors that contribute to performance aside from the size of the heart. A three legged horse would not win races even if it had a 7 kg heart. The ultimate performance of the horse is the sum of many contributory factors, and it is unlikely that measurement of only one parameter will enable us to select winners for all distances or all events, although it is true that the majority of horse sports are aerobic and so a large heart would not be disadvantageous.

Nowadays, the thickness of the ventricular walls, and indeed many other heart dimensions, can be assessed using ultrasound or echocardiography. The good news for those of us riding horses with 'average' hearts is that cardiac muscle, like skeletal muscle, does increase in size in response to training, a process known as hypertrophy. Kubo *et al.* (1974) demonstrated a hypertrophy of cardiac muscle from 0.94% body mass in untrained horses to 1.1% body mass after 2 months of training. Young (1999) demonstrated that training induces not only an increase in ventricular wall thickness but also an increase in chamber size (the inside of the ventricle where the blood flows). This means that the heart is able to pump a greater volume of blood (stroke volume) with each contraction, and can contract with greater force following training.

Cardiac output, $\dot{Q}$

Cardiac output ($\dot{Q}$) describes the volume of blood that leaves the left hand side of the heart every minute. Cardiac output is increased as the demand of the body for oxygen is increased. During maximal exercise, cardiac output may reach 240 litres/min:

$$\dot{Q} = \text{Heart rate} \times \text{Stroke volume}$$
$$240 \text{ litres/min} = 220 \text{ beats/min} \times 1.1 \text{ litres}$$

In non-elite human athletes, cardiac output increases from about 4–6 litres/min at rest, to about 16–24 litres/min during exercise, i.e. a fourfold increase above resting values, compared to a tenfold increase for horses. As well as an increase in cardiac output as a result of exercise, the *proportion* of the cardiac output received by both the heart and skeletal muscle is increased. During exercise, blood is diverted away from less active tissues such as the gastrointestinal tract and the kidney, and redirected to skeletal muscle, skin, cardiac and pulmonary circulations. Under the influence of the

sympathetic nervous system (the fight or flight control system), blood is preferentially sent to the hardest working organs. During intense exercise, the blood flow to skeletal muscle increases 70-fold over resting values (Parks & Manohar 1983).

Resting heart rate

The average resting heart rate in a Thoroughbred horse is around 30–40 beats/min when taken using a stethoscope (auscultation) or by palpating (feeling) a pulse on an artery close to the surface, e.g. under the jaw. It is not uncommon to measure heart rates as low as 22–25 beats/min in relaxed horses in quiet environments, especially if recorded with a heart rate monitor or ECG system without anyone in the stable at the time. For many years, scientists and vets have held varying opinions on the matter of whether or not the resting heart rate of a trained horse is lower than its pre-training resting heart rate. It is well established that untrained humans have true resting heart rates of around 70–80 beats/min, whilst trained distance athletes may have heart rates as low as 40 beats/min. In fact the five times winner of the Tour De France, the Spanish rider Miguel Indurain, is reported to have a resting heart rate of around 30 beats/min.

One of the reasons for the controversy over whether resting heart rate in horses changes with training is the difficulty of obtaining a true resting heart rate for a horse. Even the act of approaching a horse to use a stethoscope or a heart rate monitor may result in a degree of sympathetic stimulation that increases the heart rate above resting values, if only by 5–10 beats/min. Heart rate recordings therefore need to be made over a prolonged period of time without the presence of people or other activity to gain true resting values. This is not of course true for heart rates taken as part of a clinical examination.

Recent research carried out in Japan suggests that the resting heart rate of Thoroughbred horses does, in fact, decrease following training (Kuwahara *et al.* 1999). The theory is that as heart muscle mass increases (a process known as hypertrophy) due to training, the contractions of the heart muscle become stronger (this is referred to as an increase in myocardial contractility). Consequently more blood can be forced out of the heart with each beat, and the amount of blood necessary to supply the tissues at rest can be provided with a relatively lower heart rate. In this study, mean heart rate during the day decreased from 47 to 38 beats/min and at night from 40 to 34 beats/min, both after 7 months of training. The initial resting heart rate during the day would seem somewhat on the high side and might reflect other factors such as excitement during measurements at the start of the study. Whilst this is the first study to demonstrate a reduction in resting heart rate with training, it does need to be repeated. However, even if a genuine training effect on resting heart rate does occur in the horse, the decreases are at most likely to be in the region of a few beats/min, and so it is highly unlikely that this would be a practical way to monitor response to training or provide a basis for comparing horses.

Measuring heart rate during exercise

The measurement of working heart rates is an invaluable training aid in many disciplines and is dealt with in some depth in Chapter 18. Various methods can be used to measure heart rate.

Auscultation using a stethoscope
By counting the number of beats heard over a period of between 15 seconds (and multiplying the number of beats by four) to 1 minute, the heart rate can be estimated. A limitation of counting for only 15 seconds is that heart rate will only be estimated with a resolution of 4 beats/min, i.e. 28, 32, 36, 40, 44, 48 beats/min, etc. Counting over 30 seconds improves the resolution to 2 beats/min, i.e. 28, 30, 32 beats/min, etc. The counting period used will therefore depend on why the heart rate is being taken. This is an inexpensive and easy method; however, it can only be used when the horse is standing still (Fig. 10.1), and so it can only give us information about the heart rate before or after exercise. The great advantage of the stethoscope over other methods is that it gives vital information on the quality of the heart beat itself, enabling veterinarians to detect missed beats, abnormal rhythms (dysrhythmias) and heart murmurs. Many horses miss or 'drop' beats at rest, but have a regular heart beat during exercise. This is usually the result of second degree atrioventricular (AV) block. This occurs

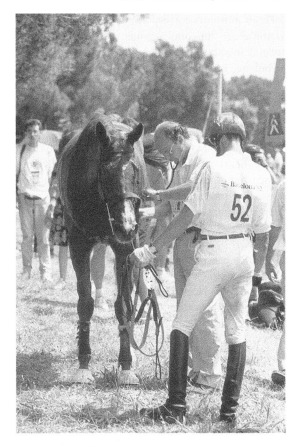

Fig. 10.1 Auscultation using a stethoscope.

when a 'P' wave is not conducted through to the ventricles, so a P wave is seen on the ECG but no QRS complex follows. The next P wave and QRS complex occur precisely in time where it would have been predicted they would occur based on the preceding and following beats. This is easily seen on an ECG and often occurs at a frequency of one beat in 3–5 in very relaxed horses before exercise. Second degree AV block has been proposed as a mechanism for control of arterial pressure in horses at rest without the need for vasodilation/vasoconstriction or changes in heart rate. If arterial blood pressure is monitored over time, in horses that demonstrate second degree AV block, the pressure is seen to increase over a number of beats, with the highest pressure just before a blocked beat. The mean arterial pressure falls as a result of the blocked beat and then increases over time until the next blocked beat occurs.

Heart murmurs correspond to sounds in addition to the clear 'lup–dup' sounds of the valves of a normal healthy heart, and are sounds caused by turbulence in the blood flow. Murmurs vary in their location (left or right side of the heart) and in their intensity (loudness) and where in the heart cycle that they appear. It is not simply a case that any murmur is bad news. Certainly a very loud murmur from the left side (the side pumping arterial blood) of the heart may almost certainly affect performance, but at present the effect on performance of the lower grades of murmurs and especially right heart murmurs is still unclear.

Palpation of the pulse in an artery

The pulse can be taken at any place in the body where a superficial artery passes over a bone. One of the easiest places to find is the facial artery as it passes over the bottom of the jawbone (Fig. 10.2a). The pulse can also be felt in the transverse facial artery (Fig. 10.2b) which is only a few millimetres in diameter, and even in the carotid artery below the jugular vein. Again, it is only possible to take a pulse in the standing horse, not during exercise. As it is often difficult to get the horse to stand still for 1 minute after exercise whilst you take a pulse, it is often necessary to listen for only 15 seconds or so and then multiply by four to obtain beats per minute. However, the longer you are able to feel the pulse, the more accurate the result is likely to be. Taking the pulse manually also requires you to dismount, unless you have help available. One of

the major disadvantages with this is that the horse must be pulled up whilst it is recovering, and recovery is actually quicker and more effective if the horse is kept on the move, coming down to rest 'through the gears'. However, the heart rate early in the recovery period (say 1–3 minutes from the end of exercise) usually gives a more accurate reflection of the work undertaken than a heart rate taken later on in recovery. The major problem is that as the horse recovers, factors other than the work previously undertaken, such as excitement start to influence heart rate.

Heart rate monitors

The majority of commercial heart rate monitors are reliable provided they are used correctly, although some perform much better than others. If there are problems with accuracy, they are likely to be at their most accurate following exercise (when the horse has sweated) in walk or trot. Often movement on the skin of electrodes and muscle electrical activity during canter and gallop can lead to inaccurate readings; a typical example is a heart rate that is similar to stride rate (100–150 per minute) and which does not increase with increasing speed.

A small unit picks up the electrical activity across the heart via electrodes placed on the skin and transmits it either through a wire or by a weak radio signal (about 1 m range) to a watch receiver (see Fig. 10.3) which calculates the number of pulses received and converts it to a rate per minute. Most

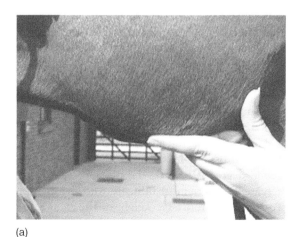

(a)

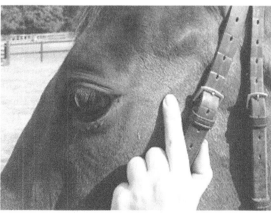

(b)

Fig. 10.2 Palpation of the pulse.

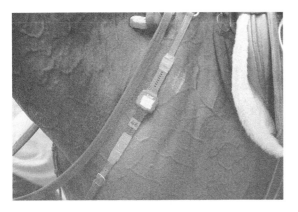

Fig. 10.3 Heart rate monitor watch receiver.

heart rate monitors display the heart rate every 5, 15 or 60 seconds. If there is a good contact between the electrode and the skin (usually this can be achieved simply by thorough wetting of the coat under the electrodes) and the equipment is looked after well (especially the electrode leads and batteries) these monitors will produce excellent results. Results are less reliable and rather more difficult to achieve on unclipped winter coats. Heart rate monitors vary greatly in price, depending on whether you want a basic one that simply displays the heart rate, or one which stores the heart rate data to be downloaded later through a computer. The correct functioning of the downloading type of heart rate monitor is easier to check than that of the non-downloading kind.

Electrocardiography

This is used to produce an electrocardiogram (ECG), a pictorial representation of the summation of electrical activity occurring in the heart. It is the most accurate method of measuring heart rate, giving information on both the heart rate and on the quality of the heart beat itself. There are essentially three different types of ECG recorder available. The traditional electrocardiogram is taken with the horse at rest; these are used to look for dysrhythmias such as atrial fibrillation. The horse is connected by leads from electrodes (the same as used for recording human ECGs) on the skin surface connected directly to the ECG recorder (see Fig. 10.4). Any movement often results in a noisy ECG signal.

The second type of system still relies on electrodes but the ECG recorder is much smaller (around 3 cm × 5 cm × 8 cm) and is attached to the horse. These recorders, often called holter monitors, are frequently left on to record a 24 h ECG to look for intermittent dysrhythmias. Originally these contained tapes but more recent versions use memory cards. The tape or card is then removed from the recorder and the recorded information is downloaded into an analyser or computer. These systems are also usually not suited to situations where there is significant movement, such as exercise.

The third type of system is a telemetry ECG (Fig. 10.4). The principle is similar to the heart rate monitor in that the electrical activity from the heart is picked up by skin electrodes and transmitted by a small unit on the horse to a base unit. The base unit displays the ECG and calculates heart rate and even, in some systems, respiratory rate using a principle known as impedance plethysmography. These systems produce excellent exercise ECG recordings but are relatively expensive.

More recently a system based on the Psion handheld computer has been developed specifically for the veterinary field. This system falls between the holter monitors and the direct attachment ECG systems with visual display (see Fig. 10.5). The electrodes are positioned and the wires connected. The ECG signal can be viewed on the Psion to verify that a good signal is being obtained. The Psion is then disconnected and the data logger attached to record the ECG. After exercise the data logger can be re-attached to the Psion and the ECG siquals downloaded onto the Psion for viewing and analysis. This system produces good quality recordings even during exercise.

ECG systems are considerably more expensive than heart rate monitors and are usually only used by veterinary clinics and research centres. However, there is now an intermediate type of system between the standard heart rate monitor and traditional ECG recording system available from Polar. The Polar NV heart rate monitor is able to work in RR mode as well as in the more common averaging modes. In the RR mode the NV monitor is able to calculate and store each RR interval (the interval between successive heart beats based on the time between each R wave in the QRS). The RR interval is the internationally recognised and

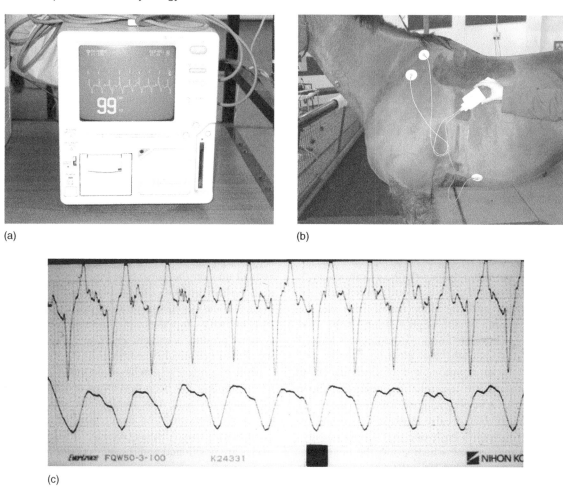

(a)   (b)

(c)

Fig. 10.4   A telemetry ECG machine: (a) receiver and display; (b) electrodes and transmitter on horse; (c) ECG and respiratory signal print-out on chart paper.

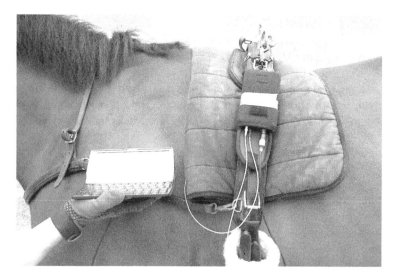

Fig. 10.5   An on-board ECG recorder that can be downloaded onto a Psion hand-held computer.

accepted way to calculate heart rate based on the ECG. In our experience the NV works in the RR mode with horses at rest provided there is almost no movement and that there is very good electrode contact. This usually requires stick-on ECG electrodes to be used. Polar also make an RR monitor system which seems to show good accuracy when compared with ECG in resting pigs, but to the best of our knowledge this system has not been evaluated in horses.

Increases in heart rate in response to exercise

Heart rate increases linearly with speed (equivalent to work) up to a maximal heart rate (HR_{max}) (see Fig. 10.6). HR_{max} is the highest possible heart rate achievable by the horse, and is shown by a plateau in the heart rate response, despite an increase in running speed. If the heart rate does not reach a plateau, the highest heart rate seen during any one piece of exercise is correctly referred to as the peak heart rate. Anything less than HR_{max} is known as a submaximal heart rate. A rough guide to the submaximal heart rates at various speeds are given in Table 10.1.

HR_{max} in the 2–3 year old racehorse is in the region of 240–250 beats/min. In humans, maximal heart rate decreases with age, according to the relationship $HR_{max} = 220$ – age in years. Although maximal heart rate also decreases with age in horses (McKeever & Malinowski 1997) there is no simple relationship available to describe the nature of the decrease over time. However, as a general guide, from previous experience, horses around 8–10 years old would be expected to have a maximal heart rate of around 220–230 beats/min, and horses over 15 years of age may be in the range 190–210 beats/min.

If a horse goes from a standing start to a full gallop, it would take about 20–30 seconds for the maximal heart rate to be achieved. Generally, horses heart rates increase in response to an

Table 10.1 Guide to heart rate at various speeds of locomotion

Gait	Speed m/s	m/min	Submaximal heart rate (beats/min)
Walking	1.7	100	60–80
Trotting	3.7	220	80–100
Cantering	5.8[a]	350[a]	100–140
	8.3[b]	500[b]	120–180
Galloping	13.3–16.7[c]	800–1000[c]	180–220

[a] Easy, showjumping canter.
[b] 'Good' canter.
[c] 'Flat out'.

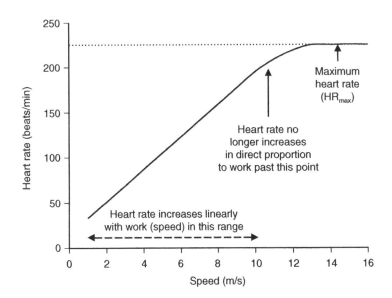

Fig. 10.6 Relationship between heart rate and speed, showing HR_{max}.

increase in work demand much more quickly than those of humans. Heart rate increases are brought about in response to an increase in sympathetic stimulation and a decrease in parasympathetic stimulation, with a concurrent increase in circulating adrenaline. This is exactly the same mechanism that is responsible for increases in heart rate as part of the classic 'fight or flight' response. Concentrations of adrenaline in the blood of horses during intense exercise can easily exceed those measured in human athletes by a factor of ten.

Standing horses can be seen to have heart rates as high as 190 beats/min purely as a result of fear or excitement. The extent to which the 'fight or flight' mechanism can raise the heart rate, and the speed with which it occurs, can be described as the 'reactivity' of the heart rate. Heart rate responses of horses are more reactive than humans, and heart rate responses of Thoroughbreds are generally more reactive than other cold-blooded types. The more reactive the breed, the more variable the sub-maximal heart rates are likely to be.

At exercise intensities producing heart rates lower than about 120–150 beats/min, the effects of excitement are often superimposed on the effects of exercise, and so the normal linear relationship between heart rate and speed may not be seen in excitable horses at these lower exercise levels. However, once the horse is in canter and gallop, you can be reasonably sure that the heart rates you see are a true indication of how hard the horse is working. Heart rate is not such a reliable indicator of the level of work during walk and trot due to the effect of excitement on the heart.

The normal heart rate response to exercise

Heart rate during exercise is directly related to work or, in real terms, speed. Therefore as speed increases, heart rate increases in proportion until maximum heart rate is reached. If a horse works at a steady speed, the heart rate should be steady. Horses' heart rates vary from between about 25 beats/min at rest to 250 beats/min during maximal exercise. At the onset of a sub-maximal piece of work, it is quite normal to see an initial overshoot of the heart rate before it settles down at a rate appropriate for the workload (see Fig. 10.7). So for

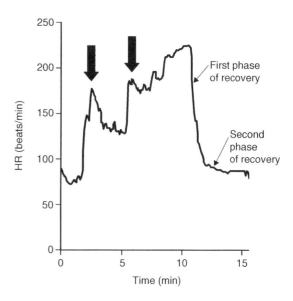

Fig. 10.7 Typical heart rate trace for a horse performing an incremental exercise test on a treadmill. Bold arrows indicate overshoot in heart rate at transitions from walk to trot and from trot to canter.

example, when going from trot at a heart rate of around 90–120 beats/min into a medium speed canter, the heart rate will increase quite rapidly, perhaps up to 160–180 beats/min and then drop back down to around 140–160 beats/min and should remain steady if the speed is kept constant and provided the ground conditions or slope does not change. In some circumstances the heart rate may not stabilise, even though the work is constant. During exercise in hot or hot humid conditions, a horse may start out trotting at a heart rate of around 120 beats/min, but if the horse's body temperature increases over time with the exercise, then the heart rate will increase slowly with the increase in body temperature. This is referred to as cardiac drift.

The heart rate overshoot at the start of exercise is a characteristic feature of the heart rate response, whereby the cardiovascular system almost over-anticipates the demand. The exuberant and rapid response of the equine heart to exercise has been suggested to account for the relatively low oxygen deficit seen in the horse at higher exercise intensities.

When a piece of work has finished, the horse should be allowed to decrease speed gradually. The rider should make sure that the horse comes down 'through the gears', and does not just flop into trot and walk. If the horse stops too abruptly after galloping, his heart will initially slow down but the rate will probably increase again, showing a similar overshoot to that observed at the onset of exercise. This results in a slower rate of recovery. If the horse warms down, you will actually find that its rate decreases more rapidly than if it is allowed to come back to walk and halt too soon. Typically, the heart rate recovery shows two phases:

(1) An initial rapid phase
(2) A second, more gradual decline towards resting values (see Fig. 10.7).

Horses defy basic physiological rules

As a general rule, the larger the animal, the lower the resting heart rate; for example, horses are bigger than humans and have a resting heart rate approximately half that of a human. Another general rule is that the larger the animal, the lower the maximal heart rate; however, horses have a maximal heart rate of approximately 240 beats/min, greater than that of a human at approximately 200 beats/min. The fact that the horse is capable of increasing its heart rate by nearly 10 times above resting is another factor contributing to the superior athletic performance of the horse. Other athletic species, such as the human and the camel, can only increase their heart rates about four times above resting values.

Stroke volume

Stroke volume increases during exercise. The maximum achievable stroke volume for a 500 kg Thoroughbred horse is approximately 1.3 litres. Generally, the bigger the heart the greater the stroke volume that will be seen at rest. Stroke volume increases in response to exercise, as stimulation of the nerves of the sympathetic nervous system directly increases the force of contraction of the heart. Stroke volumes can be increased up to 50% from resting values, but the majority of this

increase occurs in the transition from rest to walk and trot exercise, with little or no further increase once the horse is cantering and galloping. There is always the possibility that high heart rates may limit the stroke volume, as the more rapid cardiac cycle (higher heart rate) leaves less time for ventricular filling. Thirty years of studies on human athletes have failed to clarify whether stroke volume actually plateaus at higher levels of exercise or whether it continues to increase up to maximal heart rates, as it seems to vary depending upon the mode of exercise and the ability of the individual.

Maximal oxygen uptake ($\dot{V}_{O_2 max}$)

Oxygen uptake refers to the oxygen taken up by muscles, *not* the oxygen taken into the lung. $\dot{V}_{O_2 max}$ represents the maximum rate that oxygen can be used. $\dot{V}_{O_2 max}$ can therefore be considered as a measure of the aerobic capacity of an individual, but will ultimately be limited by the number of mitochondria in the muscles and the efficiency of oxygen delivery. During exercise in horses, oxygen uptake by the muscles increases by up to 35 times the resting rate. Horses have a very high $\dot{V}_{O_2 max}$ for their body mass and hence a large aerobic capacity. Maximal oxygen uptakes for ponies are usually around 90–100 ml (STPD)/min/kg and even average ability Thoroughbred horses reach 140 ml/min/kg, compared with 70 ml/min/kg for elite human distance athletes. One exception is the cyclist Miguel Indurain who is reported to have a $\dot{V}_{O_2 max}$ of around 100 ml/min/kg, making him the athletic equivalent of a pony, but still a long way behind the Thoroughbreds.

Oxygen uptake can be calculated using the Fick principle, which states that the amount of substance removed from or taken up by an organ per unit time is equal to the arterial concentration minus the venous concentration of that substance multiplied by the blood flow through the organ. For whole body oxygen uptake this can be expressed in symbols by

$$\dot{V}_{O_2} = \dot{Q} \times (Ca - C\bar{v}_{O_2})$$

where $\dot{Q}$ is the cardiac output and $Ca_{O_2} - C\bar{v}_{O_2}$ is arterial oxygen content minus mixed venous oxygen content. The mixed venous oxygen content is measured in blood taken from the pulmonary artery. If venous blood was taken from the jugular vein then this would reflect only oxygen extraction by the head and neck. Therefore the blood in the pulmonary artery is considered to represent a true mix of blood coming back to the heart from all parts of the body and so is called mixed venous blood. Mixed venous blood is therefore always much more informative when assessing anything to do with blood gas status than jugular venous blood, although the latter is much easier to collect.

Horses are capable of huge increases in oxygen uptake in response to exercise, and this is partly due to their capacity to increase cardiac output around 10 times above the resting rate. However, a larger contribution arises from the horse being able to significantly improve its oxygen carrying capacity and hence its oxygen extraction by the muscle by increasing the blood oxygen content. At the onset of exercise, or even in anticipation of exercise, stimulation of the sympathetic nerves results in an increase in circulating adrenaline. The release of adrenaline causes contraction of the spleen and the release of red blood cells (RBCs) stored within. The horse literally injects its own circulation with additional RBCs, an illegal practice carried out by some distance runners back in the 1970s who had around a litre of blood removed and refrigerated 6 weeks or so in advance of a competition. The body responded to the loss of blood cells by making more so that the level came back to normal. When the extracted blood was re-infused a few days before a race, it increased their circulating numbers of RBCs, so boosting their oxygen carrying capacity. A similar approach has been used by many professional cyclists in recent years. However, instead of adding in extra RBCs, they take a drug called erythropoetin (commonly called EPO) which stimulates the bone marrow to produce more RBCs than normal. Whereas the normal proportion of RBCs in trained human distance athletes would be around 0.4–0.45 l/l (the packed cell volume or PCV), values as high as 0.6 l/l have been measured. In recent years this led the cycling federations to set an upper limit of 0.5 l/l for the PCV before the start of competition to try and limit EPO abuse. Blood doping significantly improves the subject's $\dot{V}_{O_2max}$ (Buick et al. 1980) and therefore should improve performance in events with a large aerobic contri-

bution. As you will see below, the horse is able to achieve this and more, but legally! Splenic contraction is thought to account for the majority of the increase in oxygen uptake above resting levels, and explains why the horse is capable of such a large $\dot{V}_{O_2max}$ compared to other mammals that do not possess splenic reserves of RBCs.

Splenic reserves

At least one-third of the total number of RBCs in the horse's body are stored within the spleen and are released in response to an increase in adrenaline. The amount of RBCs in a given volume of blood is expressed in terms of the PCV which increases in a linear fashion with increases in speed. PCV at rest is approximately 0.30–0.40 l/l, rising to 0.60–0.70 l/l during maximal exercise or following injection of high doses of adrenaline. The greater the PCV, the more viscous the blood becomes, and the harder the heart has to work in order to pump it through the circulation. For example, Fedde and Erickson (1998) estimated that an increase in a horse's PCV from 0.40 l/l at rest to 0.65 l/l during exercise would double the apparent viscosity of the blood. Total mobilisation of RBCs from the spleen leads to an increase in the concentration of circulating haemoglobin, from 150 g/litre to 220 g/litre. Total RBC mobilisation occurs within about 20 s of the onset of high intensity exercise, but it takes about 1 hour for all these cells to be returned to the spleen following exercise. Blood doping would not necessarily give the equine athlete an advantage, as it would result in blood so viscous it would actually be more difficult for the heart to pump it around the body, and cardiac output would probably be reduced. Therefore horses don't need to benefit from blood doping; they do it themselves naturally by releasing stored RBCs from the spleen.

Blood pressure during exercise

Resting arterial blood pressure measured in a large artery such as the carotid in the horse is around 16.0/10.7 kPa (120/80 mmHg) as in humans. During submaximal exercise, there is usually little or no change in blood pressure, and it may even fall slightly due to vasodilation of vessels in the working muscles and skin, but during maximal exercise, blood pressures increase to around 26.7/16.0 kPa (200/120 mmHg) with mean pressures around 22.7 kPa (170 mmHg). The increases in arterial pressure in the systemic circulation are accompanied by even more dramatic increases in pulmonary artery pressure. At rest, mean pulmonary artery pressure is around 2.0–4.0 kPa (15–30 mmHg) but can increase to over 13.3 kPa (100 mmHg) during intense exercise. This response in pulmonary arterial pressure is not seen in man and has been suggested to be a consequence of the horse's high mass specific (i.e. for its body mass) cardiac output. The hypothesis is that the blood flow through the lungs is so great that the 'arterial' blood returning from the gas exchange surface in the pulmonary venous circulation overwhelms the left atrium. The left atrium is unable to keep up with the flow rate and the flow 'backs up' into the pulmonary veins. This increases the pulmonary venous pressure and this is transmitted back along the system through the pulmonary capillary beds and into the pulmonary arterial circulation. Direct measurements of left atrial pressure in horses during intense exercise as high as 9.3 kPa (70 mmHg) have been reported. Whilst some scientists have suggested this indicates that the left atrium is failing, others have suggested that the very high pulmonary venous pressures are required to help the left atrium fill the left ventricle at heart rates as high as 240 beats/min. Thus the high pulmonary vascular pressures may be a necessary part of a high cardiac output and high $\dot{V}_{O_2\text{max}}$, although the price may be the horse's predisposition to EIPH. It's often much easier to weigh these issues up in terms of evolutionary advantage: (a) run flat out for 30–40 seconds, escape and suffer a little pulmonary haemorrhage or (b) don't run as fast, don't suffer EIPH, but get caught and eaten. The choice now seems quite easy.

Matching oxygen demand and supply

In a sprint race, horses set off at near-maximal speeds. At the onset of such a race, the demand for oxygen by the muscles is near maximal, but there is a lag between the onset of the oxygen demand and the delivery of adequate levels of oxygen to the muscles. It takes a finite amount of time for the delivery of oxygen by the cardiovascular system to match the demand of the muscles. It may take 20–30 seconds to reach maximal heart rates, and a similar amount of time for full splenic contraction. This results in an oxygen 'deficit' at the onset of high intensity exercise, while the cardiovascular system catches up with the demand for oxygen by the dramatically increased activity of the muscles. Horses have generally been considered to be quite good at matching supply to demand relatively quickly, and their cardiovascular system was thought to respond faster than that of human athletes. For example, Rose *et al.* (1988) found that oxygen delivery was 95% of steady state within 30 seconds of the onset of exercise. However, a more recent study by Langsetmo *et al.* (1997) showed that below the lactate threshold the fast component of oxygen uptake was greater than in man, but both below and above the lactate threshold the characteristics of how oxygen uptake increased in response to changes in oxygen demand at the muscle level were generally similar to those in man.

The cardiovascular response to training

Cardiovascular responses to training include those factors concerning the heart itself, and those concerning the vascular system, or blood vessels. There are significant improvements in both oxygen delivery and oxygen carrying capacity as a result of training. Traditionally, we have been taught that cardiovascular 'tuning' occurs in the final stages of a training programme in response to fast work, but research shows that many adaptations occur in response to slow work carried out in the early stages of a training programme.

Increase in heart mass

Increases in estimated heart mass of around 33% using echocardiography have been shown to occur in 2-year-old Thoroughbreds after 18 weeks of conventional race training. However, the training stimulus must be of the appropriate type and duration for this to have taken place. One hour's walking a day would probably have little effect on the horse's heart. A 30 second gallop at maximal speed might also be expected to produce a different effect compared to 10 minutes cantering continuously at a heart rate of 180 beats/min. The heart is a muscle, and like any other skeletal muscle, it adapts to training demands. There are two potential ways the heart could adapt: (1) increased wall thickness and/or (2) increased chamber diameter. Increased wall thickness leads to an increased force of contraction and increased chamber diameter leads to an increased stroke volume.

In humans, weight training or power sport training tends to primarily increase wall thickness, whilst endurance training leads to an increase in chamber diameter. Throughout the course of 18 months' race training, Thoroughbreds showed both adaptations (Young 1999). Training induces increases in heart mass of approximately 0.1% body mass which leads to an increase in stroke volume, a lower heart rate at any given workload, and a greater maximal cardiac output. More blood and thus more oxygen can be delivered to the muscles.

Thomas *et al.* (1983) found a 10% increase in stroke volume after 10 weeks' training on a treadmill, where horses trotted at heart rates of 150 beats/min. However, other researchers have shown no such increases in stroke volume. It is likely that the stage of training of the horses, the age of the horses and the type of work done accounted for the differences seen.

Changes in heart rate response with training

The trained horse should almost always be able to work at any given speed with a relatively lower heart rate compared to before it was trained. For example, a horse cantering at 10 m/s (600 m/min) before training may have a heart rate of 190 beats/min, but after training may be able to canter at the same speed with a heart rate of perhaps only 170 beats/min. Trained horses are also likely to have a lower maximum heart rate during exercise, and heart rates tend to plateau at maximal heart rates of 210–220 beats/min. Fit horses also have quicker heart rate recovery after exercise. However, measurement of heart rate at any given speed, or even measurement of recovery times, does not provide a

definitive measure of 'fitness' as horses that are naturally more athletic will have relatively lower working heart rates and quicker recovery times than other less athletic horses, even when they are unfit. It is therefore difficult to separate 'fit' from 'unfit' purely on the basis of heart rate alone. It is, however, possible to use measurement of heart rate responses over time to monitor changes in fitness in individuals.

Increased plasma volume

If we drained all the blood from a horse's body and separated it into the blood and plasma components, the total volume of plasma would represent the plasma volume and the total volume of red cells the RBC volume. An increased plasma volume in response to training was shown by McKeever *et al.* (1987). A 29.1% increase in plasma volume occurred after 14 days' work on the treadmill at walking speed (1.6 m/s). By far the majority (90%) of this increase occurred within the first week, and the increased plasma volume was maintained for 6 weeks after training ceased. Thus, the increase in plasma volume (known as hypervolaemia – literally *above volume*) seems to occur in response to relatively low levels of training. Plasma volume at rest in warmblood type horses is around 50–60 ml/kg body mass. Thoroughbred horses tend to have a higher mass specific plasma volume of around 75 ml/kg at rest. A 500 kg Thoroughbred would therefore have a plasma volume of around 32 litres.

The benefits of hypervolaemia are threefold:

(1) *An increase in thermoregulatory capacity.* Imagine that you have a central heating system with just two radiators in two different rooms, but there is only enough water to fill one radiator. To have one radiator on, you have to shut the other radiator off. If you could put more water in the system, you would be able to have both radiators on. When a horse works hard, particularly in hot or hot and humid conditions, its body temperature rises more rapidly than in cool conditions. The physiological response to an increase in core temperature is to send more blood to the skin to dissipate heat. If the need to get rid of (dissipate) heat is high, the blood vessels to the skin become fully dilated and

proportionately more blood is redirected to the skin to aid heat loss. This can occur to the extent where blood flow to the muscles may be compromised. If the horse is trained and has a higher plasma volume and therefore total blood volume, skeletal muscle blood flow is less likely to be compromised in order to send sufficient blood to the skin for cooling. The extent to which horses choose to send blood to the skin or to the muscles seems to vary between breeds. Heavier breeds and types seem to choose thermoregulation over performance. Thoroughbreds appear to choose the strategy of diverting most blood away from the skin at high intensities of exercise and therefore have the capacity to reach very high body temperatures.

(2) *Hypervolaemia contributes to the increase in stroke volume.* The more blood there is in the circulation, the greater the volume of blood returning to the right hand side of the heart after circulation around the body (known as venous return). Stroke volume is directly proportional to the venous return and contributes to pre-load, a principle defined by Starling's law of the heart, 'Energy of contraction is proportional to the initial length of the cardiac muscle fibre'. A basic explanation of this is that 'what goes in, must come out'. The greater the ventricular filling (the pre-load), the more the muscular walls of the ventricle are stretched and the greater the stroke volume as a result of contraction.

(3) The increase in circulating blood volume also aids in the dilution, transport, redistribution and elimination of products of metabolism such as carbon dioxide, hydrogen ions and ammonia.

Increased total red blood cell pool

An increase in the size of the total RBC pool as a result of training is associated with an increased blood haemoglobin (Hb) content. As plasma volume increases alongside, haemoglobin (Hb) *concentration* (the amount of Hb per litre of blood) is usually not changed by training, although absolute Hb *content* (the total amount in the circulation), especially during exercise with full splenic contraction, is increased. The increase in RBC content also leads to an increase in the capacity for oxygen transport in intense exercise, but is not of any real benefit during submaximal exercise or at rest. Hb is one of the major buffers in blood, able to soak up hydrogen ions once it has unloaded its oxygen. Indeed, the presence of hydrogen ions actually aids the unloading of oxygen from Hb at the muscle capillary level of the circulation. An increase in Hb content as a result of training therefore also allows the horse to tolerate a higher hydrogen ion load.

Increased capillarisation

As a result of primarily aerobic training, the capillary network within muscle is improved. The more extensive capillary network results in a greater pressure drop across the muscle capillary bed and a slower rate of flow through the capillaries. The time taken for blood to traverse the capillary bed is called the transit time. An increased transit time of blood through the muscle as a result of training leads to improved removal of hydrogen ions, carbon dioxide and lactate. The improved removal of lactate from muscle and redistribution throughout the body leads to a delay in the time (duration and/or exercise intensity) at which the anaerobic threshold is reached. This has been used as an indicator of performance in horses. The speed at which a horse has a blood lactate of 4 mmol/l is called V_{LA4}. Thornton *et al.* (1983) showed that a 5-week training programme resulted in an increase in mean V_{LA4} from 7 to 8 m/s. Thus, on average, before training, blood lactate reached 4 mmol/l at a speed of 7 m/s, whilst after training the horses could run at 8 m/s before reaching the same blood lactate level.

KEY POINTS

- A large heart has long been thought to correspond with high athletic ability.
- The Thoroughbred heart is typically around 4–5 kg or around 0.9% of body mass.
- Training may increase both chamber size (ventricle size) and the thickness of the ventricular walls. This leads to increases in both the stroke volume and force of contraction.
- Cardiac output (stroke volume × heart rate) can increase from around 25 litres/min at rest to 240 litres/min during intense exercise.
- During exercise blood flow is diverted away from organs such as the kidney and the gastrointestinal tract to the skin and muscles. At high exercise intensities skin blood flow, and therefore thermoregulation, may be compromised to support a high muscle blood flow.
- The true resting heart rate is usually around 20–25 beats/min and there is still debate as to whether this decreases with training.
- Many healthy normal horses 'drop' beats at rest. This is referred to as second degree atrioventricular block and is related to the regulation of systemic arterial blood pressure.
- Heart murmurs are sounds associated with blood flow in addition to the normal noise associated with the heart valves.
- Heart rate is usually measured by auscultation, palpation, from an ECG or with a heart rate monitor.
- Heart rate increases linearly with effort up to maximum heart rate. Maximum heart rate is reached at around 90% of maximal oxygen uptake.
- Maximum heart rate in a 2-year-old racehorse may be as high as 240 beats/min and may decrease to around 190 beats/min by 15 years of age.
- During prolonged exercise, a slow increase in body temperature may lead to a corresponding slow increase in heart rate known as cardiac drift.
- Heart rate normally decreases rapidly at the end of exercise and this is followed by a much slower rate of recovery.
- Stroke volume can be increased by around 50% in response to exercise.
- Maximal oxygen uptake refers to the maximum rate at which the body can use oxygen during intense exercise, and this is mainly a function of oxygen delivery by the cardiovascular system and the number of mitochondria in the muscles.
- Horses can increase the number of circulating RBCs by contracting the spleen during exercise. This increases the blood haemoglobin concentration and therefore oxygen carrying capacity.
- Mean arterial blood pressure increases during intense exercise by around 70%, but mean pulmonary artery pressure may increase by 400%.
- From a fast acceleration it may only take around 20–30 seconds for a horse to reach maximum heart rate and 30 seconds to reach 95% of maximal oxygen uptake.
- Training can result in changes in heart mass, the heart rate response to exercise, heart rate recovery, plasma volume and total blood volume.

Chapter 11

Aspects of physiological stress and fatigue

One of the aims of training any horse is to produce adaptations that delay the onset of fatigue, whether this is in short-term, high intensity such as a 5 furlong (1000 m) Thoroughbred 'sprint' race or prolonged, submaximal exercise such as in endurance racing (see Fig. 11.1). A horse that becomes fatigued feels tired and will have to be encouraged to carry on exercising. The onset of fatigue does not necessarily imply the end of exercise, but it may mean that the horse has to slow down considerably in order not to become exhausted. If the horse is exhausted, it cannot continue to exercise at any intensity. Fatigue is reached when the horse is forced to either:

- stop exercising
- continue exercising, but at a lower intensity.

Fatigue manifests itself in two forms, one psychological and one physiological. Humans can use techniques to overcome the psychological aspects of fatigue and they will often have positive reasons for doing so. Human athletes are striving to reach personal goals, to beat the next guy and win the medal. Horses have no such motivation, and the horse today is almost certainly competing with the same motivation as horses of 100 years ago. This may partly explain why the considerable improvements in record times cited for human track events have not been mirrored by improved times in races such as the Derby. It is unlikely that horses are motivated by a 'will to win' to the same extent as human athletes, and they certainly cannot associate daily exercise with achieving training goals in the long term. We have to try to make sure the horse enjoys each and every exercise session, unless we can find a way to explain the principle of 'no pain–no gain' to a horse. Whilst for human athletes positive thinking may offset the psychological aspects of fatigue, the physiological aspects are impossible to ignore and will depend on what type of exercise the horse is performing. Fatigue in an equine sprinter is a completely different physiological phenomenon to fatigue in an endurance horse.

Fatigue as a result of high intensity exercise

Horses exercising maximally for short periods use anaerobic pathways as the primary means of energy production, with the resulting production of lactic acid which immediately dissociates into lactate and hydrogen ions. Remember that lactic acid production in sprinters is good in that it allows the horse to go fast by delivering ATP very quickly, albeit not economically. During high intensity exercise, all fibre types are recruited, including type IIB fibres, which have a rapid ATP turnover. Inevitably, fatigue occurs due to a combination of changes within the muscle cell, such as increases in hydrogen ions, inorganic phosphate, ammonia and ADP, and decreases in ATP, phosphocreatine (PCr) and pH. Horses may exercise maximally for a matter of seconds or minutes before fatigue occurs, depending upon the intensity of the exercise. In this case fatigue is defined as the inability to continue at maximum speed. At the point at which fatigue starts, the horse may only drop from 100% of maximal speed to 98% of maximal speed and is still running very fast, but not maximally. Let's look at each of the factors contributing to fatigue in horses exercising maximally.

1. Depletion of high energy phosphates within muscle

Muscle cells store a certain amount of ATP and PCr used to provide energy for muscular contraction in the early stages of exercise. These high energy phosphate stores should be replenished when the aerobic production of ATP gets underway. During a period of high intensity exercise the levels of ATP

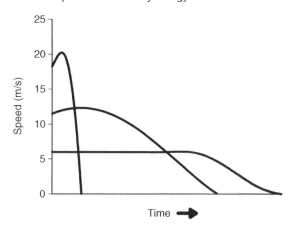

Fig. 11.1 Relationship between speed of running and time taken to fatigue.

within the muscle gradually fall, indicating that ATP is being used faster than it can be replaced. Sewell and Harris (1992) found that ATP levels in muscle decrease by 14–50% during a race, with the most significant losses occurring in type IIB fibres (up to 50%), whilst there was little loss in type I fibres. Restoration of ATP to resting concentrations following exercise takes approximately 1 hour.

2. Decrease in intracellular pH

The decrease in pH known as acidosis leads to a decrease in the aerobic capacity of muscle. Muscle cells work optimally at a pH of approximately 7.0 and decreases in pH can impair the activity of certain muscle enzymes. During interval training bouts, muscle pH can fall as low as 6.0 from 7.0 at rest and this markedly decreases the activity of phosphofructokinase (PFK), an important enzyme in glycolysis. Physical changes are seen within the cells, with mitochondria becoming round and swollen and their folded internal membranes known as cristae becoming more prominent. These physical changes are thought to be associated with impairment of the function of the mitochondria, leading to a reduction in the aerobic capacity of the muscle. The appearance of the mitochondria returns to normal during recovery following exercise. Acidosis also leads to impaired sarcoplasmic reticulum (SR) function and a reduction in the ability of the cell to transport calcium from the SR to the cytoplasm and back again.

3. Lactic acid accumulation

Lactic acid is formed via anaerobic energy pathways and quickly dissociates into lactate ions and hydrogen ions. The lactate then forms a salt with either sodium or potassium ions, and does not pose a great threat to the muscle cell. However, the hydrogen ions do pose a threat because they decrease the pH of the cell. As the lactic acid dissociates so readily, the terms lactate and lactic acid are used interchangeably. Horses are capable of tolerating higher levels of lactate than humans: blood lactates in horses can reach 35 mmol/l, compared with 25 mmol/l in humans. Repeated bouts of exercise lead to muscle lactate concentrations in excess of 200 mmol/kg dry muscle (Snow *et al.* 1985). Approximately 150 mmol/kg dry muscle is typical following fast work over a mile (1600 metres) or so. The greater the proportion of type IIB fibres a horse has, the greater the lactate accumulation will be. At low levels of exercise, peak lactate concentrations are seen immediately exercise is finished; however, lactate efflux can become saturated at higher levels of exercise, leading to accumulation of lactate and associated hydrogen ions within the muscle and a decrease in muscle pH. In this situation, peak blood and plasma lactates may not be seen until 10–15 minutes after exercise because lactate continues to leave the muscle in the recovery period until the muscle and blood concentrations are in equilibrium. Although lactate accumulation and reduced muscle pH may be seen as a bad thing, without lactate no animal would be able to sprint. Lactate is very good if you want to go fast for a short distance. The best sprinters, human and equine, produce the most lactate. It allows you to go fast, but limits for how long you can do this.

Fatigue in response to sub-maximal exercise

Exercise at sub-maximal levels relies mainly on aerobic energy pathways for ATP production. Fuel sources are mainly free fatty acids (FFAs) and muscle glycogen. Submaximal exercise at heart rates of less than 150 beats/min is usually below the anaerobic threshold and blood lactate is unlikely to increase above 2–3 mmol/l. In this situation, fatigue is likely to be due to the depletion of fuel stores (glycogen but never fat!), dehydration (loss of fluid) and marked loss of electrolytes through sweating.

1. Depletion of muscular fuel stores

Aerobic energy production utilises free fatty acids and glycogen. Lipid stores supply enough fuel for days at maintenance or to sustain low grade exercise. In endurance rides, fatigue occurs due to glycogen depletion within the liver (affecting organ systems other than muscle which are supplied with glucose by the liver via the bloodstream, e.g. the brain) and active muscle, not due to exhaustion of lipid stores. Throughout endurance, type I and type IIA fibres are recruited first of all. As the stores within these fibres are depleted, type IIB are recruited until all fibres are depleted of glycogen. When this has occurred, only very low intensity exercise can be maintained because energy is dependent upon FFA utilisation. Replacing the glycogen stores after depleting exercise may take up to 72 hours.

2. Hyperthermia

During exercise, the action of the muscles generates heat as a by-product of the conversion of chemical energy into mechanical energy. The greater the speed at which the horse runs, the greater the rate of heat production. During intense exercise, heat production increases by up to 50 times that of the resting state. At temperatures above $43°C$ the same sort of physical changes occur that are seen at low pH, i.e. swelling of the mitochondria and SR. It is likely that high temperatures impair the function of the mitochondria and the handling of calcium within the cell. The success of the horse in delaying fatigue relies on its ability to dissipate the heat that is produced during exercise, which it does by sweating – profusely! Horses can lose up to 15 litres of sweat in an hour. Fatigue can occur as a direct result of a large body temperature increase which can affect not only the muscles (weakness, fatigue) but the brain (ataxia, headache, disorientation), and as a result of the fluid losses that are necessary to dissipate the heat produced during exercise.

3. Altered fluid and ion balance

When horses sweat at rates of more than 10 litres/hour, they lose significant amounts of body water and electrolytes. An electrolyte refers to any substance that dissolves in water and carries a charge. The principal electrolytes in sweat include sodium (Na^+), chloride (Cl^-), potassium (K^+), calcium (Ca^{2+}) and magnesium (Mg^{2+}). Equine sweat is more concentrated and contains greater quantities of electrolytes than human sweat. In fact, whilst we secrete sweat which is lower in electrolyte concentration than our plasma (hypotonic sweat),

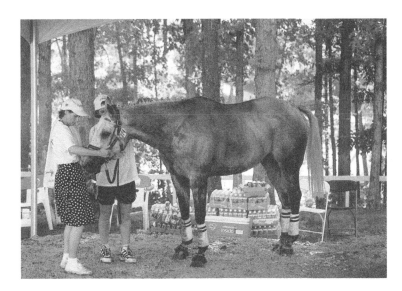

Fig. 11.2 A hot, tired and depressed horse.

the horse secretes hypertonic sweat, i.e. the horse produces sweat that is more concentrated than its body fluids. As a result, substantial electrolyte losses may occur during prolonged sub-maximal exercise. Losses of sodium, chloride, potassium and magnesium lead to an imbalance in the distribution of electrical charge on either side of cell membranes and this can disrupt the normal function of excitable tissues such as nerve and muscle. Loss of chloride ions in sweat can lead to retention of bicarbonate ions by the kidney in an attempt to maintain electrical neutrality. Retention of bicarbonate leads to an increase in blood pH known as alkalosis. Some electrolyte preparations for competition horses contain bicarbonate, and these should be avoided for endurance horses during and post-exercise as they will worsen the alkalosis.

Loss of potassium can lead to interference with the mechanisms regulating muscle perfusion because potassium is one of the metabolites responsible for vasodilation. Calcium and magnesium losses can lead to sensitisation of the phrenic nerve. This is the main nerve to the diaphragm that passes over the heart en route to the diaphragm. In its sensitised state, the phrenic nerve begins to fire at the same rate as the heart. This is known as synchronous diaphragmatic flutter (SDF) or 'Thumps', and is a contraction of the diaphragm in time with the heart but which is not related to respiratory movements. Horses most commonly get thumps in endurance competition and are always eliminated as a result. This is more likely to be because the onset of thumps signifies marked dehydration and/or electrolyte loss than because of the thumps itself. Generally horses with thumps do not appear distressed or even aware of the condition, and the condition will often disappear without intervention within a short period after exercise has been terminated. Horses with severe SDF or in which the condition does not revert spontaneously after exercise are usually treated with intravenous calcium solutions, which may also contain magnesium. Rehydration either by intravenous or nasogastric fluids may also be used.

Stress

Stress is a word that has become very fashionable. Indeed, so much is talked about 'stress' these days that the word immediately conjures up images of overworked businessmen, city financiers and the like, who are one gin and tonic away from a heart attack. Stress has had a bad press in this respect because, in truth, we could not get through one day without the main products of physiological stress, the hormones adrenaline and cortisol. Physiologists tend to regard stress not as a threat to health, but as a necessary response to daily events. To some of us, particularly the couch potatoes among us, exercise is regarded as an enormously stressful event. To an athlete, it is less so. The severity of a physiological stressor (something that induces a stress response) is largely determined by the body's previous exposure to it. In terms of animal welfare, stress is used in a very different context and is considered to occur when an animal is required to make an abnormal or extreme adjustment in its behaviour or physiology to cope with adverse effects of its environment or management. If your idea of exercise is to walk to the fridge and back, then running a mile would require you to make abnormal and extreme adjustments in your behaviour and your physiology in order to cope. The hormones adrenaline and cortisol play a major role in dealing with the stress of exercise.

Many of the responses to exercise are exactly the same as the 'fight or flight' responses seen in animals in the wild and are brought about by both direct stimulation of the sympathetic nervous system and an increase in circulating adrenaline. In fact, both adrenaline and noradrenaline are secreted from the adrenal medulla as a result of sympathetic stimulation. At rest, the plasma concentrations of adrenaline and noradrenaline are approximately 0.05 ng/ml and 0.1 ng/ml, respectively, rising to approximately 18 ng/ml and 23 ng/ml during intense exercise (Nagata *et al.* 1999). The exercise responses are simply an amplified version of the normal response to a frightening situation (see Fig. 11.3), including the following:

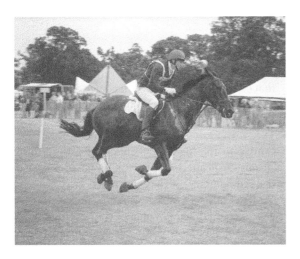

Fig. 11.3 Exercise responses are very similar to the typical 'fight of flight' responses and include an increase in circulating catecholamines, heart rate, ventilation and sweating.

- Increased heart rate and increased force of myocardial contraction leading to increased cardiac output
- Increased rate of breathing
- Splenic contraction
- Increased muscle blood flow
- Increased oxygen delivery, i.e. increased metabolic rate
- Increased mobilisation of liver glycogen and fat stores
- Increased level of circulating FFAs
- Increased sensitivity of nerves supplying skeletal muscle
- Dilation of bronchioles
- Sweating.

It's easy to relate to these responses that the body makes automatically when we think about how we feel and the changes that take place within seconds if something scares us, like a near miss in the car or a very heated confrontation.

Both noradrenaline and adrenaline (jointly referred to as catecholamines) increase in response to exercise, but tend to increase more significantly when the intensity of exercise is increased above workloads of around 60–70% $\dot{V}_{O_2max}$, i.e. round about the anaerobic threshold or a heart rate of 160–180 beats/min. Catecholamines are very important in high intensity exercise and there is a close relationship between circulating (i.e. blood) adrenaline concentrations and lactate concentrations, and also between adrenaline and high states of emotional stress and excitement. So for example, when your horse gets excited or stressed during competition this could shift metabolism away from aerobic towards anaerobic. This is simply because as we learned earlier, for high speed we need to produce lactate which is all well and good at the start of a 5 furlong (1000 metre) sprint but not so good at the start of the roads and tracks in a three-day event or a 100 mile (160 km) endurance ride. In trained horses, levels of adrenaline do not increase as much in response to exercise.

In response to both sub-maximal and maximal exercise, blood cortisol levels increase and a deficiency in cortisol actually impairs performance. Exercise results in a 2–3 fold increase in cortisol, with the peak usually occurring 15–30 minutes following exercise, and going back to pre-exercise levels within the hour. Increased cortisol concetrations in blood lead to:

- Increased glycogen deposition
- An increase in mobilisation of fat stores
- Stimulation of protein synthesis for repair of microdamage
- Increased sensitivity to adrenaline
- Increased storage of liver glycogen.

Cortisol is a 'long-term' stress hormone. All the responses initiated as a result of increases in cortisol are designed to prepare the body for long-term stress so they are geared towards sparing glycogen. Plasma cortisol concentrations are particularly high after endurance exercise (30% higher than other activities). In untrained horses, cortisol will be higher and takes longer to clear from the blood after exercise than in trained horses. Cortisol levels may peak between 10 and 30 minutes following exercise, but not return to baseline levels until 2 hours following intense exercise: recovery time seems to be related to the duration of exercise, in that prolonged submaximal exercise shows a later peak in plasma cortisol and a slower return to pre-exercise levels.

KEY POINTS

- Fatigue can be defined as either the inability to continue to exercise at all or the inability to maintain the current intensity of exercise, but with the possibility to continue at a lower intensity.
- Fatigue may have physiological and psychological components.
- Fatigue during high intensity, short duration exercise has a different basis to fatigue as a result of lower intensity, prolonged exercise.
- Fatigue in muscle associated with high intensity exercise may involve increases in hydrogen ion concentration, inorganic phosphate, ammonia and ADP, and decreases in pH, ATP and PCr.
- Fatigue in muscle associated with sub-maximal exercise is more likely to involve glycogen depletion, dehydration and marked electrolyte loss.

- Stress has a different meaning in physiology to that commonly understood; it is seen as necessary in terms of continual stimulation and challenge rather than undesirable.
- The responses to high intensity exercise are similar to the 'fight or flight' response and are closely associated with sympathetic stimulation (catecholamines). They include increases in cardiac output, respiratory rate, muscle blood flow, oxygen delivery, splenic contraction, mobilisation of fuel stores, bronchodilation, vasodilation and sweating.
- The responses to prolonged sub-maximal exercise are closely related to cortisol levels and include increases in muscle glycogen storage, mobilisation of fat stores, increases in protein synthesis, increased sensitivity to adrenaline and increased storage of liver glycogen.

Chapter 12

Thermoregulation

If your horse is turned out on a cold winter's day, the muscular effort of walking around helps it keep warm because all muscular contraction produces some heat. However, heat production by the muscles associated with exercise can become more of a problem to the horse if it becomes greater than heat loss (dissipation). The excess heat must be lost if the animal is to maintain or control its body temperature, i.e. thermoregulate. The exchange of heat by an animal with its surroundings is given by the following equation:

$$H_S = H_M - [\pm H_{CD} \pm H_C \pm H_R + H_E]$$

where H_S is heat stored in the horse's body, H_M is metabolic heat production, H_{CD} is conductive heat gain or loss, H_C is convective heat gain or loss, H_R is radiative heat gain or loss and H_E is evaporative heat loss (heat cannot be gained by evaporation). We might naturally think of H_S as being positive (when body temperature is increased) but, of course, when a horse's body temperature is falling after exercise or whilst being cooled, this represents negative heat storage.

The conversion of chemical energy available in food into energy for muscular work takes place in muscle cells with an efficiency of around 20%, with the remaining 80% of the energy released as heat. Heat production can increase 40–60 fold above resting values during exercise and is directly proportional to the rate at which oxygen is being utilised. The rate of metabolic heat production ($\dot{H}_M$) for a horse can be estimated as follows:

$$\dot{H}_M\,(kJ/min) = \dot{V}_{O_2}\,(ml/min/kg) \times 21\,(kJ)$$
$$\times 0.8 \times \text{body mass (kg)}$$

where 21 kJ is the energy contained in each millilitre of oxygen consumed and 0.8 is the fraction of this energy released as heat (remember 20% movement, 80% heat). As we have already learned, the horse is able to use oxygen at a very high rate on a per kilogram basis during exercise and so it also produces heat at a high rate. Because of its size the horse is also at a relative disadvantage when it comes to dissipating (losing) heat compared to smaller animals. This is because surface area does not increase linearly with body mass.

Heat exchange with the surrounding environment takes place predominantly across the body surface. Thus the ratio between the body mass as an index of the capacity to produce heat and body surface area as an index of the capacity to dissipate heat becomes important. If we were to take an 80 kg person, remove all their skin and lay it out, we would have a total skin surface area of around 2 m², giving a body surface area (BSA) to body mass ratio of 1 to 40 (see Fig. 12.1). If we were to take a 500 kg horse, remove all the skin and lay it out we would have around a surface area of 5 m², so for the horse the BSA to body mass ratio would be 5 m² to 500 kg or 1 to 100. Therefore although the horse is over six times as heavy as a human, it only has 2.5 times as much surface area. As far as thermoregulation is concerned, the horse has to 'squeeze' out (dissipate) 2.5 times as much heat through each square metre of body surface area as we have to. In general terms, small animals such as small birds and mice lose heat easily because of a low surface area to body mass ratio and have a high resting metabolic rate to enable them to maintain body temperature, whilst large mammals tend to have a low resting metabolic rate.

Differences in the BSA:body mass ratio exist even between breeds, with Thoroughbreds having a ratio of around 1:90 whilst heavier breeds may have a less advantageous ratio as far as heat dissipation is concerned, of around 1:120. Of course, in cold conditions the advantage is reversed and the higher ratio helps to reduce heat loss (there are few small mammals living in the Arctic). However, as

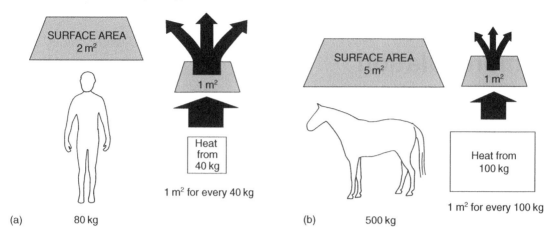

Fig. 12.1 Body surface area to body mass ratios in humans and horses.

far as a high rate of heat production and heat dissipation are concerned, the horse has one particular adaptation: 'horses sweat, gentlemen perspire and ladies glow' is a very old saying but has a sound basis. The horse is able to sweat at higher rates than any other animal.

If we were to compare the sweat rates of a human athlete and a horse, we might take a maximal sustainable sweating rate of 2 litres per hour (l/h) as a maximum for man and 15 l/h for a horse. Of course the comparison cannot be made at this level because the horse and human are of different size. If we divide by BSA, we then find that the human maximal sweat rate is equivalent to 1 l/m²/h for the human athlete and 3 l/m²/h for the horse. In fact, sweat rates are usually reported in units of ml/m²/min, and so these would equate to 17 ml/m²/min for man and 50 ml/m²/min for the horse. Hence to compensate for having a low BSA:body mass ratio and a high rate of heat production, the horse has evolved to sweat at around three times the rate that we can sweat across the same area of skin.

Whilst the horse has homeostatic mechanisms for regulating its body temperature, muscle and body temperatures, e.g. rectal temperature, do rise even with light exercise in cool conditions. For example, rectal temperatures as high as 42°C have been measured at the end of the cross-country at Burghley Horse Trials when the air temperature was only 15°C. In hot or hot and humid environmental conditions, horses find it even more difficult to keep their body temperature down because heat dissipation is impaired.

Horses are actually extremely efficient at dissipating heat produced during exercise. For example, during a 160 km (100 mile) endurance ride, if no heat were dissipated body temperature would rise by around 0.3°C/min or 15°C/h. This amount of energy would be sufficient to boil around 700 kettles! During intense exercise the rate of heat production is of course even greater. However, the exercise duration is quite short and so the actual amount of heat stored is quite small. At maximal exercise, without thermoregulation, heat storage would equate to around 1–1.5°C per minute of exercising. In fact in a Thoroughbred flat race lasting 2–3 minutes, the increase in temperature may be close to 2–3°C, suggesting that the majority of heat produced is stored rather than dissipated.

The normal rectal temperature for the horse is approximately 37.0–38.0°C: if the horse's rectal temperature reaches 40°C, which is not uncommon, then it will benefit from being cooled down. Riders should be aware of the signs of hyperthermia (overheating) to avoid the much more serious condition of heat exhaustion. The benefits of cooling are that sweating is reduced or even stopped completely in the short term and therefore fluid and electrolyte loss are reduced. Once the horse has been cooled, recovery is much quicker (respiratory rate and heart rate will decrease more rapidly) and the horse is more likely to return to its stable ready to eat, drink and rest. This is just as important whether the horse is going to have to compete the next day or start a journey home.

All mammals have elaborate thermoregulatory mechanisms, enabling them to maintain their body temperature within a large range of environmental conditions by altering heat flow between them and their environment. Heat can be exchanged between an animal and its environment by four methods (see Fig. 12.2).

(1) *Radiation.* This is movement of heat between objects without physical contact, for example, solar radiation from the sun. We are not in direct contact with the sun but we can feel its effects. This is why it feels warmer in the sun than in the shade – the difference is radiation. Animals will also emit, i.e. lose, heat by radiation to their cooler surroundings. For example, a horse may lose a lot of heat by radiation to cold stone walls compared to insulated stable walls at a higher surface temperature. In hot climates solar radiation can exceed approximately $800\,W/m^2$, which is in itself greater than metabolic heat production. As a further example of the power of solar radiation, think of the differ-ence on a frosty morning when the sun is out and then how much colder it feels when the sun goes behind a cloud. The difference is radiation. Radiation can also be reflected from the ground. Surfaces such as grass are nice to walk on in hot climates as they absorb radiation rather than reflect it. Surfaces such as sand or clay tend to reflect a lot of radiation.

(2) *Convection.* This is heat movement within a fluid. In this sense the 'fluid' could be a liquid or a gas. Convective heat transfer occurs between the horse and the surrounding air at the skin surface. Forced convection is the process whereby heat loss is increased by moving or 'forcing' air across a surface. This occurs naturally when there is a wind or we can promote forced convection using fans. The rate of heat loss is increased because colder air is continually being brought into contact with the warm surface. We can relate to the effect of forced convection. In winter, we refer to the wind-chill factor, which is how much colder a wind can make it feel: the air temperature may be 0°C, but if there is a strong wind the wind-chill factor may make it feel like –10°C. Some animals have morphological traits that max-imise convective heat losses by increasing the

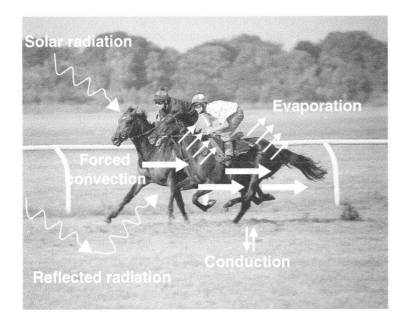

Fig. 12.2 Methods of heat exchange between an animal and its environment.

surface area available for heat transfer; for example, mules with their long ears and lean body shape. Convection also describes the movement of heat within the bloodstream.

(3) *Conduction.* This is direct transfer of heat between surfaces that are in contact with each other. For example, if you put your hand directly in contact with a warm surface it will warm up by conduction. Air has poor thermal conductivity so conductive heat transfer plays a small role in total heat balance. The horse may lose a very small amount of heat by conduction to the ground in cold weather through the feet. Conductive heat losses are only significant if the horse lies on a cold surface or if we are using cold water to cool a horse.

(4) *Evaporation.* Evaporation occurs when the molecules of a liquid gain enough kinetic energy to leave the surface of the liquid and become a vapour. In the case of the horse, the liquid surface will be the surface of the sweat layer on the coat. The addition of heat energy supplies the liquid with the kinetic energy to evaporate. Sweating and panting are the main methods of evaporative heat loss in mammals. Panting results in heat loss via the respiratory system. By increasing respiratory frequency and decreasing tidal volume, large volumes of air can be moved through the upper respiratory tract, warmed, saturated with water vapour, and then expired. This is a very important means of heat loss in some animals, particularly dogs. Horses, however, rely more on sweating and less on respiratory losses as a means of losing heat than most other mammals. This is reflected in the fact that they have sweat glands over almost every inch of their body. At high body temperatures after exercise, horses rely somewhere around 85% on sweating and 15% on respiratory heat loss to cool down. However, at rest in the stable in a hot climate horses may utilise both sweating and respiratory heat loss to similar extents. The horse is able to sweat at a faster rate than any other animal. Effective sweating depends on there being air movement over the skin and a water vapour pressure difference between the surface of the skin and the environment. Heat loss due to sweating is at its most effective in hot dry environments and is virtually ineffective when the air is saturated with water vapour, whatever the air temperature.

In cool humid conditions, heat loss can still take place by convection. However, in hot and humid conditions, both sweating and convective heat loss may be severely compromised. Following moderate to hard exercise, horses will 'blow' for anything from a few minutes up to 30–40 minutes. In the past, it was often simply assumed that the blowing was related to the 'oxygen-debt' or effectively the amount of lactate produced during the preceding exercise: because lactate is produced by anaerobic metabolism, the idea was that this had to be 'paid-back' after exercise; hence the use of the term 'oxygen-debt'. However, we now know that 'blowing' or slower deep breathing after exercise is more closely related to body temperature. Many riders are aware that a high respiratory rate (up to 180 breaths/min) and shallow breathing ('panting') are signs that a horse is hot. However, we now know that horses that have a lower respiratory rate (50–80 breaths/min) but that are breathing much more deeply (i.e. have bigger chest movements) will have much higher body temperatures. Interestingly, as these horses cool down they may well switch from the slower deep breathing (called second phase panting) into the more commonly recognised faster more shallow panting (actually called primary phase panting).

Sweating is brought about in response to two different mechanisms. The first is by an increase in circulating adrenaline due to increased sympathetic stimulation. Such stimulation may occur due to either excitement or exercise. Horses that sweat up due to excitement or fear generally sweat in discrete places, such as on the neck and between the hind legs. During exercise the first signs of sweating are usually on the horse's neck. Accumulation of sweat is often seen after exercise underneath the saddle and this has often lead people to falsely believe that this area sweats more or before other areas of the body. However, when the saddle is taken off and there is a large amount of sweat underneath, it is because the sweat that has formed during exercise cannot evaporate and so has built up; the horse has probably sweated just as much on other parts of the body but these may appear dry as the sweat there has evaporated.

Sweating can also take place simply by heating the skin. This does not involve increases in blood adrenaline levels. We know this because if a piece of skin is taken from a horse at post mortem it can be made to sweat on the bench by heating it, when we know that it has no blood supply or nerves connected to it. The complete evaporation of 1 litre of sweat dissipates the heat generated by 1–2 min of maximal exercise or 5–6 min of submaximal exercise.

Equine sweat is actually hypertonic (more salty than body fluids). Reported measurements of electrolytes in equine sweat (see Table 12.1) do vary, although all researchers agree that it is hypertonic, unlike human sweat which is hypotonic (less salty than body fluids). As a consequence, horses lose higher quantities of electrolytes when they sweat.

The precise composition of sweat may vary between trained and untrained horses and the time of exercise. For example, in one study the sodium

concentration in sweat was shown to increase during the first 15 minutes of exercise, whilst potassium and protein fell and chloride was unchanged. In the same study it was also shown that sweat composition was different in different thermal environmental conditions (McCutcheon *et al.* 1995).

Sweat composition has been analysed either by placing a patch of highly absorbent material over an area of skin and then extracting the sweat for analysis by wringing or washing with distilled water, or alternatively by sealing pouches over an area of skin. Both methods have the disadvantage that they may artificially warm and 'humidify' the area of skin that is covered and thus alter either sweat rate and or composition.

Sweating rate is most commonly measured using a ventilated capsule (Fig. 12.3). Traditionally, the ventilated capsule was made of copper and was therefore quite heavy and difficult to maintain in place and keep sealed to the coat. The principle of the ventilated capsule is as follows. A known area of skin is covered by a sealed capsule. Air is passed through the capsule at a measured flow rate. From measurements of temperature and humidity in the air entering and leaving the capsule, the amount of moisture added to the air leaving the capsule can be calculated. Provided the flow rate of air through the capsule is high enough to prevent the accumulation of sweat on the skin surface, an accurate measurement of sweating rate can be obtained. If the flow rate is too low, then evaporation rate is measured rather than the true sweating rate. Light-

Table 12.1 Equine sweat composition[a]

Electrolyte	Approximate concentration (g/l)
Sodium	3.5
Chloride	6.0
Potassium	1.2
Calcium	0.1

[a]Sweat also contains small amounts of latherin, protein, lactate and urea.

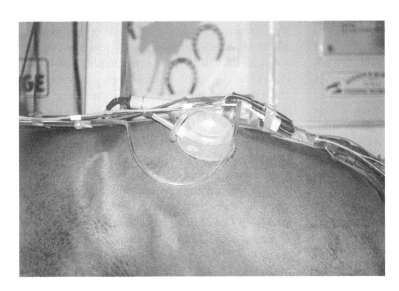

Fig. 12.3 Ventilated capsule used to measure sweat rate.

weight plastic capsules can easily be fixed to vertical surfaces such as the neck using double sided skin tape such as Blenderm, or even special skin adhesives. For a full description of the approach to measuring regional sweating rates during exercise see Scott *et al.* (1996).

Sweating rate can be as high as 10–15 litres per hour, and horses tend to sweat at twice the rate on the neck compared to over the quarters. The mechanism for this difference is not entirely clear, but it is not due to a difference in numbers of sweat glands. A study in Japan showed a similar density of sweat glands in both regions. Horses have apocrine sweat glands where each hair follicle has a sweat gland at its base. Humans have eccrine glands where the sweat gland is not associated with a hair follicle. To find the density of sweat glands in a horse's skin we therefore only need count the number of hairs per given area.

Fluid losses from sweating can be approximated by weighing the horse before and after work. As 1 litre of water weighs 1 kg, we can calculate how much fluid the horse has lost. To be really accurate, we would need to take into account any urinary and faecal losses occurring during exercise. Simply by doing one or two canters over, say, 1 mile (1600 metres) on a mild day, a horse may lose 5–7 kg (5–7 litres). A real workout on the gallops can induce losses of up to 10 litres of sweat, whilst up to 40 litres can be lost following an endurance ride. Of course, in an endurance ride horses will be sweating whilst competing and then eating and drinking during 'vet gates'. Therefore a horse in a 100 mile (160 km) race could actually lose 100 litres of fluid if it sweated at 10 litres per hour for 10 hours. Without any replacement this would be one-third of the total body water stores or around 20% of body mass for a 500 kg horse. We know horses start to have problems when dehydration starts to approach 6–7% of body mass lost. Thus, if this horse finishes the competition weighing 40 kg (equivalent to 40 litres) lighter than it did at the start, we can assume that it must have taken on board at least 60 litres of fluid during the ride (plus of course some food). This emphasises the importance of rehydration. Dehydration not only makes you and the horse feel tired and ill (remember that 90% of the effect of a hangover is simple dehydration), it also interferes with sweating. Dehydrated

horses have been shown to sweat less than normally hydrated (euhydrated) horses.

In addition to high levels of electrolytes, horse sweat contains a protein called latherin, which produces a lather on the skin. Latherin spreads sweat along the hair, so that the hair is totally coated, increasing the surface area over which sweat can evaporate. The latherin content of sweat seems to decrease during prolonged sweating. Unfit horses appear to have a higher sweat latherin content and with training the amount of latherin in sweat is reduced.

When sweating rate exceeds evaporation rate, sweat can be seen to drip off the skin. In this situation sweating does not bring about effective cooling, although as the sweat is warm it does take away a very small amount of heat. However, in relation to effectiveness of evaporation, sweat that drips only removes perhaps a one-hundredth of the heat that would have been removed if the sweat had evaporated. 'Over-sweating' is therefore wasteful of both fluid and electrolytes, and inefficient as far as cooling is concerned. One of the responses to training is actually an improved control of sweating to ensure that when the horse is hot the skin is always covered by a thin layer of sweat available for evaporation whilst reducing sweat wastage.

The knowledge of equine thermoregulation, especially in hot or hot and humid environments experienced a dramatic surge as a result of the 1992 Barcelona and 1996 Atlanta Olympic Games. Severe hyperthermia (body temperature in excess of 42°C) is more likely when there is a high ambient temperature (greater than about 25°C) and/or a high ambient humidity of about 70–90%, low wind and clear skies. British summers normally average about 20–25°C with quite low humidity (40–60%). Heavy breeds, unfit horses, horses carrying too much condition (fat horses), horses with long coats, horses not used to exercising in the heat of the day, long periods of warm-up and or exercise, and failure to allow horses to rehydrate are all risk factors for severe hyperthermia.

In some horses which exercise repeatedly in hot and hot and humid environments, the sweat glands seem to become less responsive to adrenaline, leading to a condition called anhidrosis. Anhidrosis implies a complete loss of sweating function, but this is rarely, if ever, the case. Affected animals are usually still able to sweat on the neck but at perhaps one-third of the normal rate, although sweating may be absent over much of the rest of the body. Many covered areas such as under the mane, between the hind legs, under the tail and behind the ears usually retain the ability to sweat. This may affect horses that are not native to the region, but can also affect native horses. Anhidrosis is particularly common in the southern USA in states such as Georgia, Tennessee, Florida and Arizona, especially in racehorses. Affected animals often improve when they are removed to a colder environment or during cooler winter months. Sport horses are often severely exercise intolerant when placed in a hot environment without acclimatisation.

Replacing fluid losses

Fluid losses incurred during exercise are usually effectively replaced over a period of time, either during or following exercise, by the horse drinking. Complete recovery from exercise is normally associated with a return to the pre-exercise body mass. Therefore, if we can encourage fluid intake, we should promote rapid recovery. Water and electrolytes would be gradually replaced if the horse is simply offered normal water and its normal diet, but there is a quicker and better way to replenish the body fluids lost through sweating, especially in the absence of feed intake. Replacing the lost fluid with isotonic fluid will rapidly reverse dehydration and speed recovery. In the case of eventing or endurance this will help the horse to go out and perform again the next day or after a vet gate. In human athletes a 1% reduction in body mass due to fluid loss is considered to reduce performance by 10%. Unfortunately, we don't know the relationship between fluid loss and reduction in performance for the horse. We cannot extrapolate from man because the horse has a large hind-gut which may hold around 30–40 litres of fluid that can be drawn upon during exercise and replaced afterwards. However, it seems that 3–5% body mass loss causes little problem for the majority of three-day event horses. It is important that horses that compete over the course of several days regain as much of the lost electrolytes and fluid as possible during the rest periods. Replacement of elec-

trolytes is best achieved through feeding. Whilst electrolytes can be given in water, the volume that the horse will readily consume (usually up to around 0.9 g of 'electrolytes' in a litre) will not allow a large electrolyte intake. For example, if a horse has exercised for 2 hours and lost 20 kg in mass (equivalent to 20 litres of sweat) this would be equivalent to losing around 20 g of electrolytes. To replace the electrolytes lost in the sweat we would need the horse to drink around 22 litres of isotonic fluids. A much easier way would be to put 22 g of electrolytes in the feed and provide some water.

The most effective way to replace these fluid losses during competition if there is no opportunity to feed (such as between rounds in showjumping, between chukkas in polo, or in the 10 minute box in a three-day event) is by getting the horse to drink an electrolyte solution. The idea of giving electrolytes in water to a horse before a competition is not to 'load' the body with electrolytes, as this cannot be done, but to ensure that:

- the horse is fully hydrated, i.e. not dehydrated, before the competition
- the horse is accustomed to drinking the electrolyte mixture and so will be less likely to refuse it when offered on the day of the competition because horses are always wary of a new taste when it is first offered to them.

The body monitors and controls fluid volume over the short term by responding to the sodium concentration of body fluids. If we want to encourage the horse to drink, we need to avoid decreasing the sodium concentration of its body fluid. Giving water to a horse that is dehydrated results in a dilution of the body fluids and a drop in the concentration of sodium which switches off the thirst mechanism: at the same time it signals the kidneys to excrete water until the plasma sodium concentration comes back up to normal. The important message here is that without electrolytes (principally sodium in the form of sodium chloride) either in food or actually in the water being drunk, the body cannot hold onto water. Therefore it is not possible to rehydrate simply by drinking water. Drinking lots of water may help a hangover a little bit. Drinking water and eating some food with salt in will help more, if your stomach will stand it.

However, drinking an isotonic sports drink will help your hangover the most (plus a few paracetamol).

Isotonic solutions are solutions in which the electrolyte concentration is the same as that of the body fluids (usually the plasma; iso = same). A hypotonic solution is one in which the electrolyte concentration is below that of the body fluids (hypo = below). For example, water (as it has almost no electrolytes in it) is very hypotonic, as are a large number of the rehydration products on the market for horses. The reason that they are made hypotonic is because they are drunk more readily without the need to introduce and train the horse to drink them. Hypertonic solutions (hyper = above) are ones in which the electrolyte concentration is above that of the body fluids. Hypertonic solutions will actually cause fluid to be drawn from the blood into the stomach and intestines until the hypertonic solution is isotonic or effectively until it has been diluted down. This has the effect of actually dehydrating the horse further, rather than rehydrating. The fluid, of course, is still in the horse but it is in the wrong place – in the stomach and intestines instead of in the circulation. It must get into the circulation before it can be transported to other parts of the body to replenish fluid lost. There do not appear to be any electrolyte products for horses which are hypertonic. However, there are a number of drinks for people that are hypertonic such as many fizzy drinks and orange juice. Therefore it is not a good idea to try and rehydrate on these.

The formulations of commercially available electrolyte products for giving in water are highly variable, with some manufacturers claiming their products are isotonic when they simply are not. Whether or not a product is isotonic is only related to how it is made up in solution, i.e. in water. Some manufacturers seem to be under the impression that if salts are available in the same proportions as in body fluids, then the product is isotonic, but of course it is more important that they are provided at sufficient concentration, and this means in water. It is highly unlikely that by providing an electrolyte in the horse's feed, you could overdo it and make the horse's body fluids too concentrated, unless you restricted its water intake. It is far more likely that you simply would not be providing enough salt. Administering a large single dose of electrolytes in the form of an oral paste can cause the horse to absorb water from the blood vessels surrounding the gut to dilute the concentration of the gut fluid, actually worsening the dehydration in the short term. The best solution is to give an electrolyte that is isotonic and palatable. Unfortunately, horses do not tend to readily accept isotonic salt solutions. By masking the salty water with a flavour, they can be encouraged to drink the electrolytes: apple squash seems to be a big hit with most horses. Flavouring water to mask the taste of an unfamiliar water source is a useful technique to get horses to drink when they are away from home, provided of course that they have been previously introduced to the flavoured water!

A homemade electrolyte can be made by placing 45 g of table salt and 45 g of Lite salt (sometimes also called Lo-Salt) in 10 litres of water (i.e. 90 g of electrolytes in 10 litres or 9 g/l = a 0.9% solution) according to a method first described by Carlson (1983). Table salt is sodium chloride, and Lite salt is a mixture of potassium chloride and sodium chloride in the ratio 2:1. Another recipe often used in endurance is a mixture of 2 parts salt to 1 part Lite salt. Once mixed, this would also be used at 90 g in 10 litres and would consist of 31% sodium, 58% chloride and 11% potassium. Apple squash or apple juice can be added to mask the taste of the salt in water, and apple sauce works quite well for making a paste or drench. If horses are accustomed to drinking this before the competition, they should accept it readily.

Replacing electrolyte losses

Horses lose around 10 g of electrolytes per litre of sweat, so a horse losing 50 litres of sweat in a 100 mile endurance ride will lose a total of around 500 g or 0.5 kg of electrolytes. For an endurance horse in full training, the diet may contain around 50–100 g of electrolytes per day, so following competition it could take around 5–10 days to fully restore the electrolytes lost in a single competition. In reality this means we probably have little chance of preventing an electrolyte deficit occurring by providing electrolytes in water during competition. For example, even if we could persuade our horse to drink 100 litres of isotonic fluid, that would only replace 90 g of electrolytes (0.9 g electrolytes per litre of isotonic fluid × 100 litres). It is therefore important to think of the electrolytes that we give in water as a way of effectively rehydrating the horse, not as a way of replacing lost electrolytes. This must come through the diet or perhaps also from feeding or in pastes or drenching during a competition itself. Even if our horse ate four meals during the ride, each of which contained 50 g of electrolytes, we would still have replaced only 290 g of the total loss of 500 g. This example illustrates the importance of having horses on an adequate and balanced (in terms of relative proportions of the different electrolytes) electrolyte intake during training. A horse that starts a competition with depleted electrolyte stores is more likely to run into trouble, e.g. tying-up, thumps, than a horse that starts with full body electrolyte stores.

Mixtures of 1 part salt to 1 part Lite salt or 2 parts salt to 1 part Lite salt, besides working well in rehydration solutions, can also be fed in the diet during training or competition at around 30 g per feed, or in homemade pastes or drenches. When calculating how much to give in the form of a paste or drench, it is probably worth increasing the dose by 50% to allow for loss during administration because some will not be swallowed and fall on the floor, so if you were going to aim to give 30 g in a single drench, then increase this to 45 g.

Assessing environmental thermal stress

Accurate assessment of environmental conditions to determine the environmental thermal load is an essential step towards proper management of competitions in hot or hot and humid conditions. This can be carried out months or even years before a competition based on climate records. Monitoring should also be carried out in the period immediately before and during competition. This approach enables the assessment of the range of conditions likely to be encountered, as well as the pattern of change throughout a typical day. This may help in trying to schedule competition periods to avoid the most thermally stressful parts of the day.

Environmental thermal stress can be estimated or quantified in a number of different ways: personal experience, measuring the temperature and humidity, estimating radiation and air movement, and by using heat indices.

Personal experience

How thermally stressful is it today, today compared with yesterday, and today compared with a previous competition? There is a danger in this approach because shade, full hydration, relative inactivity (at least compared to competitors and horses) and acclimatisation can all lead to underestimation of the level of thermal stress.

Measurements of temperature and humidity

This is an improvement, but it is difficult to weigh up warm and humid versus hot and dry. Very cheap equipment for use in homes or offices may be highly inaccurate, more so for humidity than temperature. Readings of temperature and humidity are meaningless unless taken in the shade, and the devices should not be stood in cars or on hot surfaces. They should be placed above the ground, out of direct sunlight and where air can circulate around them.

Radiation and air movement

A further improvement on measurements of shade temperature and humidity is some form of estimation of radiation and air movement. On days with clear skies radiation will be very strong, and on still days there will be little cooling from air movement. These data can be collected with either very simple equipment read manually or with more sophisticated logging equipment. A problem arises with a more comprehensive assessment of the factors that contribute to thermal stress, and that is interpretation. How would we compare a hot, dry day with little wind and partly cloudy versus a hot, humid day with moderate wind but no clouds in the sky? This is where attempts have been made to develop different heat indices.

Heat indices

Various heat indices are used by different countries and different weather bureaux around the world to give people warning of the risk of sunburn and/or heat stroke. It is not always apparent how these indices are calculated, and they are designed primarily for people either during recreation or work, not exercise. Therefore these have generally not been useful for management of equestrian sport.

1. Comfort Index

The Comfort Index was the first heat index adopted by the Federation Equestre Internationale (FEI). The Comfort Index was calculated by adding shade temperature in degrees Fahrenheit to percentage relative humidity. The attractiveness of this index is that it is easy to make the necessary measurements using simple, relatively inexpensive and widely available equipment, and the calculation can be done quickly by anyone. The main problem with the Comfort Index is that it can be misleading for many combinations of temperature and humidity, especially as it makes no allowance for radiation or air movement. Its use is now actively discouraged.

2. Wet Bulb Globe Temperature (WBGT) Index

The WBGT Index, which was developed and initially used for military applications, was adapted for equestrian competition before the 1996 Atlanta

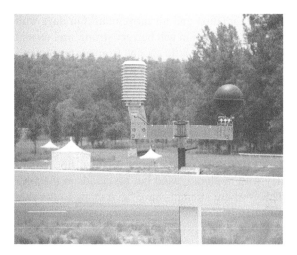

Fig. 12.4 Equipment for measurement of the wet bulb globe temperature (WBGT) index. The screen containing humidity and temperature sensors is on the left.

Olympic Games. The WBGT Index takes into account temperature, humidity, radiation and air movement (see Figs 12.4, 12.5a,b). The index comprises two parts: the wet bulb component and the globe component.

The wet bulb component is obtained by measuring the wet bulb temperature in the shade, ideally inside a proper meteorological screen. The wet bulb temperature is a function of both ambient temperature and relative humidity. In hot dry conditions evaporation of water from the wick surrounding the bulb of the thermometer causes the wet bulb temperature to fall. In this situation there would be be a marked difference between a conventional dry bulb temperature and the wet bulb temperature. However, in hot and humid conditions, there would be less evaporation from the wick, and when relative humidity is 100% no evaporation can take place and the dry bulb and wet bulb temperatures would be equal. The wet bulb temperature can also be calculated from measurements of temperature and relative humidity using sensors rather than conventional thermometers.

The globe temperature component comes from the temperature inside the centre of a 20 cm copper globe painted matt black. When radiation is strong the globe temperature is increased, but wind will cool the globe and decrease the temperature. The globe temperature is therefore a balance of the heating and cooling effects of radiation and wind. The globe shape ensures that the measurements, particularly radiation, are omnidirectional (from all directions).

The WBGT Index is calculated as

$$\text{WBGT Index} = 0.7 \times \text{wet bulb temperature}\,(^\circ\text{C}) \\ + 0.3 \times \text{globe temperature}\,(^\circ\text{C})$$

Thus the weighting is more in favour of the wet bulb temperature component of the index. Although the components of the WBGT Index are measured in degrees Celsius, the Index itself does not have units. The WBGT Index should ideally be measured at more than one site, especially for competitions such as three-day events where the course may run over a large area. The equipment should always be sited at the approximate height from the ground of the horse's trunk. Equipment for monitoring weather and environmental conditions is often sited 3–4

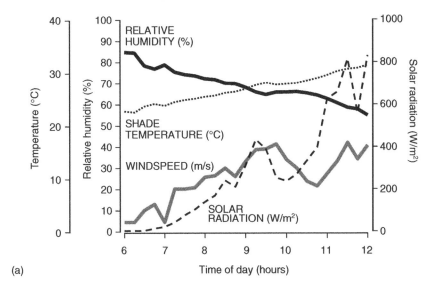

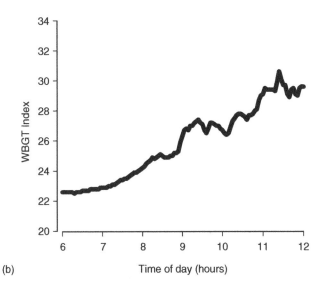

(a)

(b)

Fig. 12.5 (a) Variations in shade temperature, relative humidity, solar radiation and windspeed in a 6 hour period. (b) The same environmental data expressed as WBGT Index.

metres from the ground. At this level factors such as wind and ground radiation may be very different to that at 1 metre, i.e. the level of the horse, and be less accurate.

The advantage of the WBGT Index (compared to the Comfort Index) is that, based on treadmill and field investigations and experience from real competition, it accurately reflects the severity of the environmental heat load imposed on both the horse and the rider.

Interpretation of the WBGT Index

If the WBGT Index has a disadvantage, it is the fact that it is not linear. The implications of increasing from 20 to 25 are much less severe than increasing from 23 to 28. For this reason, guidelines were drawn up for the use of the WBGT Index in the management of the 1996 Atlanta Olympic Games speed and endurance test for humid heat acclimatised horses at three- and four-star level (from Schroter *et al.* 1996).

- *WBGT Index under 28.* No changes to the FEI recommended format should be necessary except in unusual circumstances.
- *WBGT Index 28–30.* Some precautions to reduce heat load on horses are advised:
  — reduction in phases B and C
  — addition of a 10 minute cooling stop on phase C
  — extension of phase X (10 minute box) to 15 minutes with provision of shade and adequate ice and water for cooling
  — provision of cooling after phase D.
- *WBGT Index 30–32.* Additional precautions to those for WBGT Index 28–30 necessary to prevent overheating of horses are needed:
  — reduction of phase B
  — reduction in distance of phase C and inclusion of two cooling stops
  — 15 minute phase X with provision for cooling
  — reduction in length and jumping efforts of phase D
  — provision for cooling after phase D.
- *WBGT Index 32–33.* Further modification of course and competition as above and in addition:
  — strict veterinary monitoring of horses at all possible opportunities (cooling stops on phase C (×2) and phase X)
  — compulsory provision of shade for horses held on course.
- *WBGT Index 33+.* These environmental conditions may not be compatible with safe competition and further veterinary consultation is required before continuing.

It must be stressed that these guidelines may not apply for a different set of conditions. For example, at Badminton unseasonally warm Spring weather one year led to a WBGT Index of 25 on cross-country day: even some of the fit horses at this level began to experience difficulties with the conditions until they were cooled adequately. The fact that a WBGT Index of 25 could produce a problem is a result of the fact that before the event the weather had been cold and so none of the horses would have been acclimatised, even to warm conditions. The highest WBGT Index reported by Schroter *et al.* (1996) was 34.7. One of the authors (D.J.M.) experienced these conditions which occurred during the speed and endurance test at the 1995 North America Young Riders Championships near Chicago. Based on the information that had already been gathered as part of the research leading up to the 1996 Atlanta Olympic Games, cooling stops were introduced and the course altered. As a result, there were no significant problems for horses resulting from the highly thermally stressful conditions; however, a number of riders were taken to hospital and treated for heat stroke. Thus, whilst at a WBGT Index of 33 or more, horses may be able to cope with a two-star speed and endurance test, it was considered that riders may not. Because the horse and rider must be considered equal, that is injury could occur due to fatigue, weakness or disorientation on the part of either the horse or the rider, the WBGT Index recommendations were set with this in mind.

The WBGT Index does not need to be obtained using sophisticated and expensive equipment. A Stevenson type screen (a white ventilated housing), a wet bulb thermometer and a 20 cm globe with the bulb of an ordinary thermometer at its centre are all that are required. An even simpler approach would be to measure wet bulb temperature and dry bulb temperatures and to estimate the globe temperature as shade dry bulb temperature plus 12°C.

Acclimatisation and acclimation

The thermoregulatory systems of the body adapt according to prevailing environmental conditions. Rapid transition between extreme environments usually results in an acclimatisation response which induces physiological changes enabling the animal to cope better with such conditions. The extent of the response depends on the difference in the environments and on the duration and nature of exercise training undertaken. Similar changes, but with slower progression, can be observed when there is a gradual transition from one environment to another. The International Union of Physiological Sciences distinguishes between thermal acclimation and thermal acclimatisation as follows:

- *Thermal acclimation* is defined as the process of adaptation that takes place under artificial or laboratory conditions.

- *Thermal acclimatisation* is defined as the adaptation that occurs under natural conditions.

A considerably greater amount of information exists concerning the response of humans to acclimation to heat or heat and humidity. Responses reported following acclimation of human subjects have included, though not always, an increased plasma volume, decreased body temperature at rest and during exercise, decreased exercising heart rate, improved skin blood flow, an increased stroke volume, more appropriate distribution of cardiac output between skin and muscle capillary beds, lowered threshold for the onset of sweating, improved sweat distribution, increased sweat output, decreased sweat electrolyte content and reduced glycogen utilisation.

A number of studies have clearly shown that the ability of both man and horses to perform a standardised exercise test in hot humid conditions is reduced compared to that in hot dry or cool conditions. In man it is clear that a period of acclimation or acclimatisation is beneficial.

Acclimatisation

Only one study has been undertaken concerning acclimatisation of horses to thermally stressful environmental conditions (Marlin *et al.* 1996a). A group of European horses were flown to Atlanta for a period of 4 weeks during July–August. The change in the WBGT Index during the period in which the horses were exercising was from 21 in Europe to 27 in Atlanta. Measurements were made of body mass, plasma volume, rectal temperature, respiratory rate, and water and feed intake. In addition, blood samples were collected for haematology and clinical biochemistry. During acclimatisation, the horses lost approximately twice the amount of body mass for undertaking the same work as in the climate from which they had travelled. Resting respiratory rate was elevated from arrival in Atlanta, but there were no significant changes in resting rectal temperature or heart rate. Plasma volume was unchanged, although there was a trend for the horses with the lowest mass specific plasma volume (ml plasma/kg body mass) to show an increase after 14 days. Because horses were flown to Atlanta, it was difficult to separate the effects of transport from those changes relating to initial exposure to the climate. However, it was clear that there was an improvement in the demeanor (appearauce and behaviour) of all horses from day 1 to day 10 of acclimatisation. Furthermore, white blood cell counts in all horses were higher during the acclimatisation period compared to the control period in Europe. While this may have initially been an effect of transport, the elevation persisted until the horses had been in Atlanta for around 3 weeks and may indicate a stress response related to acclimatisation. As is often the case with 'field studies', it was difficult to demonstrate unequivocally a beneficial effect of acclimatisation. However, subjectively the horses appeared markedly improved by 14 days in Atlanta, and all horses remained clinically normal and healthy throughout.

Acclimation

To date there have been only two studies of acclimation of horses to humid heat. These were carried out by the University of Guelph and the Animal Health Trust. Both studies will be described.

Geor *et al.* (1996) at the University of Guelph exposed six Thoroughbred horses to 33–35°C and 80–85% RH (WBGT Index ≈ 32) for 4 hours per day for 22 consecutive days. The exposure consisted of 1 hour of passive exposure, i.e. non-exercising heat exposure, 1 hour of exercise on a treadmill (20–65% $\dot{V}_{O_2,max}$) and a further 2 hours of passive exposure. Exercise was discontinued when rectal temperature (T_{rec}) reached 41.0°C. With acclimation there was a small decrease in resting T_{rec} which was maintained during exercise. By day 10 of acclimation there was a significant decrease in heat storage during exercise, although this and other physiological adaptations were apparent by 5 days. Following acclimation, the decrease in body mass associated with exercise was reduced from around 2.7% to 2.0% body mass. Maximal oxygen uptake did not change following acclimation. It was concluded that 'three weeks of exposure to, and exercise in, hot and humid ambient conditions resulted in a progressive reduction in thermal and cardiovascular strain. Furthermore, the reported physiological adaptations are consistent with an improved thermal tolerance (heat acclimation).'

The Animal Health Trust study investigated the

response of five horses of mixed breed to a 14 day period of acclimation at 30°C and 80% RH (WBGT Index ≈ 29) (Marlin *et al.* 1996b). The horses were exposed for 100 minutes per day, of which 80 minutes was active (exercise) and 20 minutes was passive. The horses lived in stables at about 7°C for the remainder of the time. Three different types of training were used throughout the acclimation period to represent the type of activity that a horse would undergo in preparation for competition and included: seven sessions consisting of a single bout of low intensity exercise (about 30% $\dot{V}_{O_2max}$), three sessions consisting of two bouts of medium intensity exercise (about 80% $\dot{V}_{O_2max}$) and three sessions consisting of two bouts of high intensity exercise (95% $\dot{V}_{O_2max}$). Horses completed the low intensity exercise on alternate days, with medium or high intensity days in between. To determine if an acclimation response had taken place, the horses underwent a competition exercise test (CET) on the treadmill designed to simulate the speed and endurance phase of the three-day event competition before and after acclimation.

Before acclimation when the CET at 30°C 80% RH was undertaken, none of the horses could complete the full test and were stopped when pulmonary artery temperature reached 43.5°C. After acclimation, the horses were able to exercise for a mean time of 16% longer before the pulmonary artery temperature reached 43.5°C, and thus did more work. Following acclimation, resting T_{rec} was significantly lower by day 6 than at the start of acclimation. In the CET, T_{rec} remained lower throughout, except during the later stages of recovery. Heat storage following acclimation was therefore greater, although the horses had done more work; however, projection of values for pre-acclimation heat storage to the same exercise time did not fully account for the greater post-acclimation heat storage.

Coincident with the increased heat storage was a lower body mass loss following acclimation (3.8% versus 2.1%) and a change in sweating response. However, there was no apparent change in either the sweat rate–skin temperature or sweat rate–core temperature relationships. As reported by Geor *et al.* (1996), no change in $\dot{V}_{O_2max}$ occurred with acclimation. Plasma volume and total body water were also unchanged following acclimation. Because the

horse already has a high mass specific plasma volume (about 60–70 ml/kg) it may be that there is little possibility for a further increase. However, as in the acclimatisation study (Marlin *et al.* 1996a) there was a trend for two horses with low plasma volumes to show an increase post-acclimation. It was concluded that physiological changes indicative of an acclimation response and of an improved heat tolerance were observed.

The main findings from the two acclimation studies and the single study of acclimatisation of horses to hot humid conditions are as follows:

- Acclimation of fit horses to hot humid conditions does not alter $\dot{V}_{O_2max}$
- Acclimation results in a reduction of resting body temperature
- Sweat losses are reduced for the same exercise following acclimation, but this probably reflects lower body temperatures rather than a change in sweating sensitivity
- Plasma volume remains unchanged in the majority of horses but may increase in individuals with an initially low mass specific plasma volume
- Heat storage may be increased or decreased
- Acclimation effects are apparent by 5–10 days, with little further change between 14 and 21 days
- Passive exposure is not essential for acclimation, and animals can continue to live at relatively cool ambient temperatures
- Following acclimation, horses may be able to tolerate higher body temperatures
- Acclimation may partially restore the reduction in performance seen in unacclimated individuals exercising in hot humid conditions.

These findings were formulated into recommendations which were circulated to all teams sending horses to compete in Atlanta. These were the following:

- The majority of horses are likely to benefit from a period of acclimatisation to hot humid conditions before the games
- For unacclimatised horses, the risk of developing severe dehydration, heat stress, heat exhaustion and related medical conditions is greater than for acclimatised horses
- Training in hot dry conditions before departure may offer some benefit but is unlikely to fully

prepare horses for competing in a hot humid environment

- Effective acclimatisation is likely to take place after approximately 14 days of training
- Begin acclimatisation training by exercising lightly and early in the morning; progress to more intense exercise in the late morning
- Monitor rectal temperature and water intake morning and evening and before and after exercise
- A small percentage of horses may show an adverse reaction to acclimatisation. This could include: little or no improvement in heat tolerance after 10 days; reduction or loss of sweating ability despite high body temperature (anhidrosis); large increases or decreases in water intake: marked body mass loss; reduced feed intake.

Management of competitions in thermally stressful environments

Today, competitions such as the Olympic Games, World Equestrian Games, World Championships and racing can take place at almost any time of the year and in a wide variety of climates. The initial reaction to the announcement that a competition is to be held in thermally stressful conditions, for example the summer Olympic Games in Atlanta in 1996 or the endurance rides that now take place regularly in the United Arab Emirates, is to say these competitions should simply be moved. However, the need to attract large audiences for competitions such as the Olympics means, inevitably, that scheduling will be in months of good weather. To minimise the risks of heat related illness and injury there are steps that can be taken to protect both the horse and the rider.

- *Avoidance.* If it is not possible to move a competition to a cooler region or to a different time of year, then time of day can have a large influence on environmental thermal stress. The most thermally stressful time of the day is commonly between 12 noon and 3 pm. Morning usually offers the best opportunity to avoid severe thermal stress. Air and ground temperature are at their lowest just before dawn. This advantage offsets the higher humidity associated with low air temperature. Afternoon and evening are less desirable for competition because heating of the ground means that air temperature is slower to fall in this period.

- *Monitoring of the thermal heat load* before and during the competition using the WBGT Index. This will aid in determining the severity of the environmental heat load and allow appropriate management strategies to be developed in advance.

- *Education* of riders, grooms, team officials and competition officials.

- *Reduction in distance and/or effort.* The effect of thermal stress is to make horses work harder. Therefore a four-star three-day event speed and endurance test in thermally stressful conditions may approach the effort of a five-star competition. It therefore makes sense to try and reduce effort by reducing speed, distance and jumping efforts. Phase A can be reduced as less time will be required for physiological warm-up. Phase B should be reduced because, being a high intensity phase, a great deal of heat is generated. Phase C should be maintained in time but the horse needs to be aided in cooling down. Phase D may need some reduction in distance and this must also take into account jumping efforts. Testing difficult fences should be placed in the early to middle part of the course and certainly not in the latter part. In showjumping and dressage the actual period of competition is relatively short and so reduction of the competition itself is not required. However, these horses may be at risk of effects on performance and/or heat exhaustion as a result of prolonged warm-up.

- *Acclimatisation.* Competitions should be organised on the basis that horses will need to acclimatise in advance and adequate provision made for horses to arrive well in advance.

- *Shade.* Providing plenty of shade at the start of the course, around the course or main arena and after competition, plays an important role in reducing the heat stress on horse and rider. Remember that it is easy to suffer from heat stroke from being outside in very hot conditions, especially if in full sun. The risk of heat stroke can be reduced by avoiding full sun as much as possible. For arena competitions such as showjumping and dressage, horses should be warmed-up in the shade if possible, wait to go into the arena in the shade, and return to the shade to be cooled after competition (see Fig. 12.6). For horses in the speed and endurance test, shade on course to be used in the event of holds and shade in cooling areas and the 10 minute box can significantly aid recovery and cooling.

- *Cooling stops.* In the speed and endurance test the use of cooling stops is one of the most important approaches to reducing the risk of heat related injury and illness (see Fig. 12.7). Reduction in body temperature not only reduces the potential impact of high temperature on coordination and strength, but also reduce fluid and electrolyte loss.
- *Veterinary monitoring.* With the extension of the 10 minute box to 15 minutes, two inspections of horses should be possible, one at the end of phase C and the second at around 10–12 minutes. This will enable horses that gave cause for concern at the end of phase C to be re-examined and to pick up horses that may have failed to show recovery or deteriorated since finishing phase C.

Thermoregulation in the cold

Before 1990 there were only around 30 scientific publications dealing directly with the responses of

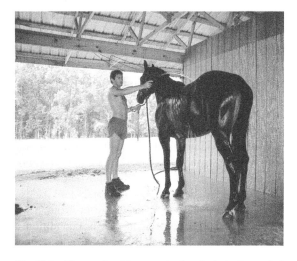

Fig. 12.6 Horses should return to the shade to be cooled after competition when there is strong solar radiation and air temperatures are high.

horses to hot or cold climates, and these were approximately equal in number. Between 1990 and 2000 there were around 80 papers published in direct relation to thermoregulatory responses of horses to heat, but only a further 15 papers on cold responses. However, there are some important considerations to be borne in mind in relation to exercising in cold conditions.

- Warm-up serves both physiological and psychological purposes. From a physiological point of view, we warm-up horses to minimise injury and maximise performance. In a very cold climate, decreased environmental temperature could reduce the increase in muscle temperature normally associated with warming-up, which has implications for reduced muscle strength. It has even been suggested that exercise in the cold can increase the risk of exertional rhabdomyolysis in susceptible horses. To avoid these effects, in very cold climates the warm-up period should be longer and consist of longer periods of initially low speed work.
- In very cold conditions the ground is likely to be harder and possibly more uneven. This could lead to increased risk of orthopaedic injury. In fact, anecdotally it is reported that the use of ice or snow spikes for racing on snow does lead to a higher incidence of orthopaedic injury. This is probably an unavoidable consequence of competing on rough, hard or slippery footing.
- Very cold environmental conditions may affect metabolism, with a greater shift towards aerobic and anaerobic glycogen utilisation compared to the same intensity of exercise in temperate conditions. The shift is mediated by increases in circulating adrenaline and noradrenaline released in response to cold. In fact, the same increases in catecholamines also occur in response to heat. The implication is that even at relatively low intensities a greater reliance on glycogen may bring about an earlier onset of fatigue due to marked glycogen depletion, particularly in moderate to prolonged exercise.
- *Laminitis.* Anecdotally, it has been suggested that the consumption of large volumes of very cold water can lead to laminitis, especially if these are consumed after exercise when the horse is hot.

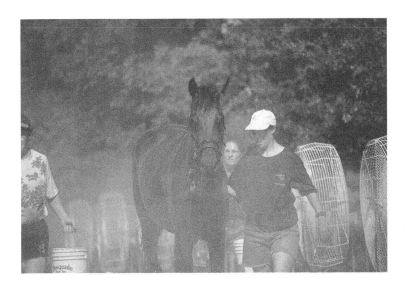

Fig. 12.7 The introduction of cooling stops has been one of the most important strategies for reducing the risk of heat related injury and illness.

Most horse people would avoid offering ice cold water to horses after exercise if at all possible but there is little scientific evidence that consumption of cold fluids leads to the condition.

- *Water intake.* Ponies living outdoors in a very cold climate have been shown to drink more water when the buckets and water were warmed compared to ice cold. However, in summer the ponies drank almost equal volumes of ice cold and warm water.
- *Energy for maintenance.* Even with a good layer of fat and a thick coat for insulation, horses and ponies living in very cold climates will need to expend energy to keep warm. Therefore to maintain their body mass and condition they will need to increase their feed intake. It has been estimated that horses need to increase their energy intake by 1% for every 1°C decrease in environmental temperature below 0°C, i.e. at −10°C they would need a 10% increase in energy from feed.
- *Effects on the respiratory system.* At −25°C, respiratory rate is lower at rest and during and after exercise. This might have implications for the overall level of minute ventilation, especially if the horse was unable to maintain ventilation by increasing tidal volume. The most likely reason why horses reduce their respiratory rate is either to allow more time for warming inspired air or to reduce respiratory heat loss, or even a combination of both. Remember that horses effectively hypoventilate during intense exercise based on

the increase in arterial carbon dioxide tension, and therefore any further decrease would be expected to have a negative effect on performance. However, ventilation does not seem to have been measured in horses exercising in very cold conditions. Breathing very cold air, especially during exercise, is known to exacerbate human asthma and may well induce pulmonary inflammation and asthma in athletes regularly training in such conditions. Whether this occurs in horses is currently unclear, although it has been shown that airway temperature is reduced in horses exercising in Finland in very cold conditions. Remember that previously we considered the inspired air always to be warmed to body temperature and fully humidified. In addition to inflammation, one study on Standardbreds racing in Quebec by Lapointe *et al.* (1994) reported that the incidence of EIPH was highest in cold conditions (81% of horses racing), intermediate in temperate conditions (65%) and lowest in warm conditions (50%). A mask was even developed in the 1970s for horses racing in cold climates with the aim of reducing epistaxis (visible bleeding at the nostrils) by warming inspired air.

Therefore competing in the very cold can potentially carry as many risks as competing in very hot or hot and humid conditions, but scientific knowledge in the former is currently less advanced.

KEY POINTS

- For every unit of energy made available for muscle contraction, 4 units are released as heat.
- Heat production during exercise is proportional to exercise intensity measured as oxygen consumption.
- Body temperature is a balance between heat gain (production ± environmental) and heat loss (to the environment).
- Heat can be exchanged by the horse with its environment by the processes of radiation, convection, conduction and evaporation.
- At high body temperatures, around 15% of total heat dissipated may be via respiration.
- Increased ventilation after exercise is primarily driven by increased body temperature.
- Horses can sweat at rates of 10–15 litres/hour.
- Sweating can be stimulated by the sympathetic nervous system, by adrenaline and by directly heating the skin.
- Equine sweat is more concentrated than other body fluids and is referred to as being hypertonic.
- Horses have apocrine sweat glands where each hair follicle has a sweat gland associated with it.
- Equine sweat contains a protein called latherin which helps the sweat to spread along the individual hairs, creating a greater surface area for evaporation.
- When sweat rate exceeds evaporation rate, sweat is seen to drip from the body surface.
- Anhidrosis is a disorder of reduced and sometimes absent sweating in response to a suitable thermal stimulus.
- Increasing fluid loss above 5% body mass is likely to have a noticeable impact on performance.

- Rehydration cannot take place with water alone, but requires sodium either from the diet or in water.
- Isotonic fluids are the same concentration as body fluids and are effective at rehydration without associated feed intake.
- Environmental thermal stress can only be assessed by taking into account shade temperature, relative humidity, radiation and air movement (wind).
- Acclimatisation is thermal adaptation in response to a change in the natural environment (for example flying a horse to a hotter climate), whilst acclimation is the process of adaptation to an artificially created environment (such as in a treadmill laboratory).
- Information on acclimatisation and acclimation of horses is limited compared with in man, but around 14 days is considered a minimum length of time to get a suitable effect.
- Studies have shown that after acclimation or acclimatisation to thermally stressful conditions of elevated temperature and/or humidity, horses have an improved exercise tolerance, reduced or increased heat storage, reduction in resting rectal temperature and reduced fluid loss.
- Steps that can be taken to manage horses competing in thermally stressful hot or hot and humid conditions include avoidance, education of riders and officials, reduction in effort, acclimatisation, provision of shade, inclusion of adequate facilities for cooling, cooling stops, more frequent and detailed veterinary monitoring, and stricter criteria for continued participation of horses in the competition.

Chapter 13

Introduction to biomechanics

Biomechanics is one of the youngest branches of equine exercise physiology: it can be split into two aspects, kinematics and kinetics. Kinematics is the study of movement, describing the three-dimensional linear and angular displacements of the limbs, whilst kinetics is the study of forces that are generated or absorbed to cause or resist movement. The pioneer of equine biomechanics and the man responsible for producing the first moving pictures was Muybridge (1899). His pictures, taken using a series of cameras to capture the sequence of limb movements in horses, were the first to show that there was indeed a moment of suspension in the trot stride where the horse was completely off the ground. We can study kinematics using cameras, video or specialised tracking equipment, and we can study kinetics using devices known as force plates and accelerometers. Before advances in computer technology the main obstacle facing scientists interested in gait analysis was that many measurement techniques required laborious and time-consuming methods of data acquisition. Many advances in both data acquisition and processing have been made since the 1980s, enabling scientists to conduct larger, more detailed studies within any given time frame. A further drawback of being involved in a 'new' and rapidly expanding field of research was that the variations in terminology used by different scientific authors often led to difficulty in interpreting each other's results. To facilitate comparisons of research findings, standard terminology for the description of overland kinematics was proposed by Leach *et al.* (1984), and was later updated by Leach in 1993. In 1989, Clayton published a paper giving standard terminology that could be used to describe aspects of the jump sequence (Clayton 1989a).

Much of the early work in biomechanics resulted in descriptive studies aimed at characterising various aspects of 'normal' equine locomotion.

With a wealth of information now available relating to the kinetics and kinematics of normal horses, scientists are now able to apply these findings with a view to developing methods of performance prediction based on biomechanical characteristics, and also to develop sensitive and quantitative systems for lameness detection. The study of equine gait is also necessary, not only to develop systems of lameness detection, but for testing the efficacy of treatment strategies, for example remedial shoeing. Thus, biomechanics research can make a significant contribution to equine welfare.

There are some serious challenges faced by the biomechanics researcher to achieve these aims. In performance prediction, the idea is to talent-spot elite youngsters. We would all like to be able to spot Olympic event horses and Derby winners, and it would be much better if they could be spotted at an early age, preferably before the onset of a training programme, so that we needn't waste time and effort training unlikely candidates. If we are to do this, we need to know first of all what it is about a great horse that makes it great. With that established, we then need to know whether or not these characteristics will be evident in young horses. In other words, is a horse born with good movement or can horses develop good movement over time? Happily for us, it seems that many aspects of an individual's gait are established in horses as young as 12–18 months (Back *et al.* 1994). Of course, spotting a horse with all the right biomechanical credentials is still only half the battle in finding the perfect sports horse. As discussed in Chapter 19, elite performance is likely to result from a combination of many factors including cardiovascular and muscular characteristics, fitness, management and health, in addition to biomechanical characteristics.

To be able to quantify lameness, scientists need to develop gait analysis systems that are objective and more sensitive than a simple visual appraisal by a clinician. Much of the early work aimed at quantifying lameness merely served to demonstrate that the visual system of an experienced vet is actually a very fine diagnostic tool! Whilst we are heading rapidly towards the point where techniques of gait analysis rival the clinician in terms of producing reliable diagnoses, such techniques are not likely to become commonplace in equine veterinary practices unless they are capable of producing results rapidly and without the need for a specially trained technician to both acquire and interpret the data.

Studying the gaits

To study the gaits we need to ensure that the measurements we obtain are reliable and reproducible. For certain applications, they should also be sensitive enough to detect the timings of events that are indiscernible to the naked eye, such as the time elapsed between heel lift-off and toe lift-off at the end of stance. For example, the trot of an elite horse may be aesthetically pleasing, but to find out exactly what it is about the trot that makes it 'elite' requires sensitive and accurate equipment. To provide valid data, the equipment itself should not actually interfere with or restrict the gait in any way during the period of recording. The most useful equipment for gait analysis would enable both field and treadmill measurements to be taken.

Kinetics and force plates

By applying Newton's third law, 'to every action there is an equal and opposite reaction', we can study the forces the limb applies to the ground by using forceplates, and hence the forces the ground applies to the limb. Forceplates in one form or another have been used extensively in equine biomechanics research for the last 20 years. One type of forceplate (the Kistler forceplate) is a large aluminium sandwich, usually measuring around 900 mm × 600 mm, in each corner of which there is a piezoelectric force transducer. Each transducer produces an electric charge when it is deformed. Once the forceplate has been calibrated with a known force, the resultant electrical signal can be correlated with the level of force applied to the plate.

Forceplates give valuable information about the stance phase of each limb, how much weight is borne by each limb, and how much each limb is responsible for the overall propulsion of the horse in a particular gait. The difficulty with forceplate measurements is that many attempts are needed to get the limb of interest to strike the forceplate approximately centrally to obtain a good recording. Only one foot at a time should hit the forceplate, and it should hit the plate centrally rather than near the edge. The forceplate should be covered with the same surface as the rest of the track so that the horse is not able to distinguish the forceplate and therefore does not alter its gait in any way on approach, or try to avoid the forceplate altogether. The faster the gait, the longer the stride length and the more attempts necessary to get a good hit on the plate. At the canter it may take 20 runs over the plate to get one successful hit. It would be possible to have a series of forceplates in a line to increase the number of successful hits per run; however, a single forceplate system is likely to cost in the region of £50 000. It is possible to build larger forceplates, but if more than one foot struck the plate at the same time it would not be possible to separate the signals. Forceplates potentially have a future in lameness detection, but obviously it is not ideal to have to run a lame horse time and time again to obtain the necessary data. Some horses, for instance those with structural asymmetries, tend to bear weight asymmetrically when standing, and this is detectable by measuring the vertical ground reaction forces under each limb individually. Lame horses may behave in the same way, shifting their weight to favour the lame or injured limb when standing, and this would also be detectable using forceplates.

The forceplate may be a useful tool in determining the symmetry of the right and left limb pairs in weight bearing and propulsive actions, but it can still only provide data relating to the stance phase. Forceplate data are perhaps most useful when they are used in conjunction with a kinematic technique such as high-speed cinematography. One of the great strengths of the forceplate is in assessing foot balance by following the ground reaction forces (GRFs) throughout the stance phase. Traces can be taken before and after corrective trimming and shoeing to monitor the effects of the remedial farriery on the stance phase.

The forceplate measures the force applied to the plate in three directions, giving three different types of 'GRFs' as follows (see Fig. 13.1):

- The mediolateral (F_x) force acting from side to side of the limb, or across the path of the horse
- The craniocaudal (F_y) force acting from front to back of the limb, in the direction of travel
- The vertical force (F_z) acting perpendicular to the ground.

Of the three forces, most attention is paid to the F_z and F_y traces. This is partly because the F_x values are highly variable, even between runs of the same horse, and are therefore not studied to the same extent as the F_z and F_y traces. The F_z trace represents the degree of weight bearing of a limb, whilst the F_y trace represents the extent to which the limb propels and decelerates the horse throughout each phase of stance.

Figure 13.2 shows generalised F_z and F_y traces plotted against time. Forces are given in Newtons, but to enable comparisons to be made both between horses and between gaits, forces are often normalised to N/kg body mass, with the time-scale expressed as a percentage of the total stance duration of that limb, the latter allowing for variations in stride frequencies between horses. When the foot is on the ground during the first half of stance it has a decelerative or braking effect on the horse, and during the second half of stance it has an accelerative or propulsory effect. Consequently the F_y trace shows two phases, with the first phase corresponding to the braking phase of the limb and the second phase corresponding to the propulsive phase of the limb. The time of crossover between the two phases occurs approximately when the cannon bone is vertical, and this instant in time is often referred to as mid-stance. The relationship between each phase defines the major role of the limb, whether it is predominantly braking or propulsive. The peak amplitude of the F_z trace increases with increasing running speed.

Kinetics can also be studied using accelerometers which, as the name suggests, measure accelerations and decelerations produced during limb movement. Accelerometers can be attached to various parts of the horse's limb or to the hoof wall and thus have the advantage over the forceplate in that unlimited strides can be measured consecutively. Accelerometers vary greatly in their size and hence in the degree to which they might influence the horse's gait. As they record continuously throughout stance and swing, interpretation of the intervals between accelerative peaks can provide a certain amount of kinematic data (stride frequency and duration) in addition to the kinetic data. Their ori-

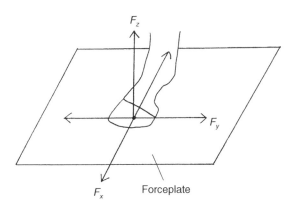

Fig. 13.1 The three orthogonal ground reaction forces measured during stance (when the foot is on the ground) using forceplate analysis.

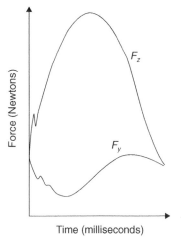

Fig. 13.2 Generalised ground reaction force (GRF) traces.

entation on the hoof or limb is important if information concerning forces in a particular direction is needed, e.g. vertical, and if this is the case they will only be accurate when the accelerometer axis is orientated in that direction.

Recently, an exciting area of development in equine biomechanics has involved the use of inverse dynamic analysis (inverse dynamics refers to the estimation of the forces that cause an observed motion). Inverse dynamic analysis combines kinematic, forceplate and morphometric data to determine the net joint power. Calculations of net joint powers enable scientists to define the roles of joints, and to recognise changes in the roles of the joints that may occur due to lameness. It may also be used to predict the impact of surgery or remedial farriery on the joint function. At the time of writing, net joint powers had only been established for normal horses in walk and trot (Colborne *et al.* 1998; Clayton *et al.* 1998).

Studying kinematics

One of the easiest and most accessible methods of studying kinematics is with a video camera. One of the main benefits of this approach is the relatively low cost and instant replay, making simple videography one of the more likely methods of gait analysis to be used by veterinary practices to aid lameness diagnosis. Standard home VHS cameras capture at 25 Hz (or 25 frames per second) but more expensive professional equipment made specifically for movement analysis may capture at up to 200 Hz. Skin markers can be placed on the horse to make it easier to measure particular joint angles and linear distances directly from the video or, alternatively, software programmes are available that enable sequential 'stick diagrams' of the limb movements to be produced.

Cinematography uses film rather than videotape and has been more commonly used than videography in the past; however, the high cost of film has led to videography becoming more popular. High-speed cinematography is available with frame speeds of up to 1000 frames per second. The major problem with both videography and cinematography is that only one or two strides may fall within the calibrated field of view of the camera at any

given time. There are several ways to increase the number of strides that can be measured in sequence: we can capture the data from a moving vehicle travelling along-side the horse, we can pan the camera to increase the field of view, or we can film the horse on a treadmill.

Moving the camera alongside the horse generally introduces too much camera movement and is rarely used for research. Camera panning increases the number of strides that can be kept in view and provides more information than a stationary camera. Running the horse on a treadmill allows all strides within the period of exercise to be recorded, but there may be differences in how the horse moves with a rider in the field and, of course, it cannot be used to study jumping! Cinematography is expensive but it is also very accurate and produces vast quantities of data. Recent advances in data processing and in computer analysis of data have greatly reduced the time taken to interpret cinematographic data, thus increasing its popularity with researchers. Other techniques that have been used for many gait analysis studies are those in which anatomical markers are placed on the horse and 'tracked'. There are two commonly used types of system, those which use passive light-reflecting markers and those which use active markers that are detected on-line. All the methods that use skin markers require a correction factor to be applied for the displacement of the markers due to skin movement. Skin markers are placed over the centres of rotation of the joints in question, but inevitably the skin moves as the limb is moved. Studies have been carried out to quantify the extent of skin displacment and it has been found to be greater over the proximal joints than the distal joints. As long as the degree of displacement is known it can be accounted for in any measurements that are made.

Stride length and stride frequency

The stride length (SL) is the distance travelled by the horse's centre of mass during one stride, or the distance between successive prints of the same foot. The SL can be measured quite easily by running the horse over a raked sand surface so that the footprints are visible and measuring the distance between successive hoofprints from the same foot or by examining video footage. The number of strides per unit time is known as the stride frequency (SF).

$$\text{Speed (m/s)} = \text{SL (m)} \times \text{SF (strides/s)}$$

and

$$\text{Stride duration (s)} = 1/\text{SF (strides/s)}$$

When horses increase their speed within any gait, they tend to accomplish this by first increasing their stride length, and then their stride frequency. As the horse increases its speed from walk through to gallop, its stride length increases from approximately 2 metres at the walk to approximately 6–7 metres for a Thoroughbred at the gallop. For many years horsemen have taught that a horse can be judged by its walk alone and that a good walk, i.e. one with a large stride length, signifies a good long stride at gallop. This is largely true. There ought to be a strong correlation between stride length at the walk and at the gallop, because the lengths of the limb and trunk largely determine stride length. Horses have increased in size throughout evolution, gaining in speed also. Whilst larger animals have long stride lengths, they are not capable of producing stride frequencies as high as smaller animals; in other words top speed is achieved as a result of a compromise between large SL and large SF. Maximal SF for a horse is approximately 2–2.5 strides/s (2–2.5 Hz) compared to the maximum SF for a mouse of 8 strides/s (8 Hz).

Thoroughbred horses, which have been selectively bred for speed tend to maximise SF by adopting a low, straight action known as 'daisy-cutting'. This is in contrast to the rounder, more elevated action of the Warmblood breeds. Thus, Warmbloods are well adapted for dressage and showjumping, and the Thoroughbred is supremely adapted for speed, being able to gallop a mile (1600 metres) at 18 m/s, equivalent to covering a mile in $1\frac{1}{2}$ minutes.

The gaits

A gait is a particular pattern of footfalls; the main gaits are the walk, trot, canter and gallop. Gaits fall into two main types, symmetrical and asymmetrical. A symmetrical gait can be defined as 'any gait in which the placements of the left and right fore and hind limb pairs are evenly spaced in time'. By this definition, walk and trot are symmetrical and canter and gallop are asymmetrical.

Walk

The walk is a four-beat gait with footfalls occurring in the following order: left hind (LH), left fore (LF), right hind (RH), right fore (RF). In this gait, at least two limbs are in stance phase at any one time and there is no period of suspension in the gait. With speed comes stability. Think of riding a bicycle. The slower you go, the harder it is to stay upright. The same applies to the horse: the slower the gait, the more limbs must be in contact with the ground at any one time to maintain stability. At the faster gaits the horse has fewer limbs in contact with the ground, yet manages to maintain stability simply due to its forward momentum. This may also explain why dressage horses that do not go positively forward into a good rein contact tend to have more difficulty than others in remaining truly straight, particularly in walk. As riders we are always taught that 'the hind limbs are the horse's engine', but forceplate studies of normal walks have shown that, contrary to popular belief, the forelimbs are every bit as responsible for generating propulsive forces as the hind limbs. Figure 13.3 shows the typical ground reaction forces in the fore and hind limb during walk. Notice that there is a dip in the F_z trace, reflecting the period of bilateral support of a fore and hind limb, respectively, which serves to reduce the weight bearing of the forelimb momentarily. Also, as the swinging limb carries some upward momentum through late swing, this tends to unweight the contralateral (opposite) stance limb. The amplitude of F_z for the forelimbs is greater than that of the hind limbs, demonstrating that the forelimbs play a greater role in weight bearing than the hind limbs. The F_y trace clearly shows that in walk, a substantial portion of the driving force for forward movement is provided by the forelimbs. This would seem to make sense when we consider that, in the walk at least, the spine is relatively flexible and does not form a rigid link between the 'engine' and the forelimbs. In faster

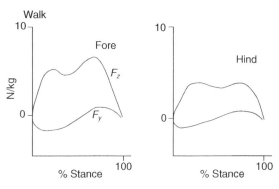

Fig. 13.3   Walk GRF traces.

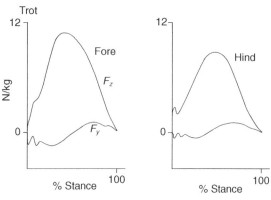

Fig. 13.4   Trot GRF traces.

gaits the spine is held more rigidly by the musculature and so the forward thrust provided by the hind limbs is more effectively transmitted to the forehand.

Studies of the walk of dressage horses have shown that few actually achieve a regular four-beat rhythm in walk, with horses either showing lateral couplets, i.e. shorter time between the lateral footfalls (Clayton 1995) or diagonal couplets, i.e. shorter time between the diagonal footfalls (Deuel & Park 1990). The loss of regularity would appear to contradict the FEI definition of the walk, which states that 'the pace should remain marching and vigorous, the feet being placed in regular sequence'. Similarly, FEI definitions state that there should be no change in tempo (equivalent to stride frequency) when moving from the collected to the extended gaits. However, a study of 11 elite dressage horses at the Atlanta Olympics (Hodson *et al.* 1999) showed that the stride duration of the extended walk was indeed shorter than that of the collected walk (1.05 seconds compared to 1.16 seconds), but of course the degree of the difference would be too small to be discernible by dressage judges. If we take these findings to a logical conclusion we may decide that we ought to have tracking systems and computers doing our dressage judging, but that would then not enable us to reward such qualities as 'presence' and 'submission'.

In the study of Hodson *et al.* (1999) it was also found that both the collected and extended walk strides had a longer stance duration in the hind limbs than in the forelimbs, which probably reflects what riders refer to as 'impulsion'. Impulsion is synonymous with the more scientific expression

'impulse', where impulse = force × time. Impulse is increased by increasing either the stance duration or the forces applied by the limbs, not just in the walk but in other gaits also.

Trot

The trot is a two-beat gait, with footfalls in the following order; LH and RF together, followed by RH and LF together. Trot diagonals are named left and right according to the forelimb of the diagonal, so the right diagonal would refer to the right forelimb and the left hind limb. The trot should have a period of suspension in between the stance phases of each diagonal pair.

Figure 13.4 shows the typical ground reaction forces obtained during trot in normal horses. In trot, the magnitude of the peak vertical force (F_z) of the forelimbs is greater than that of the walk, approximately 11 N/kg as opposed to 6 or 7 N/kg for walk. There is only one peak in the F_z force at trot, reflecting the single loading and unloading phase in stance as the palmar tendons absorb and then give back energy like a spring. Again, the forelimbs bear more weight than the hind limbs, but the role of propulsion has shifted more to the hind limbs as shown by the greater area under the second part of the F_y trace for the forelimbs compared to the hind limbs.

The fact that the trot is a symmetrical gait with the hind limbs generating the majority of the propulsive forces may explain why many dressage and showjumping trainers use trot more often than any of the other gaits when carrying out the early ridden work of a young horse: this and the fact that most riders use 'rising trot' so that their seat is up off the horse's back 50% of the time. One of the major characteristics of a 'good' trot is the degree of advanced placement of the hind limb of each diagonal pair; in other words, a 'good' trot is one in which the hind limb impacts with the ground slightly ahead of its diagonal forelimb. In a good working trot the hind limb will actually strike the ground around 0.03 seconds (3/100ths of a second) in advance of the forelimb, giving the impression of 'lightness' of the forehand to an observer. On moving from the collected to the extended gaits, the extent to which the hind limb 'oversteps' (correctly termed overtracking) the print left by the ipsilateral forelimb (i.e. forelimb on the same side) is increased, thereby increasing the stride length. The normal walk of a good horse will demonstrate overtracking by 10–20 cm. In the collected trot horses 'undertrack' as the hind feet are lifted in a more rounded fashion and are placed behind the prints of the forefeet. In all other trots, working, medium and extended, overtracking occurs. The FEI also states that the horse is judged according to the ability to maintain the same rhythm throughout transitions between collected, medium and extended trot; in fact, even elite dressage horses tend to have a higher stride frequency when performing extended trot than collected trot. For example, a group of FEI level dressage horses studied by Clayton (1994a), had stride frequencies of 77 strides/minute (1.28 Hz) in collected trot and 83 strides/minute (1.38 Hz) in extended trot; however, the increase in stride frequency on moving from collected to extended gaits is less in an elite horse than in a horse performing at the lower levels.

Canter

Canter is a three-beat gait with one period of suspension. The order of the footfalls depends upon which 'lead' the horse is on. If the horse is on the right lead, the right fore and right hind are the last of each fore and hind limb pair to hit the ground. Thus, the right lead canter sequence of footfalls is LH, RH and LF together, followed by RF. This is followed by a period of suspension before LH impacts again. As the speed of the canter increases, the diagonal pair 'dissociate' such that the hind limb

impacts in advance of the diagonal forelimb. When this happens the gait is no longer three-time but four-time and becomes gallop.

Figure 13.5 shows the typical ground reaction forces produced by each limb in a right lead canter. The roles of the limbs as determined by GRF analysis show that the non-lead hind limb has the largest propulsive element of all the limbs. The non-lead hind limb tends to propel more than the lead limb as it is responsible for turning the downward action at the end of the suspension phase of the stride into forward motion across the ground. The non-lead fore is the first one down of the forelimb pair and shows more weight bearing and more propulsive action than the lead forelimb. In fact, the lead forelimb hardly propels the horse at all, as it is the last limb to leave the ground before the next suspension and therefore much of the energy for 'take-off' has already been produced by the time the lead fore impacts.

The collected canter often does not have any suspension phase at all. As the horse moves from the collected to the extended canter the degree of

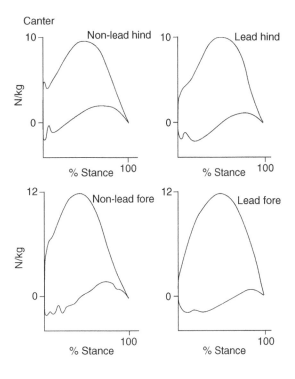

Fig. 13.5 Canter GRF traces.

suspension within the stride and the stride length increase. Kinematic analysis has demonstrated another contradiction to textbook definitions in that the collected and extended canters of elite horses are four-beat gaits, not three-beat gaits. A study of dressage horses competing at the Seoul Olympics in 1988 (Clayton 1994b) showed that the speed of the collected canter was actually slower at 3.3 m/s than the speed at which most horses would normally make the trot-to-canter transition, and thus the energetic cost of the collected canter may be greater than that for a horse moving freely in canter. The Olympic dressage horse has stride lengths of up to 4 metres in the extended canter (moving at speeds of approximately 6.5 m/s) and those horses with longer strides tend to receive higher marks for this movement.

Gallop

Gallop is a four-beat gait. The sequence of footfalls for a right lead gallop are LH, RH, LF, RF. To change lead at the gallop, horses will often change behind first, so that the footfalls become RH, LH, LF, RF. This is known as a rotary gallop and it puts the left fore at great risk of an over-reach injury being inflicted by the left hind limb. Usually rotary gallop only lasts half a stride before the horse also changes lead in front to complete the lead change within one whole stride. Frequent changing of leads during a race is thought to be a sign of lameness or fatigue. To date only the kinematics, but not the kinetics, of the gallop stride have been studied in any great depth. The horse increases its stride length at the gallop both by increasing the degree of suspension within the stride as a percentage of stride duration and by decreasing the amount of time which the lead hind and non-lead fore spend in bipedal ('two-legged') support. In other words, a good galloping horse spends as much of the stride time as possible travelling forward in the suspensory phase and as little time as possible on the ground!

Gait transitions

Various factors are thought to influence the point at which transitions between gaits are made. It is likely that in any given situation, a combination of the following factors determine the point at which the transition is made.

The rider

In ridden horses the rider determines when gait changes are made and indeed when transitions within a gait are made, e.g. from a working to an extended trot. There is no evidence to suggest that there are any significant differences in spatial (in space or location) and temporal (over time) kinematics from the ridden to the unridden state as long as the rider can maintain their balance without interfering with that of the horse. The only influence of a rider with a good riding position is that of additional weight. This causes a slight increase in flexion of the joints of the hind limbs compared with the free running horse at the same speed. As yet, scientists have not begun to investigate the possible positive effects of an experienced rider on gait characteristics, such as increasing the activity of the hind limbs or helping the horse to work 'in balance'.

Energy cost

When given free choice, horses will usually select a gait that uses the least energy at any given speed, so the transition from trot to canter would be made at the point at which it became more expensive (in terms of energy) to trot fast than to canter slowly. If the rider asks the horse to increase the stride length in trot to increase the speed, the horse may actually be using more energy than if it moved up to canter (Hoyt & Taylor 1981). Horses therefore make transitions between gaits to minimise the energetic cost of transport.

In general terms, the energetic cost of transport (the energy required to move 1 kg of body mass 1 metre and measured in terms of either heart beats or ml of oxygen used, i.e. ml O_2/kg/m) is highest for walk, lowest for trot and canter and then higher at gallop (see Fig. 13.6). The most economic way to cover a distance is at trot and/or canter. However, this does not take into account other important factors that need to be considered, such as energy

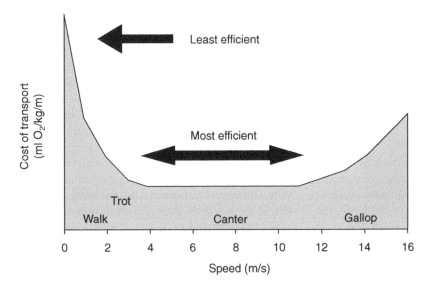

Fig. 13.6 Relationship between energetic cost of transport and speed.

supply and thermoregulation. Thus a fast canter may be economical in terms of the absolute amount of energy required, but be limited in distance by fatigue, exhaustion of energy stores, e.g. glycogen, and thermoregulatory constraints, including dehydration and hyperthermia. Recently, Preedy and Colborne (2001) have developed a method for determining mechanical energy conservation and efficiency in equine gait, taking into account all potential and kinetic energy components of each of the body segments.

Froude number

Imagine that the body is moving over the limb in an arc, like an inverted pendulum. The body is subject to several forces. One is the centripetal force, which is directed radially inwards towards the centre of rotation and which restrains the tendency for the body to leave the arc. This force can be expressed in terms of Newton's second law as $F = ma = mv^2/r$, where m is the mass of the body in the arc, v is its tangential velocity (normal to the radius of the arc) and r is the radial distance from the centre of rotation. The approximate inverse of this is also sometimes called the centrifugal force, referring to the equivalent force tending to throw it out of the arc. This is, however, an inertial force that is directed radially outwards. Consistent with Newton's third law, these two forces are not an

action–reaction pair, because the centrifugal force depends on the motion of the body within a non-inertial reference frame, whereas the centripetal force is described with reference to its own rotating frame. In biomechanics, the non-inertial reference frame is normally used, considering both the classical Newtonian forces as well as suitably defined inertial forces.

The body is also subject to the force of gravity. The force of gravity is the same whatever the speed and is not linked in any way to the direction of motion. However, it has been proposed that as soon as the centripetal force becomes equal to the force of gravity, the animal moves up to the next gait. The Froude number is given by the ratio of the forces of inertia to the gravitational forces acting on the animal's leg. Upward gear changes correspond to a Froude number of 1.0. Horses shift from walk to trot at a Froude number of 0.7–0.9. As soon as there is a Froude number of more than 1.0, there is a moment of suspension in the stride. A suspensory phase, in effect, increases the stride length by adding a 'jump'.

Peak vertical force

Another factor that is thought to govern the point at which a transition is made is the peak vertical force through the limbs. Horses switch gait when the vertical force reaches a critical amount. However, if the horse carries a rider, it will not switch gait at the crossover of the trot and canter efficiency curves, but at the point at which the force through the limb reaches a maximum level.

The jump stride

There is a great deal of variation in the kinetics and kinematics of the jump stride as there are so many variables that influence it, including factors such as the speed of approach, the height of the fence, the influence of the rider in the approach and over the fence, and the effect of related obstacles.

The jump stride itself includes a take-off, a suspension and a landing phase. The foot placements of the jump begin with placement of the trailing hind at take-off and end with placement of the trailing hind on landing. In the approach to the fence, the horse orientates its body such that the forelimbs are used as struts to elevate the cranial trunk and the hind limbs rotate underneath the body, often being placed closer to the fence than the forefeet and providing a propulsive force for take-off. If the forelimbs slip on take-off the hind limbs are not able to generate the same degree of vertical lift and the horse is more likely to hit the fence. As we saw earlier increasing the stance time of the hind limbs can increase 'impulse', and so the stance time of the hind limbs in take-off is greater than that of a normal approach stride. The higher the fence and the slower the speed of approach, the more likely it is that the horse will show hind limb synchrony. In other words, the horse alters the timing of the hind limb placements such that they land and push off on take-off at the same time, having been placed close together on the ground in front of the fence. In a horse jumping at high speed, there is little hind limb synchrony and the horse tends to 'jump out of its stride' with a considerable spatial, i.e. distance, separation of the hind limbs. Hind limb synchrony is rarely seen in hurdlers and steeplechasers on take-off.

GRF analysis of the limb placements during the jump stride show that the roles of the hind limbs and the forelimbs are very similar to the roles they play in the canter stride; thus the jump stride is to a certain extent a canter stride with a more signifi- cant period of suspension. The non-lead forelimb shows the greatest peak vertical force of all the limbs, as it did in the canter stride, although the actual peak vertical force is greater than the canter stride whilst the lead forelimb has a large retard- ing component, converting some of the forward momentum into vertical lift. The hind limbs show very little deceleration and lots of acceleration, more so than in the normal canter stride. The approach and take-off phases pre-determine the path of the horse's centre of gravity during suspen- sion. During the airborne phase the horse starts to unfold the forelimbs in preparation for landing and raises the head and neck, to aid what is essentially a forward rotation on descent into a backward or anticlockwise rotation to bring the hind limbs to the ground. Horses jumping at speed may be unsuc- cessful in their attempts to reverse this rotation on landing, resulting in the classic 'crumpling' type falls seen in steeplechasing and hurdling.

On landing the aim is to transfer the vertical movement into a forwards, horizontal movement, whilst minimising the concussive forces on the limbs and preparing for the next stride. The non-lead fore impacts first, usually at an angle of approximately 90° to the ground. The lead fore impacts at an angle of about 68° to the ground. The fact that the non-lead fore lands almost upright means that it has little decelerative effect on the horse and most of this role is taken by the lead fore. However, the non-lead fore bears the brunt of the landing force and consequently a large peak vertical force. Large peak vertical forces would be expected in showjumpers landing over large (1.40 metres and above) fences. Consequently showjumpers tend to suffer from concussive related joint problems in the distal forelimbs. The first hind limb down on the landing side (the non-lead hind) shows the majority of the propulsion as it aims to create the forward push-off for the next stride.

Studies of elite showjumping horses show that a good horse tends to have a lower velocity in the approach stride. Good horses also place their hind limbs closer to the fence on take-off (Deuel & Park 1991) and they are able to return to the overland stride pattern quicker after the fence, which may reduce the time taken between fences, a critical factor in timed jump-offs. Successful showjumpers also tend to locate their hind feet closer to the vertical projection of the total body centre of mass, which gives them better vertical velocity (Colborne *et al.* 1995).

Spinal kinematics and back problems

Since the 1980s there have been a number of research studies investigating both spinal kinematics and the incidence of back problems in horses. Now that equine 'sports therapy' has become a part of everyday life in most competition yards, riders are far more likely to blame a back problem for their horse's loss of performance than, say, distal limb lameness. Perhaps this is a result of the recent surge in number of practising equine chiropractors, sports massage therapists, etc. There is no doubt that back pain can be responsible for significant loss of performance, and may even be responsible for the onset of behavioural problems such as napping and bucking, but that does not necessarily mean that the back is the source of the problem. Horses with subtle limb lameness and multilimb lameness are often quite difficult to diagnose, as chronic conditions often result in the horse making compensations in their gait whilst continuing to work for a prolonged period of time. Such compensations often lead to an array of musculoskeletal problems of which back pain may be one, whether or not it is the root cause, and gait modifications which require a skilled clinician to interpret correctly. In 1980, Jeffcott published a study of 443 horses with back problems in an attempt to pinpoint the causes. Soft tissue injuries and vertebral lesions were the two main causes, accounting for around 80% of the cases. Some of the horses were found to have dental and behavioural problems rather than primary back problems, and in some of the horses no clear diagnosis could be made.

Rider awareness of the function of the spine in locomotion, and of aspects of management such as saddle fitting, can only be a plus as far as the welfare and performance of the competition horse is concerned, provided they do not take this to the extreme and call in a 'back person' before they think of calling the vet. Besides, it is illegal in the UK for anyone other than a qualified veterinary surgeon to make a diagnosis, and no practitioner should treat an animal without veterinary referral, a fact of which not all owners (and some practitioners!) seem to be aware.

The spine has evolved to perform certain functions, including acting as a support and framework for muscles and ligaments, and transmitting the propulsive forces of the hind legs through to the forehand of the horse. In contrast to smaller animals such as the cat, horses tend to hold their spine fairly rigidly, particularly when travelling at high speed. As a consequence of this, horses tend to negotiate turns in canter and gallop by adducting, i.e. bringing towards the midline, the inside limb and tipping the thoracic cavity within a 'sling' formed by the scapula and pectorals of each forelimb. It is really only when they begin ridden work that horses are asked to truly 'bend' around turns and circles, something that the free running horse would not necessarily need to do. The types of movement seen within the spine are shown in Fig. 13.7 and can be defined as follows:

- Dorsiflexion refers to the dipping of the back, otherwise known as lordosis
- Ventroflexion refers to the arching of the back, otherwise known as kyphosis
- Lateral flexion is side-to-side movement of vertebrae
- Axial rotation is the rotation of vertebrae around the spine's longitudinal axis.

The subject of 'how much movement occurs in the equine spine' has been of much interest for many years, largely due to the implications this has for riders and trainers. Post mortem studies have been performed to try and determine the range of movement possible within the spinal column. Unfortunately these studies require that the musculature bringing about the movements be dissected away, and so what is measured is not a true reflection of what occurs in live horses. Two such post mortem studies were conducted in the 1980s. Jeffcott and Dalin (1980) performed a post mortem study in which they removed all the musculature just leaving the ligaments intact. Townsend and Leach (1983) performed a similar study in which the spinal musculature was again removed, but the rib cage left intact. In both experiments the spines were fixed at either end and forces applied in various directions. Both studies found that the maximum

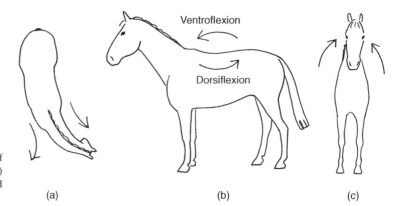

Fig. 13.7 Three different types of movement seen in the vertebrae: (a) lateral rotation; (b) dorsiflexion and ventroflexion; (c) axial rotation.

(a)   (b)   (c)

amount of dorsoventral movement occurred at the lumbosacral joint. Most of the 'rounding' of the back that is seen in the horse over a fence or even the arched back of the bucking rodeo horse largely stems from flexion of this joint. There was found to be a wide range of dorsoventral movement within the T_1–T_2 joint and the least amount of dorsoventral flexion was found to occur between L_2 and L_6.

There would appear to be scope for axial rotation and lateral bending throughout the spine, but the degree of lateral bend lessens as you move towards the latter part of the lumbar region. If we consider the spine to be rather like a toy train made of lots of little wooden carriages representing the vertebrae, only small lateral rotations of each carriage are necessary to allow the train to bend round tight turns. In the same way, the smallest degree of flexion within each vertebra summates to produce a significant degree of 'bend' within the spine as a whole.

Audigie *et al.* (1999) studied kinematics of the equine back in sound trotting horses using skin markers placed at specific points along the dorsal midline of the trunk. They found that the back extended (dorsiflexed) during the first half of each diagonal stance and flexed (ventroflexed) during the second part of each diagonal stance phase, with ranges of motion of less than 4°. They concluded that at a slow trot, trunk muscles act mainly to limit flexion–extension movements of the back rather than to induce movements.

Bow and string theory

The bow and string theory suggests how the spine is affected by the limb muscles and how the spine supports the mass of the horse (Badoux 1975). The equine spine is likened to a bow and string, see Fig. 13.8. The vertebral column, the pelvis and the epaxial muscles correspond to the bow. The bow is kept under tension from the string, which is taut. When the bow is under tension the horse's back is better able to carry load from above. The string corresponds to the sternum and the abdominal muscles. Imagine what occurs when the limb muscles contract. When the protractors of the fore-limb and the retractors of the hind limb contract the bow is bent in such a way as to ventroflex or arch the back. When trying to picture this you must imagine that the muscle is contracting when the limb is load-bearing. In contrast, when the re-tractors of the forelimb and the protractors of the hind limb are contracted, the bow goes slack and dipping or dorsiflexion occurs. The more powerful the retractor muscles of the hind limb and the greater the degree of flexion of the lumbosacral joint, the greater the tension that is placed on the bow. The bow and string analogy helps us to understand why we place so much importance on engagement of the hind limb to bring about a 'rounded top line'.

An individual's conformation and the nature of the sport in which it takes part can have a bearing on

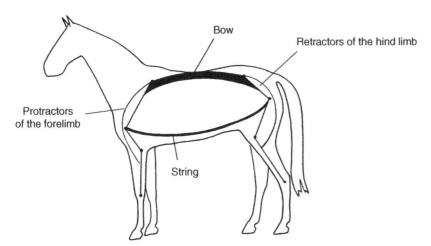

Fig. 13.8 The bow and string.

the type of back injuries seen. Sway backed horses tended to get intermittent soft tissue injuries. A sway backed horse has a 'weakened bow' and so is less able to support the load of a rider effectively. Short backed horses may be more likely to suffer from conditions such as 'kissing spines' where the tips of the dorsal spinous processes impinge on each other during dorsiflexion, whereas longer backed horses are more prone to soft tissue strain. Across the various disciplines, horses that are required to jump at speed have a higher incidence of back problems as a population than other types of sports horses.

It is often useful in cases of true 'back problems' to see the horse and rider combination together, as problems in rider position and back pain in the rider can often manifest themselves as problems in the horse, if the horse is only ever ridden by that one particular person. A combination of effects such as poor conformation, poor foot balance, an ill-fitting saddle and a rider who is not able to get the horse to engage the hindquarters sufficiently

can lead to an overt lameness, when any one of these factors on their own would not be severe enough to cause a significant loss of function. A typical scenario might be one in which a low level hind limb lameness leads to loss of activity of the hindquarters, causing the horse to carry itself in a hollow outline, i.e. with the spine in extension. This leads to a weakening of the 'bow', with the fore-limbs becoming more responsible both for load bearing and propulsion, leading to increased con-cussion of the forelimbs and bilateral forelimb lameness. As the horse is equally lame in both fore-limbs, it goes unnoticed for months or even years, and the shuffling, inactive gait is then thought to be 'normal'. Too often, people consider lameness to be simply an idiosyncratic gait, claiming that the horse 'has always moved like that'. In this age of advanced diagnostic techniques and a myriad of treatment approaches, should we not bite the bullet and ask ourselves whether or not in fact the horse has 'always been lame'?

KEY POINTS

- Biomechanics includes the study of kinematics and kinetics. Kinematics is the study of move-ment, describing the linear (movement in a hor-izontal plane) and angular displacements of the limbs, whilst kinetics is the study of forces that are generated in order to cause movement.

- Kinematics is studied using cameras, video or specialised tracking equipment, whilst kinetics is studied using devices known as forceplates and accelerometers.
- Many aspects of an individual's gait are estab-lished in horses as young as 12–18 months.

- Ground reaction forces obtained using force-plates give us information regarding the degree of load bearing of a limb, and the extent to which the limb propels and decelerates the horse throughout each phase of stance.
- As the horse increases its speed from walk through to gallop, its stride length increases from approximately 2 metres at the walk to approximately 6–7 metres for a Thoroughbred at the gallop.
- Various factors are thought to influence the point at which transitions between gaits are made. It is likely that in any given situation, a combination of the following factors determine the point at which the transition is made: rider influence, Froude number, energy cost, and peak vertical force through the limb.
- The jump stride is very similar to a canter stride in terms of the roles of each limb.
- What riders refer to as impulsion, scientists call 'impulse', and it is usually obtained by increasing the duration of stance of the hind limbs.
- The equine spine is capable of movement in three planes, dorsoventral flexion, lateral bending and axial rotation to varying degrees.

Part III

Applications of Exercise Physiology

Chapter 14

The demands of equestrian sport

Eventing

Eventing includes any competition that consists of dressage, showjumping and cross-country tests. British eventing is governed by the British Horse Trials Association. International competitions are known as CCIs (Concours Complet Internationale) and are run under FEI (Federation Equestrian Internationale) rules. Horses are allowed to compete in affiliated events from the beginning of the calendar year in which they become 5 years old. Competitions are one-day, two-day or three-day events. In one- and two-day events the dressage test is first and the cross-country test is last. In three-day events the dressage is first and the showjumping is last. Events are scored on a penalty basis, the penalties incurred for each 'phase' or 'test' are added together and the competitor with the lowest total penalty score is the winner. Penalties for a knockdown in the showjumping are 5 for the first knockdown and 10 for the second, with 10 penalties for first 'disobedience', i.e. a refusal or a run-out. Horses are more heavily penalised for refusals or run-outs in the cross-country, with 20 penalties for the first refusal and 40 penalties for the second. The cross-country phase is an extended 'speed and endurance' phase consisting of roads and tracks, steeplechase and cross-country jumping. Two-day events have a modified steeplechase and roads and tracks.

There are several grades of competition starting with the easiest 'intro' classes, and progressing through to pre-novice, novice, intermediate and advanced classes. Horses are graded from three to one depending on the number of points they accrue throughout their career. Points are awarded for placings at novice competitions and above, but not for placings in pre-novice or intro classes. Grade 3 horses have less than 21 points, grade 2 horses have

between 21 and 60 points, and grade 1 horses have 61 or more points. Only horses without any points are eligible to compete in intro and pre-novice competitions. Only grade 3 horses may compete at novice level; grade 2 and 3 horses may compete at intermediate level, and grade 1 and 2 horses may compete at advanced level.

Selecting the event horse

All sorts of horses compete successfully up to novice level, but if you intend to go on beyond novice level, you need a horse with a fair amount of natural athletic ability. Many of the top level event horses are full or three-quarter Thoroughbred, and many are not terribly big horses. One of the best event horses in recent years was Charisma, only 15.2 hands (157.5 cm). Often, horses in the range 15.2–16.2 hands (157.5–167.6 cm) are easier to manoeuvre and can more easily negotiate tricky distances. Usually small, wiry looking horses actually have excellent bone circumference to body mass ratios, and stand up well to hard and fast work. The most common types of injuries in event horses are soft tissue injuries such as tendon and ligament damage. When selecting youngsters to compete in eventing, it pays to select those individuals with good conformation in order to avoid putting any unnecessary strain on the connective tissue structures of the distal limb.

Physical demands of eventing

The dressage test in intro and pre-novice competitions is of similar standard to preliminary competitions in pure dressage. The showjumping phase consists of 8–12 obstacles of maximum height 0.95 metres for intro and 1.05 metres for pre-novice. The cross-country is a course of between 1600 and 2800 metres with 18–25 jumping efforts to be ridden at a speed of 450 metres/min (7.5 m/s). The maximum height of fences is 0.90 metres in intro and 1.00 metre for pre-novice.

In novice horse trials, the dressage test may include movements such as 5 metre loops, lengthened strides, give and retaking reins in canter, rein back and 10 metre half circles. Maximum height of the showjumping fences is 1.15 metres. The cross-country phase of the novice competition is between 1600 and 2800 metres in length, with 18–28 jumping efforts of maximum height 1.10 metres to be ridden at 520 metres/min (8.7 m/s). As penalties are given for exceeding the allowed time for cross-country, any horse that is near to its top speed at 520 metres/min, such as cobs or heavier part-breds, may find it difficult to progress beyond novice level successfully.

In the intermediate horse trials dressage test, horses may be asked to do movements such as shoulder-in, medium trot, lengthened strides in canter, canter 15 metre circles, counter-canter, half-pirouettes in walk and travers in trot. The showjumping maximum height is 1.20 metres and the cross-country maximum height is 1.15 metres. The cross-country course is between 2400 and 3620 metres with 22–32 jumping efforts to be ridden at 550 metres/min (9.2 m/s). At advanced level the dressage test may also include collected canter, half pass in trot and flying changes. This would be equivalent to advanced medium in pure dressage as this is the first level at which flying changes are introduced. The maximum height for showjumping is 1.25 metres whilst the maximum height for the cross-country is 1.20 metres. The cross-country course is between 3250 and 4000 metres with 25–40 jumping efforts to be ridden at 570 metres/min (9.5 m/s).

Whilst the size of the jumps and the number of obstacles are similar for all one-day events within a certain class of competition, events vary considerably in terms of the physiological demands they place on a horse. Some cross-country courses are on near flat terrain, whilst others involve steep uphill and downhill gradients. Firm going may predispose to lameness in some horses, whilst soft going (after rain or even sand) can increase the effort by up to 30% and may also cause muscle and tendon injuries. You need to know what to expect before you take the horse to the competition and

select the events for young horses according to their level of skill and fitness training.

Three-day events are graded in terms of difficulty between one-star and four-star. There are only three four-star events per year in the world and these are Badminton (May), Burghley (September) and Rolex Kentucky in the USA (April). The dressage test in a four-star event would contain any of the movements required at advanced level. Day 2, the speed and endurance test, consists of two phases of roads and tracks (phases A and C), a steeplechase phase (phase B) (see Fig. 14.1) and finally the cross-country phase (phase D). Horses may cover a total distance of about 25.6 km (16 miles) during the speed and endurance phase. Phases A and C are ridden at a speed of 220 metres/min (3.7 m/s), usually in an active trot over a distance of between 4400 and 5500 metres in phase A and 6600–8800 metres in phase C. There is a compulsory 1-minute hold between phases A and B. The steeplechase involves riding at an average speed of 690 metres/min (11.5 m/s) over a course of up to 3105 metres (1.9 miles) including no more than ten steeplechase type fences. Unless the event horse can truly 'jump out of its stride' without decelerating too much in the approach to a steeplechase fence, the horse may well have to gallop at something nearer 800 metres/min (13.3 m/s) to make the time.

Following the second roads and tracks phase (phase C) there is a compulsory 10-minute halt

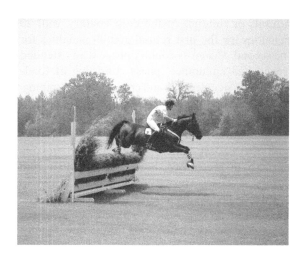

Fig. 14.1 The steeplechase phase of a three-day event.

before phase D, during which a panel consisting of a veterinary surgeon and two officials inspect the horse. The panel has the right to withdraw from the competition any horse which is unfit to continue. Phase D consists of a cross-country course of between 6840 and 7980 metres (4.3–5.0 miles) including a maximum of 45 jumping efforts of maximum height 1.20 metres. The course is ridden at a speed of 570 metres/min (9.5 m/s). There used to be a rule in three-day events that all horses had to carry a minimum of 75 kg (to include rider and tack) when on the speed and endurance phase. This meant that small riders would have to carry large amounts of lead in weight cloths to make up the load. Clayton (1997) demonstrated how the additional load caused the leading forelimb to land closer to the fence and also increased fetlock and carpal (knee) extension on landing. This was thought to increase the risk of suspensory desmitis and superficial digital flexor tendon strain; as a result the Minimum Weight Rule was abolished in 1998. The showjumping phase consists of a 500–600 metre course of 11–13 elements (up to 16 jumping efforts) of a maximum height 1.20 metres to be ridden at 375 metres/min (6.3 m/s).

In international competitions horses are subject to a veterinary inspection before the start to check that they are fit to compete and then on the morning of the final day to check that they are still sound following the cross-country. As part of this process horses are trotted approximately 40 metres and back on a hard, level surface.

Physiological and biomechanical demands of eventing

A study by Deuel (1995) carried out during the dressage test of the Barcelona Olympics showed that horses with longer stride lengths and faster speeds in the extended canter tended to receive higher marks, although unfortunately this was also correlated with non-completion of the cross-country phase! Possibly the horses that truly excel in the dressage test are unlikely to also excel in the cross-country test. This may be because the dressage judges will look for an elevated gait with large vertical displacement of the body, whereas to excel in the speed and endurance phase a horse should have an economical, ground covering stride.

On the first phase of roads and tracks (phase A), typical heart rates are approximately 100–120 beats/min, i.e. completely aerobic. The first phase of roads and tracks acts as a warm-up opportunity for the steeplechase phase, so there is no need to trot or canter horses around for long periods of time before starting phase A. However, walking the horses for 20 minutes or so before the start will enable them to stretch and may help to keep them relaxed. A short period of canter during the first roads and tracks itself can be used to try and achieve full splenic contraction, thereby maximising the aerobic energy contribution on phase B. Deuel and Park (1993) showed that horses in the steeplechase phase of the Seoul Olympics three-day event had an average speed of 726 metres/min (12.1 m/s), with the higher placed horses having speeds of between 780 and 858 metres/min (13.0–14.3 m/s). Superior performance in this phase was also associated with a long stride length.

On the steeplechase (phase B), heart rates could be anything from approximately 170 to 220 beats/min (see Fig. 14.2), indicative of a fair degree of anaerobic activity as is also evident from blood lactic acid concentrations as high as 25 mmol/l at the end of this phase. The second phase of roads and tracks (phase C) is designed to allow the horse to recover from the steeplechase before tackling the cross-country. Adequate recovery, of course, depends on the fitness and athletic ability of the horse, but other factors may also play a role. A good strategy is to finish the steeplechase, carry on in

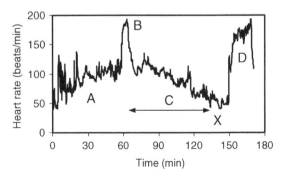

Fig. 14.2 A typical heart rate trace from Burghley three-day event speed and endurance phase. A, roads and tracks; B, steeplechase; C, roads and tracks; X, 10-minute box; D, cross-country.

canter bringing the speed slowly down until the horse is in a trot, and eventually bringing the horse back into a walk. Some riders are able to do this over the whole of the second phase of roads and tracks so that the horse walks into the 10-minute box. Soft going on phase C due to sandy soil or heavy soft ground can slow recovery as can hot or hot and humid conditions.

On the cross-country phase, heart rates can fluctuate anywhere between 140 and 200 beats/min (see Fig. 14.3). Anaerobic pathways supply the bursts of energy required to negotiate the obstacles, including jumping, turning and acceleration, but the extent of anaerobic contribution will depend on how athletic and how fit the horse is and also on how the horse is ridden. A rider who changes pace quickly coming into a jump and then kicks on hard coming away from jumps to make up lost time will demand greater anaerobic contribution from their horse than the rider who maintains a steady pace round the whole course. Experienced horses are likely to complete the cross-country phase with a

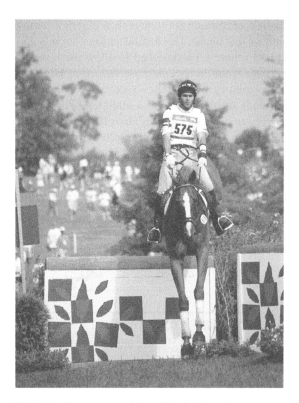

Fig. 14.3 Cross-country (phase D) of a three-day event.

steadier heart rate than a novice horse, as the experienced horse and rider are more likely to go in a good rhythm. A horse that pulls strongly and fights the rider will use up a lot more energy than the horse that simply 'cruises' around the course. On completion of cross-country, blood lactate levels are usually anywhere from 3 to 30 mmol/l.

Fitness for horse trials

Event horses are required to excel in three very different phases of competition. The event horse requires a good aerobic capacity, coupled with suppleness, power and agility. The training programme of the three-day event horse is probably one of the most intensive of any equine sport in that it requires the horse to be trained up to advanced medium level in dressage, and also be talented and skilled enough to jump in three quite different jumping tests (steeplechase, cross-country and showjumping).

It is often stated that 'event horses can't showjump'. Certainly, in comparison to top level showjumping, eventers do not jump nearly such demanding tracks in terms of fence height and spread or technical difficulty. With the emphasis on success in the cross-country test, it is the different style of jumping and the degree of care necessary by the horse that seem to present problems in the showjumping phase. Event riders often seek help from pure showjump trainers to try and improve, although many horses have reached top level competition despite a weakness in this phase. The cross-country is the only aspect of a one-day event that requires specific fitness training. A Thoroughbred would not require much specific fitness training to compete in events up to novice level, because much of the skill training that would be necessary to prepare the horse for the showjumping and cross-country would provide sufficient fitness. Once horses are competing at intermediate level and above, specific training would be required for the cross-country phase and/or speed and endurance test.

Endurance

Endurance racing in horses is the equivalent of marathon running in human sport. The maximum distance covered in competition is 160 km (100 miles) at average speeds of up to 20 km/h (12.5 m.p.h.) in some desert races. Average speeds are very much dependent on the environmental conditions, terrain and ground conditions. Shorter distances such as 100 km (62.5 miles) may be covered at speeds of 500 metres/min (8.3 m/s), only 20 metres/min less than novice eventing cross-country speed. Many people assume that endurance horses never need to go above a trot – this is quite wrong.

In the UK rides are organised by the Endurance GB (EGB). International endurance competitions are run under FEI rules. The majority of top level endurance rides are race rides (gated rides) where there is no optimum time and it is literally the first horse over the line that wins (subject to passing the final vetting). Set-speed rides, in contrast, are performed in an optimum time, with awards being given according to the average speed achieved and the horse's condition as judged by the officiating veterinary surgeon at the veterinary inspections. The ultimate in endurance competition is the 100 mile (160 km) ride.

Under EGB rules, horses have to complete a series of progressively difficult set-speed rides to qualify for the ultimate test of 100 miles. Rides are graded from the shortest bronze buckle rides, through to silver stirrup and finally gold stirrup. Horses must be at least 5 years old to compete in bronze buckle rides (and they are considered to become 1 year old on the 1st January following the year in which they were foaled). The maximum competitive distance for a 5-year-old is 416 km (260 miles). The bronze buckle qualifiers (BBQ) are held over 32 km (20 miles), and ridden at a speed of between 6 and 8 m.p.h. (i.e. between 160 metres/min and 213 metres/min). Riders competing in BBQs are not required to have a 'crew' as back-up. The bronze buckle finals (BBF) are held over 48 km (30 miles) at the same speed, but for these a helper is compulsory.

Silver stirrup qualifiers (SSQ) are held over 64 km (40 miles) to be completed at a minimum speed of 10.4 km/h (6.5 m.p.h.) excluding the half-way halt of 30 minutes with a vetting at 20 minutes. The silver stirrup finals (SSF), for which horses must be aged 6 years or above, are over 80 km (50 miles) to be ridden at a minimum speed of 10.4 km/h (6.5 m.p.h.) with a halfway halt of 30 minutes with a vetting at 20 minutes. There are compulsory 30-minute halts halfway on the route of most set-speed rides of over 30 miles in one day.

Horses may only attempt a gold series ride provided they have successfully completed 1 × BBQ, 1 × BBF, 2 × SSQ and 1 × SSF (or an endurance ride (ER) organised by an approved endurance riding society of 80 km (50 miles) at minimum speed of 10.4 km/h (6.5 m.p.h.) or more, i.e. a total of 288 km (180 miles) in competition. It may therefore take 2–3 years to get a horse to gold series level. Once a horse has achieved gold series status it is eligible to enter any category of ride, including race rides.

Gold series rides are held over a minimum of 96 km (60 miles) at a minimum speed of 10.4 km/h (6.5 m.p.h.). Some of the most difficult rides in the UK are the Golden Horseshoe (160 km over 2 days), the White Rose (160 km in a day) and the Tattersalls ride (140 km in a day). Only gold series horses, i.e. those that have done a qualifier of 64 km (40 miles) at a minimum speed of 11.2 km/h (7 m.p.h.) are eligible to compete in the Golden Horseshoe. To win a gold award, the horse must complete the 160 km (100 mile) ride with no penalties at a minimum speed of 12 km/h (7.5 m.p.h.) and a pulse rate not exceeding 56 beats/minute after 20 minutes and after 30 minutes at the finish. There are also silver and bronze awards.

At endurance rides or 'race rides' run over a variety of distances, the winner is the competitor with the fastest total time taken (excluding the compulsory halts) and whose horse passes the final vetting. In this case it is the horse with the fastest time that wins. The minimum speed for these events (unless otherwise stated) is 9.6 km/h (6 m.p.h.).

Selecting the endurance horse

A very good endurance horse is the equine equivalent of the marathon runner, a lean, wiry individual who covers the ground effortlessly. The endurance horse should resemble an almost two-dimensional, rather than a three-dimensional figure, i.e. as angular as possible, not barrel-shaped, as this sort of shape enables them to lose heat more easily. They are usually quite small, around 152.4 cm (15 hands), a factor that also contributes to effective heat loss. The bigger the horse, the more difficult it becomes for them to lose heat, as big horses have a relatively lower surface area to body mass ratio. They should have excellent lower limbs and feet, and be capable of extending their gaits easily. It is imperative that the endurance horse has as near perfect foot balance as possible, with well trimmed and well shod feet. The endurance horse should be capable of a 4–5 m.p.h. walk (120 metres/min). Horses with naturally bold, forward thinking temperaments are best. Many of the top endurance horses are Arabs or Anglo-Arabs. Thoroughbreds are also successful, but are less likely to have such good feet as the Arab. However, more and more breeds are being introduced into endurance. One of the reasons endurance has become so popular is that anyone with a well conformed horse that moves reasonably well can compete seriously provided they do sufficient preparation.

Physiological demands of endurance

It has been estimated that aerobic energy pathways contribute 95% or more of the total energy cost for an endurance ride. Good endurance horses should have a naturally high aerobic capacity. This means muscles low in type IIB fibres, small fibres, good capillary supply and a large heart with relatively thin walls to give a large stroke volume. In peak condition an endurance horse should be able to work at 170 beats/min before reaching the lactate threshold. Throughout the course of an endurance ride blood lactates do not usually reach more than 10 mmol/l, and this is often only the case as a result

of a fast finish. Heart rate on average for the whole ride would be in the region of 120–140 beats/min (see Fig. 14.4). For a horse in a 160 km (100 mile) ride in warm conditions, around 100 litres of sweat may be lost. Therefore to have a horse that drinks readily and frequently is considered an advantage. Large amounts of electrolytes are also lost and muscle and liver glycogen stores can become depleted. A horse that is able to relax and eat well in the vet gates is also essential.

Veterinary inspections

Veterinary inspections are held before the start of the ride; at major rides this might be the day before the ride. At both gated rides and set-speed rides the heart rate and other parameters are taken in the vetting/trot up area. At bigger, international rides these parameters may be taken in the stable. After an initial resting examination, each horse is then trotted up (see Fig. 14.5). Any abnormalities in the normal gait are noted for a comparison to be made at later inspections, and any horses considered lame are eliminated.

Set-speed rides have veterinary checks, one at the halfway halt and one at the end of the ride. At set-speed rides the clock stops when you arrive at the vetting area and you 'present' 20 minutes after arrival at the halfway halt. If your horse is found to have a pulse rate of more than 64 beats/min (or the rate set on the day) at the time it is presented to the vet, it is eliminated. At race rides there are compulsory vet 'gates', where the clock runs until you 'present'. Pulse monitors are allowed in competi-

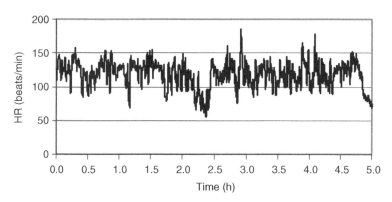

Fig. 14.4 Heart rates during an endurance ride.

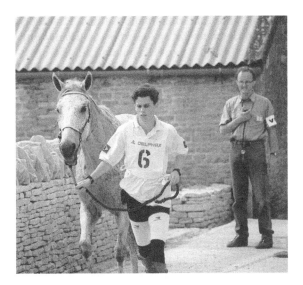

Fig. 14.5   Trotting up at the vet gate.

tion so it is possible to 'warm-down' into the vet gate. The principal member of the crew must be present at veterinary inspections.

At each vet check or gate the horse has a brief clinical examination that will include an evaluation of general condition in terms of lacerations and wounds, hydration status, and shoeing state. The horse also has to effectively perform a very short 'exercise test', which actually gives far more information about their physiological state of recovery than simply the absolute heart rate. The 'exercise test' consists of a heart rate measurement being taken before trotting in hand a set 30 metres away from the vet and back. As soon as the horse sets off, the clock starts and the heart rate is then taken exactly 1 minute after the horse set off on the trot course. In practice, this means the horse trots for 25–30 seconds, and then has 30 seconds or so to recover before the second heart rate reading is taken. This test is called the Ridgeway Test or the Cardiac Recovery Index. In set-speed rides any horse whose heart rate is over 64 beats/min at the second reading is eliminated. In race rides the horse will normally have to be presented to the vet within 20 or 30 minutes of arriving at the vet gate in accordance with the decision of the veterinary commission. If the horse fails the heart rate test only it may be re-presented to the vet. Rules regarding the re-presentation of a horse that fails the heart rate test

do vary slightly but are always published in the ride schedule and riders are notified of these at the briefing. If the horse fails on pulse then it is allowed to re-present providing there is time within the original 30 (or 20) minutes. For example if a horse presents at 20 minutes and the vetting took 4 minutes, the horse would have 6 minutes to re-present. A horse can literally fail at 28 minutes and walk straight back in and pass.

The Ridgeway Test is a fair test, as horses which trot faster, with higher heart rates, will have a longer time to recover, and horses which trot slowly have less time to recover, so individual differences in speed of trotting will balance out. Also, it is very easy for riders to practice this procedure outside the competition. When the horse has passed the vet gate of an endurance ride, it moves into a 'timed hold'. The hold time starts at the time at which the rider has requested to present the horse for the veterinary inspection, provided of course this was subsequently successful. A final vetting is also completed at the end of both set-speed rides and race rides. In set-speed rides the horse presents 30 minutes after completing the ride. In race rides the horse can present before 30 minutes have elapsed, but in this case is only allowed one presentation.

In contrast to eventing and many other equestrian disciplines, it is not uncommon for top riders to only have one top level horse at a time. The time input to the training of just one horse and the time spent in the saddle during competition usually means that riders are unlikely to be able to keep more than two horses at top level at any one time. Last but not least, the skill of the crew can contribute significantly to the performance of horse and rider on the day. A good crew will be skilled in keeping horse and rider fed, watered and adequately cooled throughout the race, and will have experience with that particular horse to know what to do in the event of loss of a shoe, etc.

Racing

Flat racing

Horseracing in the UK takes place both on the flat and over fences. Flat races are run mainly over anything from 5 to 16 furlongs (1000–3200 metres), and never over more than 23 furlongs (4600 metres). Within flat racing, there are sprinters (running under 1600 metres (1 mile)), middle distance horses (running around 1600–2400 metres (1–1½ miles)) and stayers running at 1900 metres (1¾ miles) and above. Top horses can do 5 furlongs (1000 metres) in under 60 seconds (16.6 m/s), 1600 metres (1 mile; 8 furlongs) in 99 seconds (16.2 m/s) and 1900 metres (1¾ miles; 14 furlongs) in 176 seconds (15.9 m/s) (Fig. 14.6). The fastest race time ever for a horse race in the UK was set in 1960 by Indigenous at Epsom on firm going who ran at an average speed of 18.7 m/s (1122 metres/min; 42 m.p.h.) over 5 furlongs (1000 metres). Most of the big prize money is for the prestigious middle distance races such as the Derby (2400 metres; 1½ miles).

Race times are strongly correlated with ground conditions or 'going', with firm ground producing the best times. Horses may be suited to a particular sort of going as a result of their conformation or their top speed. For example, a horse which has very upright forelimb conformation may be more likely to suffer concussion-related injuries on firm ground, and a horse with a higher, rounder action may have the advantage on soft ground. Horses with a relatively low top speed but lots of stamina will have the advantage over faster horses if ground conditions are soft or heavy. Flat racehorses are trained over short distances (usually no more than a mile (1600 metres)) and often uphill. During training horses will usually spend more of their time

walking and cantering than trotting. Fast work (three-quarter to full speed work) is usually only performed twice a week. Swimming may be incorporated into the horse's training programme to add variety to the work or to reduce concussive forces on the limbs whilst allowing the horse to maintain fitness during a period of injury.

Racing on turf takes place between March and the end of October. Thoroughbreds can begin their career on the flat as 2-year-olds when they can run in races of between 5 and 8 furlongs (1000–1600 metres). They are not allowed to race more than 5 furlongs (1000 metres) before the Derby in early June, and can only race over more than 6 furlongs (1200 metres) after August. The race preparation of the 2-year-old therefore takes place between the yearling sales in the October of the horse's first year and a few months of their second year. Thoroughbreds are all aged on the 1st January; hence the Thoroughbred breeding season is manipulated to try and produce foals as early as possible in the year so that they are as physically mature as possible by the time they get to the racetrack as 2-year-olds. Following a period of basic training and introduction to starting stalls, 2-year-olds may be doing some cantering work by the January of their second year. Pattern races or group races are the elite races in flat racing. Pattern races are divided into groups 1, 2 and 3, with the 'classics' the ultimate races in the flat racing calendar in Great Britain being group 1 races. The 'classics' are made up of the 1000

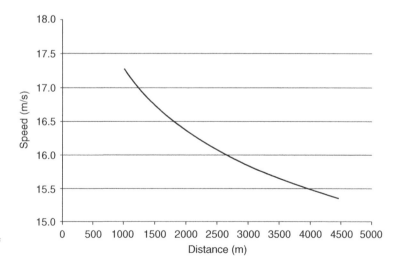

Fig. 14.6 Relationship between average running speed and race distance.

Guineas at Newmarket (for 3-year-old fillies) over 1 mile (1600 metres), the 2000 Guineas for 3-year-olds (colts and fillies) at Newmarket over 1 mile (1600 metres), the Derby for 3-year-old colts and fillies at Epsom over 1 mile 4 furlongs (2000 metres), the Oaks at Epsom for 3-year-old fillies over 1 mile 4 furlongs (2000 metres), and the St Leger at Doncaster for 3-year-old colts and fillies over 1 mile 6 furlongs and 132 yards (2920 metres).

National Hunt racing

National Hunt racing includes hurdling, steeple chasing and National Hunt flat races known as 'bumpers'. National Hunt races are held over longer distances than flat races; hence horses need rather more stamina and less top speed (running at speeds between 11 and 14 m/s). Steeplechasers are generally taller and bigger than flat racehorses, whereas horses bred for hurdling tend to be smaller and lighter than 'chasers. There are two types of National Hunt horse, those that have been specifically bred for the job and those that have entered National Hunt via flat racing. Many horses make the transition from flat to National Hunt via hurdling.

Steeplechases are held over distances between 2 and $4\frac{1}{2}$ miles (3200–7200 metres), with fences no lower than 4 feet 6 inches (1.37 metres) in height. Hurdles are over distances of $1\frac{3}{4}$–3 miles (1900–4800 metres) with hurdles no less than 3 feet 6 inches (1.07 metres) from the top bar to the bottom bar and give when hit. The hurdler will jump faster and flatter than the steeplechaser, the object of the exercise being to take as flat a trajectory as possible and maintain speed through the air. Horses cannot hurdle until 1st July in the year in which they are 3 years old, and cannot steeplechase until they are 4 years old. A horse that is bred specifically for National Hunt racing will probably be left a little later than the flat horse before being backed. For these horses that have not raced on the flat there is an opportunity to run in National Hunt flat races known as 'bumpers'. These are confined to 4-, 5- and 6-year-olds who have never raced 'under rules'.

The National Hunt season extends from November to May, although National Hunt racing runs to a lesser extent all year round. The main races of the National Hunt racing calendar are the Cheltenham Gold Cup ($3\frac{1}{2}$ miles (5600 metres)) held in March, the King George V Gold Cup at Kempton on Boxing Day, and the Grand National ($4\frac{1}{2}$ miles (6800 metres)) at Aintree in April. The best record in the Grand National was Red Rum, who won it three times in 1973, 1974 and 1977; he was also second in 1975 and 1976. Incidentally, Red Rum showed some form on the flat and over hurdles before his steeplechasing career. He dead-heated in a 5 furlong (1000 metres) seller in 1967 as a 2-year-old, was beaten by a short head over a mile (1600 metres) in 1968 and was second in the Lancashire hurdle in 1969, 4 years before he won his first Grand National. Winning speeds for the National average 750 metres/min (12.5 m/s or 28 m.p.h.), but can be nearer 650 metres/min (10.8 m/s or 24 m.p.h.) if the going is heavy.

The jumping element of National Hunt racing brings with it the risk of a whole different set of injuries to flat racing. Many of the injuries sustained by flat racehorses are incurred as a result of the training programme, whilst National Hunt horses are far more likely to be injured during the race itself. Jumpers tend to be susceptible to soft tissue injury, particularly tendon injury, whilst flat horses are more prone to bucked shins and fractures of the distal forelimb. National Hunt horses are trained over longer distances than flat racehorses and at lower speeds. The National Hunt horse will probably spend more time being exercised per day than the flat horse.

The best National Hunt horses are excellent jumpers, but it has been known for horses to do well in certain races despite the fact that they have made jumping errors such as taking off too early, too late, or pecking on landing. Whilst the National Hunt horse does not have to jump cleanly like the showjumper or cross-country horse, a good National Hunt jumper will be able to negotiate the fences without slowing down too much on approach, and landing in a balanced manner to achieve a fast getaway from the fence. Possibly due to the limitations of the measurement techniques for investigating jumping at speed, there is very little published research relating its kinematics; therefore we have a lot still to learn about what it is that makes a good National Hunt horse in terms of conformation and biomechanical characteristics.

Showjumping

The British Show Jumping Association (BSJA) is the governing body for the sport of showjumping throughout the UK. Showjumping is a test of gymnastic ability, power and, in some classes, speed. Horses receive penalties for either knocking fences down or for 'disobediences' such as refusing or running out. Horses also receive time penalties if they do not complete the course within the maximum set time. In jump-offs, horses are jumped either over slightly bigger fences or against the clock or both. Horses normally jump at speeds of between 300 and 450 metres/min.

Many top showjumpers are tall (167.6 cm; 16.2 hands plus) warmblood types bred specifically for the sport. Courses vary enormously in height and technical difficulty, but at top level the horse will be jumping courses up to 1.60 metres in the first round at speeds of between 300 and 400 metres/min (6.7 m/s). Horses are graded according to the prize money they have won: grade A, £1800+; grade B, £800 to £1799; or grade C, nil to £799. Ponies (animals standing up to 148 cm without shoes) are graded JA (£600+), JC (£50–£599) and JD (nil to £49). Ponies are not allowed to jump over 1.50 metres at any time.

The energy for showjumping is supplied by a combination of aerobic and anaerobic pathways, with the anaerobic component being synonomous with the powerful muscle contractions involved in the jump itself (Fig. 14.7). During such powerful contractions, the blood flow to certain areas of the muscle may actually cease transiently as blood is forced out into the venous circulation. A study by Art *et al.* (1990b) of the physiological response of horses to showjumping showed that heart rates start at approximately 150 beats/min at the beginning of a round and steadily increase throughout the round. Peak heart rates may reach over 190 beats/min and blood lactates may reach about 10 mmol/l, indicative of the significant anaerobic contribution. Due to the short duration of each showjumping round (often less than a minute) and the requirement for powerful muscular contractions, showjumpers are one of the few types of equine athlete that would not really benefit from more than a small amount of aerobic training.

Dressage

Dressage horses are required to perform dressage tests in walk, trot and canter, of duration 4–8 minutes. Within each of these gaits are specific gait types varying according to stride length, namely collected, working, medium and extended gaits (in order of increasing stride length). The exception is the walk, which does not have a 'working' variation. In a dressage test horses are required to perform

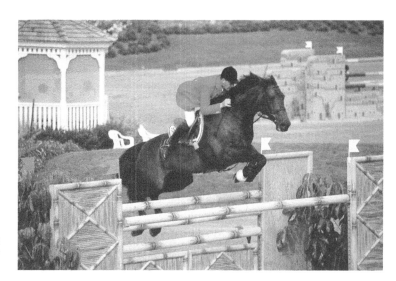

Fig. 14.7 In showjumping, the jumping efforts rely totally on anaerobic energy pathways.

up to 30 separate 'movements' which are given a score 1–10 (zero would be given if the movement were not actually performed). In addition there are marks awarded according to 'overall' qualities of the test, namely, freedom and regularity of paces, impulsion (i.e. the desire to move forward, elasticity of the steps, suppleness of the back and engagement of the hindquarters), submission (attention and confidence, harmony, lightness and ease of the movements, acceptance of the bridle and lightness of the forehand), rider's position and seat, correctness and effectiveness of the aids.

Horses from 4 years old embark on a progressive skill training programme, and are awarded points according to their performance in affiliated competitions run by 'British Dressage'. The number of points awarded is directly correlated to the total score the horse achieved for the test, with a maximum of 7 points awarded for a score of 67+.

Horses may compete at the level they are graded or higher as follows: preliminary (up to 37 points), novice (up to 74 points), elementary (up to 149 points), medium (up to 249 points) and advanced medium (up to 324 points). Advanced competitions are open to any horse. Horses tend to always work at home at one grade higher than that in which they are competing.

Little work has been carried out on the physiological demands of dressage, although Clayton (1989b) recorded heart rates of horses performing Grand Prix dressage tests of total duration 7½ minutes at an average speed of 2.34 m/s. Heart rates rarely exceeded 150 beats/min and higher heart rates did not necessarily correlate to work at the higher speeds, e.g. extended canter. These results suggest the dressage horse works primarily aerobically, but does not exclude the possibility that some lactate may be produced in the muscles during certain movements. Twelve per cent of the time was spent in medium and extended trot and canter. In comparison, a study of horses competing in the dressage test of a one-star three-day event showed mean heart rates during the test of 92 beats/min in environmental conditions of 33°C shade temperature, 49% RH, 45°C black globe temperature, 0.5 m/s windspeed and a WBGT Index of 30.7. Following warm-up, mean loss of body mass was 1.7 kg (0.3% body mass). Mean body mass loss as a result of the test itself was 2.3 kg (0.4% body mass) and

rectal temperature increased from 37.3 to 38.3°C after the warm-up and to 38.8°C by the end of the test. Plasma concentrations of sodium and total protein, and blood packed cell volume were all increased compared to before the test. It is likely that in cool conditions these changes would be much less, but higher level tests, i.e. top level pure dressage, in cool conditions could result in changes similar to these.

Clayton (1993) has suggested that during training dressage horses should work in concentrated periods approximately equal to the duration of the test (determined by the level at which the horse is working) with rest intervals in between where movements such as circles and lateral work (to develop suppleness) are performed. In the work periods, frequent transitions between and within gaits should be performed, and brief (up to 12 second) bursts of extended trot and canter included.

A useful addition to the exercise programme of the dressage horse is passive stretching. These exercises should be performed following thorough 'warm-down' in walk, yet whilst the muscles are still warm following the main exercise period. A suitable time would be on return to the stable about 20 minutes following the end of the main work session. A carrot can be used to encourage the horse first to bring its nose to its knees, between its legs, then to its ribs, and finally to its flank (either side). Forelimbs can also be raised, stretched (forwards) and held for a couple of seconds before releasing. If these stretches are carried out correctly on a daily basis, they can help to improve a horse's range of movement, as well as being a useful indication to the rider as to the horse's suppleness at any point in the training schedule.

Polo

Polo is thought to be one of the oldest ball games and originated over 2000 years ago in ancient Persia. It is played on a grass pitch 300 yards (274 metres) long by 200 yards (183 metres) wide with four players on each of two teams. Polo involves short bursts of fairly high intensity exercise. The 'ponies' used are usually around 152.4 cm (15 hands), often Thoroughbred types. Each game consists of four (occasionally six) chukkas. The actual

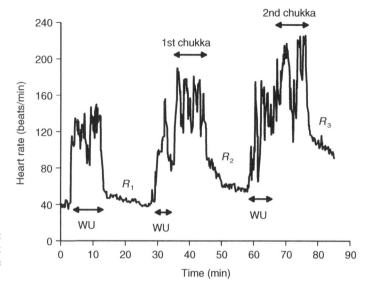

Fig. 14.8 Heart rates during a polo match: WU, warm-up; R, recovery period. Note that heart rate recovery becomes slower after the second chukka.

playing time in each chukka lasts 7.5 minutes, but with the watch stopped for penalties or the ball going out of play, the time may extend to 10 minutes or more. Players must change ponies every chukka, so you can compete with two ponies, riding one in the first and third chukkas and the other in the second and fourth. However, at the higher levels of polo, players will have a fresh pony for each chukka. Exercise intensities constantly change throughout the chukka; horses work at heart rates of approximately 170 beats/min but may reach

maximum heart rates for short periods of time (Fig. 14.8). In one study of low-goal polo it was found that around 16% of total playing time was above 90% of maximum heart rate and that peak heart rates in individual horses during play ranged from 203 to 222 beats/min (Martin *et al*. 1999). Given its profile and popularity, it is perhaps surprising that there is so little information published on the demands of polo. Preparation for polo usually involves lots of canter work (often performed as ride and lead exercise) and skill training.

KEY POINTS

- One-day events consist of a dressage test, a showjumping test and a cross-country test in that order, with competitions at all levels from intro to advanced.
- Three-day events consist of dressage, a speed and endurance test made up of phase A (roads and tracks), phase B (steeplechase), phase C (roads and tracks) and phase D (cross-country). Three-day events are organised at four international levels, 1-star CCI*, 2-star CCI**, 3-star CCI*** and 4-star CCI****.
- The maximum speed eventers are required to produce is 690 metres/min in the steeplechase

phase of a 4-star three-day event, when they will be working at heart rates between 170 and 220 beats/min.
- The ultimate competitive endurance test for horses is 160 km (100 miles) in a day.
- There are two main type of endurance events, set-speed rides and race rides. In set-speed rides, riders must complete within a set-speed range; in race rides the winner is the first horse and rider over the line (subject to successful vetting).
- Horses must be 'gold series' horses before they can compete over 100 miles, having completed

$1 \times$ BBQ, $1 \times$ BBF, $2 \times$ SSQ and $1 \times$ SSF (or equivalent).

- Satisfactory completion of an endurance ride is dependent upon veterinary inspections at vet checks (set-speed rides) and vet gates (race rides). The veterinary inspection includes the Ridgeway Test (or cardiac recovery test) whereby the horse's heart rate is recorded before a 30 second trot-up and then 1 minute after the start of the trot-up.
- Flat races are held over 5–23 furlongs (1000–4600 metres) with sprinters running less than 8 furlongs (1600 metres) and stayers running over 14 furlongs (2800 metres) or more. Flat horses race at speeds between 15 and 17 m/s.
- National Hunt racing includes National Hunt flat races (bumpers), hurdling and steeplechasing. Steeplechasing involves bigger fences (4 feet 6 inches or 1.37 metres) and longer distances (up to $4\frac{1}{2}$ miles or 7200 metres) than hurdling, and steeplechase horses are, on average larger than flat racehorses and hurdlers. National Hunt racing involves speeds of between 11 and 14 m/s.
- Showjumping at top level involves jumping obstacles of approximately 1.60 metres at speeds of approximately 450 metres/min. Showjumping involves both aerobic and anaerobic energy production.
- Dressage is a predominantly aerobic sport with horses' heart rates rarely reaching 150 beats/min. The average speed in a dressage test is less than 3 m/s and the duration of the test may be up to approximately 8 minutes.
- Polo involves bursts of high intensity exercise, producing mean heart rates of approximately 170 beats/min and occasionally reaching maximum heart rate during 'chukkas' of between 7.5 and 10 minutes.

Chapter 15

Training principles

Horses are natural athletes

Before we put all the theory into practice and embark on a training programme, it is encouraging to know that all horses have the potential to respond favourably to training. Remember that we have already learned that horses are born with a capacity for sprinting, but we also know that with appropriate training they can also excel at endurance events. As individuals, they vary in the extent to which they are or can be trained to be suited to different sports, but all horses have inherent athletic capabilities that are far superior to most other mammals and even to other athletic species such as the dog, human and camel. On a purely biomechanical level, horses have an energy efficient gait, with relatively little vertical displacement of the body at high speeds, compared with dogs or cats. They also have well developed biological springs in the form of the tendons that act as energy saving devices by storing energy during tendon loading in stance which is returned to the limb on lift-off.

On a physiological level, they have a very high aerobic capacity even when scaled for their size, i.e. per kg of body mass, as shown by the average and extreme values of $\dot{V}_{O_2max}$. As we have seen in Parts I and II, there are a number of factors which contribute towards the high $\dot{V}_{O_2max}$ of the horse of around 160 ml/min/kg, including high muscle mass (for example 200 kg for a 500 kg horse), splenic contraction (nearly doubling the number of circulating red blood cells during intense exercise) and high cardiac output (~240 litres/min during maximal exercise). The heart is usually large, around 1.0% of body mass, and may be as much as 1.3–1.4% in elite animals. The heart rate has a tremendous dynamic range, being able to increase from around 25 beats/min at rest to around 245 beats/min during maximal exercise. They have a high muscle:bone ratio and large proportion of the total body mass is muscle. In peak condition, they may have as little as 4% body fat. Horses are unusual in that they excel in both aerobic and anaerobic activities; not only do they have an abnormally high $\dot{V}_{O_2max}$ but they have a much greater percentage of type II fibres and a high anaerobic capacity (compared to human athletes), and can tolerate lactate concentrations in blood of over 30 mmol/l. They also have a high thermal tolerance, being able to dramatically reduce skin blood flow to increase muscle blood flow and tolerate muscle temperatures of 46°C, pulmonary artery blood temperatures of over 43°C and rectal temperatures of over 42°C. Not only can they tolerate high body temperatures, they have also evolved to have the highest sweating rate of any animal. They can rapidly increase their blood adrenaline concentrations to 10 or 20 times those of human athletes. However, the key to unlocking all this potential really comes down to training. Without training we are at best likely to achieve a mediocre performance and at worst, induce serious injury.

Training objectives

All athletes need to perform some form of training programme to prepare for their chosen sport. Regardless of the sporting activity, the aims of a training programme will include all or a combination of the following basic objectives:

(1) To increase stamina ('endurance') or aerobic capacity
(2) To increase speed
(3) To increase muscular strength
(4) To delay the onset of fatigue as a result of exercise, i.e. as a result of the increase in aerobic capacity and $\dot{V}_{O_2max}$ (see Fig. 15.1)

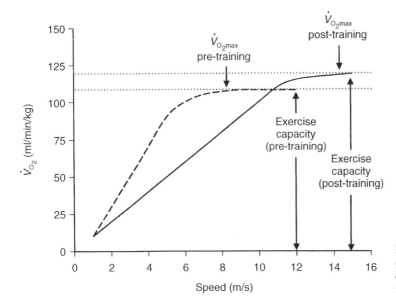

Fig. 15.1 Improvement in $\dot{V}_{O_2max}$ and exercise capacity with training. Exercise capacity represents maximum speed reached at the point of fatigue.

(5) To reduce the risk of musculoskeletal breakdown as a result of exercise
(6) To improve biomechanical skill and neuromuscular co-ordination
(7) To maintain the horse's willingness to work.

The training programme for any equestrian discipline will be aimed at achieving all of these objectives to a varying degree. For example, the racehorse trainer will spend a lot of time trying to improve the horse's speed and stamina, but very little time improving biomechanical skill.

If we include a final aim 'to improve the chance of winning' then it is clear that we must also start out with the right material. In order to perform well in a sprint race, a horse must have inherited certain characteristics that enable him to sprint, such as suitable conformation, a high proportion of type II (and especially type IIB) fibres and a competitive temperament. No amount of training is going to increase the top speed of an inherently slow horse, and no amount of skill training will turn a nondescript dressage horse into a medal winner. Training can, however, maximise your horses' performance and enable them to realise their full genetic potential, whatever that may be and however modest. When training a horse you never have a truly blank page as you are always starting with a unique mix of physiological and biomechani-

cal raw ingredients governed by the horse's individual genetic make-up. In addition, previous injuries or disease may also have an impact on how close you can get to a horse's individual genetic potential.

The extent to which training influences performance varies depending upon the sport. In a sport such as dressage, it is unlikely that the fitness of the horses competing will have a major bearing on final placings, but in a sport like endurance the degree of training of the cardiovascular and musculoskeletal systems is highly likely to influence the placing. As a general rule, the less technical the competition the greater contribution fitness training makes at the end of the day.

Training specificity

Fitness training should be specific to:

(1) The sport
(2) The individual horse.

Sport specific training means that you should mimic the competition as far as possible. It also means essentially that you should prepare for endurance competitions by training at low intensities for prolonged periods of time and for sprinting sports by training at high intensity for short periods of time. You should simulate the likely stresses and strains to which the horse will be subjected but without actually reproducing the competition workloads which are likely to increase the risk of musculoskeletal breakdown. For example, racehorse trainers may gallop horses two or three times a week, but if the horse is going to race over 1600 metres (1 mile) then they may only be 'worked' (galloped at race pace) over 800–1200 metres (4–6 furlongs).

Part of the skill in training is being able to walk the tightrope between adaptation and breakdown – being able to produce a horse fit enough to do the job, whilst subjecting them to minimum wear and tear along the way. Anyone can get a horse fit, but a good trainer can do it with minimal risk of injury and hence can produce a horse that wins not just that season but every season (see Fig. 15.2).

Training should be specific to the individual. In other words, training programmes should be tailored to the individual with a degree of flexibility. If the racehorse trainer has all his horses do exactly the same work every day, the horse with

natural stamina may never get to improve its speed or vice versa. The trainer should be sensitive to the individual horse's weaknesses and work specifically to improve them. A 'weakness' could be anything from a certain aspect of conformation such as poor feet in the racehorse (which may be improved by farriery), a tendency for a sore back (which may be helped by paying particular attention to the horse's outline, saddle fitting), a predisposition for tying-up (which could be addressed by a change to a high fat diet and never allowing complete rest days), or anything which needs to be borne in mind throughout the training programme. This is where the skill of the trainer can make a difference in minimising the impact of such weaknesses on the overall performance. Jenny Pitman writes in her autobiography about a horse she had managed to buy quite cheaply because he was a known box-walker. Box-walkers are difficult to keep 'weight on' and therefore not very easy to train. After buying the horse a goat as a stable companion he stopped box walking and was sold at a profit after he won every time out! Being aware of even minor behavioural idiosyncrasies may be the difference between get-

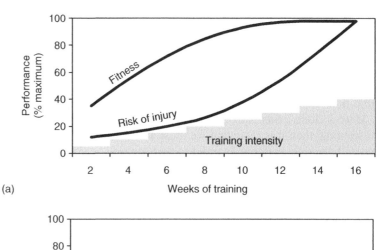

Fig. 15.2 (a) Relationship between training intensity, fitness, performance and injury risk. Note that the risk of injury increases as the training intensity increases. (b) If a low training intensity is maintained over a prolonged period, one might expect that the risk of injury would not increase with time (dotted line); however, the duration of training also has an implication for increasing risk of injury through wear and tear.

ting an okay performance from a horse and getting an outstanding performance. These things come with experience of training and managing horses.

Identify the challenge

The first thing to do when designing a training programme is to identify the demands of the competition. For example, the novice eventer will have to gallop at 520 m/min for 5 minutes, and the endurance horse might have to travel at around 16 km/h (10 m.p.h.) for 160 km (100 miles). Will these horses need to improve their stamina, their speed, their strength or all three (see Fig. 15.3)? Stamina can be translated as aerobic capacity, whilst speed and strength are associated with anaerobic capacity. No sport relies purely on one to the complete exclusion of the others, but you need to identify which is the most important. Sports may be described as being 50% aerobic and 50% anaerobic, meaning that 50% of the energy required to do the job is provided aerobically. This method of describing the contribution of each energy pathway is known as energy partitioning (see Chapter 2). The good news is that nearly all horse sports are predominantly aerobic, so we know that the first thing to do in the training programme of any horse is to improve their aerobic capacity.

As a rough guide, to improve aerobic capacity one should train at around a heart rate of 150–180 beats/min. To improve aerobic and anaerobic simultaneously, you should train above 150–180 beats/min (see Fig. 15.4). For racehorses you will need to train nearer 200 beats/min to train both aerobic and anaerobic capacity. Whilst human athletes such as weightlifters may train specifically for improvement in anaerobic capacity, it is actually quite difficult to specifically improve anaerobic capacity in horses. Just about all the work we do with horses tends to improve aerobic capacity and probably to a lesser extent anaerobic capacity, even

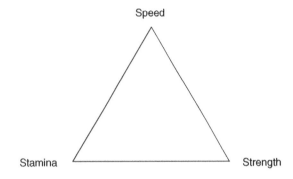

Fig. 15.3 Speed, strength and stamina triangle.

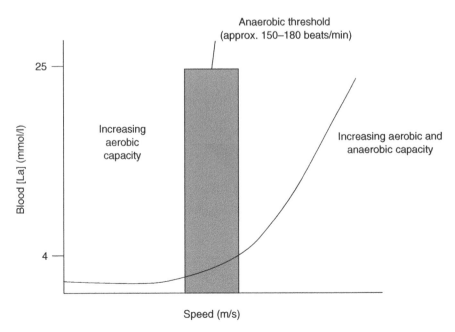

Fig. 15.4 Optimum training thresholds.

if we are specifically aiming to improve the anaerobic component of the performance. It is far more difficult to train for pure increases in strength and speed in horses than it is in humans. The main reason for this is that the strength training for a human weightlifter and speed training for a human 100 metre runner involves large amounts of work in the gym with weights. The only real equivalent for strength training in horses might be very short interval work with repetitions of 100 metre sprints or draught work pulling a very heavy weight.

In any horse sport, the percentage of the total energy requirement that is provided by aerobic pathways tends to be greater than for the equivalent sport in humans. Human athletes running over 100 metres in 10 seconds (a true sprint) work about 95% anaerobically. The equivalent of a true sprint in horse sports might be barrel racing where the horse works flat out for 10–12 seconds and which is probably nearly 90% anaerobic. Even in Quarter horse races over 400 metres the anaerobic contribution falls to around 80% because the horses are working for around 20 seconds.

The contribution of aerobic ATP synthesis is greater in horses than humans exercising maximally for similar duration. One reason for this may be because horses are able to increase their rate of oxygen consumption faster at the onset of exercise under certain circumstances than humans; furthermore, horses also have a much higher maximal oxygen uptake. In the first few seconds of a race all the energy comes from ATP and PCr stored within the muscle. This is quickly supplemented with energy from anaerobic glycolysis and lactate formation. The amount of anaerobic energy needed at the start will therefore depend on how quickly the aerobic pathways can be accelerated. Therefore the faster you can accelerate the aerobic pathways up to full speed the lower the potential contribution from anaerobic pathways. At the onset of exercise, oxygen demand exceeds oxygen delivery because it takes a certain amount of time to match supply with demand for the following reasons:

(1) Aerobic means of energy production take longer to accelerate than anaerobic means
(2) The cardiovascular system, responsible for delivering oxygen to working muscle, takes a certain amount of time to respond fully to a

rapid increase in demand for blood flow at the muscles.

As a result of this delay, an oxygen deficit occurs at the onset of exercise (Fig. 15.5). However, horses are better than humans at matching supply to demand early on in an exercise bout and so their overall anaerobic energy demand for any given piece of work tends to be lower than that for humans. Horses reach 95% of their maximal oxygen uptake after only 1 minute of maximal exercise (Rose *et al.* 1998).

Training intensity, frequency, duration and volume

Training intensity is a measure of the rate of energy expenditure during an exercise period and is largely determined by the speed of travel, but also by factors such as ground conditions (heavy, soft ground may increase work by up to 20–30%), load carried (increased load = increased work), terrain (horses will have to work harder going uphill) and air resistance (headwinds make work harder). The duration of the workload is given by the time spent exercising in any one session, and the frequency describes how many times that piece of work was carried out in a given time-scale. The ideal training programme for a horse is given by the correct intensity of work, lasting the correct duration and carried out with a frequency that allows sufficient time for recovery between training bouts but induces a

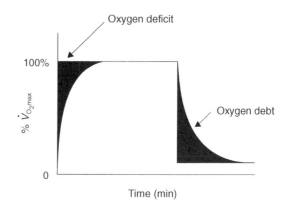

Fig. 15.5 Oxygen debt and oxygen deficit.

training response. The volume of work to be done in any given time-scale is thus given by

$$\text{Intensity} \times \text{Frequency} \times \text{Duration}$$

Knowing this all the trainer has to do is administer it. Sounds easy doesn't it?

Unfortunately scientists are not yet able to 'prescribe' the correct combination of the above factors, and to a large extent a trainer has to work it out for themselves, as any one prescription could not possibly work for all horses in all situations for all disciplines. Too high an intensity may produce the wrong type of training response (e.g. an increase in speed when an increase in stamina was desired), too low a frequency (e.g. galloping only once a week) may produce no training response, whilst too high a frequency may increase the risk of injury, and exercising for too long at a low intensity may use up energy and result in body mass loss, concussive injury but no increase in fitness.

Many other factors relating to the individual horse determine how much work needs to be done. Factors such as temperament, type or breed, inherent ability, inherent weaknesses and also those factors relating to the training situation, such as availability of gallops, frequency and timing of any qualifiers, climatic and environmental conditions, may all have an effect.

Training intensity is given by the rate of energy expenditure which correlates with the speed of running. How hard does a horse have to work to get a training response? In the early stages of training the horse will not have to work particularly hard for a training effect to occur, but later in the programme the horse will have to work much harder to get the same increase (see Fig. 15.6).

The intensity of the exercise can be most accurately judged by measuring the oxygen uptake of the muscles ($\dot{V}_{O_2}$). (Sometimes when $\dot{V}_{O_2}$ cannot be measured, for example in real competition, the heart rate or percentage of heart rate max is used instead to estimate the intensity.) When working at 100% $\dot{V}_{O_2\text{max}}$ (when heart rate will also be at a maximum), the horse is working at its maximum aerobic capacity. The horse can run or work at speeds above its $\dot{V}_{O_2\text{max}}$ (sometimes termed supramaximal exercise intensities, e.g. 130% $\dot{V}_{O_2\text{max}}$) but when doing so the horse has to meet the extra demand for energy entirely from increases in anaerobic energy generation.

Humans working at 10–20% of their maximal oxygen uptake ($\dot{V}_{O_2\text{max}}$) do not see improvements in either strength or endurance; however, when training at 50–90% $\dot{V}_{O_2\text{max}}$ a significant increase in aerobic capacity is seen. It is likely that in the initial stages of a work programme, working at intensities of only around 40% $\dot{V}_{O_2\text{max}}$ (approximates to trotting at 220 metres/min and heart rates around 100–130 beats/min) will produce training induced improvements in aerobic capacity over a period of 3–4 weeks, but as training progresses this intensity

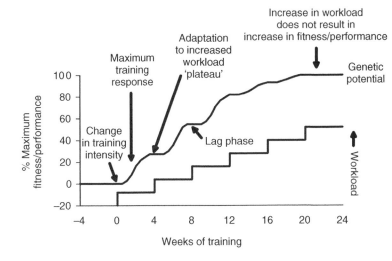

Fig. 15.6 In the early stages of training the horse will not have to work particularly hard for a training effect to occur. In the latter stages of a training programme an increase in workload may not produce an increase in fitness.

will have little effect on fitness and horses will probably need to work at intensities of around 70% $\dot{V}_{O_2max}$ (about 160 beats/min) or more to continue improving fitness. As the intensity of work increases throughout a training programme the volume of work done should decrease.

As the horse works harder (usually equivalent to faster, but could equate to the same speed up a steep hill) even though the majority of energy will still be obtained from aerobic pathways, more and more will be obtained from the anaerobic breakdown of glycogen to lactate. Because anaerobic breakdown of glycogen is rapid but less efficient than aerobic breakdown, the faster the horse goes, the faster the muscle glycogen stores are used up. The relationship between speed and glycogen breakdown is therefore not linear. This means that high intensity workouts should not be performed every day or the horse will not have sufficient time to replenish glycogen stores. A reduced muscle glycogen concentration before competition will almost certainly have a negative effect on performance, whether in events requiring short sprints or jumping or endurance.

Tapering for peak performance

Reducing training intensity before a major competition allows time for total tissue repair and full restoration of muscle glycogen stores. A taper period of 2 weeks has been shown to bring about a marked increase in muscle strength in human swimmers. Also there is a marked increase in the maximal shortening velocity (speed of contraction) of type II fibres following tapering. Although no studies have been done in horses which demonstrate the value of tapering, it may be a useful tool to apply in equine training programmes. Certainly, many endurance horses tend to perform a decreased volume of work before competition. Tapering ensures that glycogen stores in muscle are at a peak and that any minor damage to muscle fibres has had a chance to be repaired before the big day. Human runners and swimmers who reduce their training by about 60% for 15–21 days show no losses in $\dot{V}_{O_2max}$ or endurance performance. As well as physiological benefits there may well be psychological benefits of tapering in equine athletes.

Overtraining

Overtraining in human athletes is defined as a loss of performance despite the maintenance of an intense training effort. The symptoms of overtraining in human athletes are highly individual and are not fully understood, but is recognised as an important cause of loss of performance. Frequently the initial signs of overtraining are psychological changes such as mood swings, loss of appetite and anxiety. Whilst it is clear that overtraining occurs in human athletes and many racehorse trainers have the impression that something along these lines often occurs with horses in training, to date studies in horses have not been able to demonstrate the clear presence of a similar syndrome.

The symptoms of overtraining in human athletes include:

- Loss of performance, muscle strength and or co-ordination
- Decreased appetite and weight loss
- Increased muscle tenderness
- Head colds and allergic reactions
- Mood swings
- Increased resting heart rate and increased heart rate during submaximal exercise.

Overtraining in human athletes is thought to be the result of a combination of emotional (psychological) and physiological factors. Overtraining in human athletes is also associated with a steady increase of the heart rate during steady state exercise at an intensity where a stable heart rate would normally be expected, or an unusually high heart rate for any given piece of work. Strenuous training is associated with an increase in the circulating level of cortisol which in turn leads to suppression of immune responses. Highly trained and overtrained human athletes are thus particularly susceptible to infections. However, a number of researchers have tried to demonstrate immune suppression and other proposed indicators of overtraining in racehorses in training, but without success. To minimise the risk of overtraining, human athletes often use a cyclic training procedure whereby alternate easy, moderate and hard periods of training are performed. Many trainers structure their week on this basis in any case, such that in any one week there are two days of each type of work, with an easy day always following a hard day. For a horse that needs to maintain peak fitness for a long period of time, such as a racehorse, the training programme would be based on weekly cycles of easy, moderate and hard work. Riders and trainers also often use the approach of increasing volume and intensity up to competition, followed by a period of reduced volume and or intensity of training before gearing up for the next competition. In this way the horse is only maintained in full work for the shortest period needed, helping to reduce wear and tear.

If overtraining does truly exist in the horse, the failure to clearly demonstrate it to date most probably points to a psychological syndrome (boredom, stress, aversion) or the adverse effects on performance of undiagnosed subclinical conditions (mild lameness, respiratory disease) rather than a measurable or quantifiable physiological phenomenon.

Detraining

A great deal of knowledge of both human and equine detraining comes from clinical cases, where forced cessation of training has occurred due to injury or illness. In humans enforced detraining leads to a reduction in aerobic capacity and in level of skill, but muscle strength is unchanged even after several weeks. In other words, aerobic capacity is lost before anaerobic capacity. Losses of skill, including agility and flexibility, occur quickly, a fact which is often neglected because these skills are so quickly regained, but this can be dangerous because decreased flexibility leads to injury.

Studies of detraining in horses give conflicting results, suggesting that the rate and extent of loss of aerobic capacity depend on the level of fitness of the individual. It has been shown that horses maintain fitness following cessation of training longer than humans and require less work to maintain a relatively high level of fitness. In theory a lay-off of a couple of weeks (providing it was not due to injury of the structures being trained) should not set the horse back in its training programme apart from the inevitable loss of suppleness.

KEY POINTS

- The aims of training may include combinations of the following: increases in aerobic capacity, anaerobic capacity, speed, strength, biomechanical skill, co-ordination; delaying the onset of fatigue; decreasing the risk of injury; maintaining the horse's willingness to work.
- The importance of these factors will vary between different sports and activities.
- In training the horse, the aim is to get as close to the individual horse's genetic potential as possible.
- The impact of fitness as a result of training is greater the less technical the sport, i.e. it is low in sports such as dressage and high in sports such as endurance and racing.
- Training should be tailored to be specific to different sports and individual horses.

- Sport specific training means reproducing the demands of competition within training, but at a reduced duration or frequency.
- It is necessary to identify the demands of competition in order to construct an appropriate training programme.
- Nearly all horse sports are predominantly aerobic.
- Human athletes improve anaerobic capacity by short sprinting or work in the gym. It may be difficult to maximise anaerobic capacity in horses.
- Training intensity is determined by the rate of energy expenditure, which usually correlates with speed of running.
- Training intensity may also be influenced by factors such as ground conditions, weight carried,

terrain, air resistance and thermal environmental conditions.

- Training volume = intensity × duration × frequency.
- Increases in fitness are greater and occur more rapidly in the early stages of a training programme than towards the end.
- The intensity of a piece of exercise or work can be expressed as $\dot{V}_{O_2}$, percentage $\dot{V}_{O_2max}$, heart rate or percentage of maximum heart rate.
- When a horse is working at an intensity equivalent to maximal oxygen uptake, this is the maximal aerobic rate of working and any further increases in work (speed) must come totally from anaerobic energy pathways.
- Anaerobic energy pathways are gradually recruited from around 60–70% $\dot{V}_{O_2max}$.
- The minimum intensity to elicit a training response in a horse is probably around 40% $\dot{V}_{O_2max}$.
- Tapering is the process of reducing training volume before competition. In human athletes tapering has been shown to significantly improve performance and is carried out over a period of 2–3 weeks before competition with a reduction of around 40%.
- There are currently no studies of the effects of tapering on performance in horses.
- Overtraining is well defined and recognised in human athletes, but has not yet been clearly demonstrated scientifically to occur in horses.
- Detraining is the response to reduction in training volume or cessation of training.
- Horses detrain relatively slowly compared with human athletes.

Chapter 16

Training facilities

Training and racing surfaces

A wide variety of surfaces are used for training and racing horses throughout the world. Undoubtedly turf is one of the most suitable surfaces on which to exercise horses, but it is not durable enough to stand up to everyday use and is an inconsistent surface which varies enormously with environmental conditions. Increasingly, horses are trained on a range of surfaces, with many horses spending much of their time training on synthetic all-weather surfaces. To understand the desirable properties of a training or racing surface, we should consider the effect that the horses have on the surface and vice versa.

Hoof–surface interaction

In terms of the interaction between the hoof and the surface, we can think of the stance phase as comprising three subphases, a decelerative phase, a load-bearing phase and a propulsive phase. In the decelerative phase of the stance, the horse's limb is in front of the vertical and some deformation of the surface is required (but without break-up) to prevent slipping. 'Hard tracks' allow little deformation, and horses may slip if light rain wets the surface or turf growth is lush. A certain amount of slippage is normal and acceptable. This is borne out by the increased degree of injury seen using 'toe grabs' as they do not allow the foot to slip.

In the load-bearing phase, vertical impact forces are at a maximum, resulting in maximal compression or deformation of the surface. The foot of a galloping horse may penetrate the surface by 3–7 cm in this phase.

In the propulsion phase, the tip of the hoof rotates into the surface as horizontal forces come into action propelling the horse forwards. The propulsion phase ends with a flick of the hoof when it is unweighted, which may create divots if the soil or surface deforms or fails. If the surface deforms in this phase, 'kickback' of the surface occurs. Kickback is undesirable in both training and racing surfaces because high kickback is extremely unpleasant and off-putting for the horses and riders travelling behind.

A surface must be able to withstand both impact forces and shear forces. A material such as concrete has a high impact resistance, whereas wood chips have a low impact resistance and absorb the energy transmitted from the horse to the ground. The advantage of this is that concussive forces up the limb are reduced; the disadvantage is that less energy is returned to the limb to aid forward movement and thus the energetic cost of locomotion on a highly absorptive surface is high. A material with a low impact resistance makes the horse work harder, because more energy is lost to the surface each time the foot hits the ground. A surface with a high impact resistance is a 'fast' surface, and one with a low impact resistance is a 'slow' surface.

A surface with a low shear resistance, e.g. sand, allows the toe to penetrate on impact but moves on push off. A surface with a high shear resistance, e.g. firm turf, does not allow the toe to penetrate and increases the risk of slipping. The ideal surface has an intermediate shear resistance, which is low enough to allow the toe to penetrate as the hoof breaks over, but not so low as to slide away from the hoof as it pushes off at the end of the stance phase. Turf is pretty near perfect in this respect. Sand, which has a low shear resistance, can be stabilised by the introduction of fibres. The fibres act like a root system, increasing the shear resistance of the sand, and any kickback can be reduced by covering the surface with loose sand, watering and rolling.

There are a wealth of all-weather surfaces available for horses, incorporating components such as polypropylene fibres (long and short), washed silica sand (washed to remove dust and therefore do not create dust when ridden on), polyethylene fibres (long and short), PVC granules, polyester fibres, chopped rubber, and wood fibre. Many 'artificial surfaces' are wax coated to eliminate both dust and the need for watering. Wood chip surfaces are normally cheaper than synthetic surfaces but by their nature are less hard wearing, usually only lasting about 5 years. Synthetic surfaces are designed to be dust free with minimal kickback and minimal 'tracking' (i.e. horses do not easily cut out a track in an arena), not to change their properties significantly when subjected to both high and low temperatures, to require no irrigation and minimal maintenance.

Training gallops

Sufficient distance should be allowed to provide a warm-up canter (or there should be a separate warm-up facility) and sufficient pull-up. Rising ground is desirable, because horses can be worked harder at lower speeds, the vertical impact on the forelimbs is reduced, and it is easier to pull up. The width should be at least 3–4 metres; the wider the better. If there are sharp turns, wood fibre is not really an option because of its relatively low shear resistance. If running a gallop up a hill, it should be run diagonally rather than straight down; otherwise you can end up creating a river bed, with the bottom end saturated, and migration of surface material down the slope. By building a gallop across a hill, water runs off the track, not down it.

Kickback can be reduced by watering, using a surface which is bonded by oil or monofilament fibre, covering with loose sand and rolling, or by using a large particle material, such as wood chips or rubberised fibre which kicks up but does not go very high. The danger of using very large particle material is that strain injuries and even back injuries are more likely because the particles move underfoot during the stance phase of the stride. This is one of the disadvantages of large pieces of wood chip and may be a problem when such a surface is newly laid, although many trainers find

wood chip to be a satisfactory surface once it has settled in.

Racing surfaces

Thoroughbreds race on turf in Europe, South Africa, Australasia and South America. There are 59 racecourses in Great Britain (60 if you count Newmarket twice because it has two flat courses, the Rowley Mile and the July course), between them holding 1000 fixtures each year. The number of race days varies between courses from as few as 10 up to 30. Following the loss of so many days' racing due to bad weather, it was deemed necessary to pursue the idea of running on all-weather surfaces. In addition to being able to race all year round, all-weather courses stand days of racing at a time. Currently there are three all-weather surfaces in the UK; the first all-weather race was at Lingfield Park in October 1989 on an Equitrack surface. Southwell racecourse followed in November 1989 and Wolverhampton in December 1993, both of which are Fibresand surfaces. Lingfield has recently been updated with a new 'polytrack' surface. Whilst the introduction of all-weather surfaces has allowed the flat racing season to extend it has not attained the same status as turf racing.

Turf courses in Britain overlie conditions from sand to heavy soil. Typically, the soil 70–150 mm below the surface forms a compact layer on racetracks. Plants need to be pretty resilient to withstand all the bruising they receive during racing. Grass species such as perennial rye grass are quite resilient, whereas bents and fescues cope with occasional use, their advantage being that they require little fertiliser or irrigation, although they do not tolerate high wear. Ideally, grass should have a couple of weeks without use to recover from a meeting.

As the water content of turf increases, so does the shear damage, resulting in divots being cupped out of the surface. On very wet tracks, hooves may sink up to 200 mm below the compact top layer of the surface. This limits propulsion, slows down race times and tends to increase the risk of muscular injuries rather than skeletal injuries. Particular damage is done to a racing surface on the bends, and at the end when horses decelerate. The worst damage is usually 2–3 metres in from the rail. Where there are jumps, troughs will be formed in front of fences and mounds behind.

The state of the going is announced by the clerk of the course in advance of the race day and at intervals before the race itself, as the state of the going can change in an afternoon. There are seven official states: hard; firm; good to firm; good; good to soft; soft; heavy. Contrary to what one might expect, the number of injuries suffered on soft and heavy going is actually less than on hard or firm ground; this is probably because the average speed is reduced on softer going and it is speed which tends to correlate with injury rate.

All-weather surfaces are generally firmer and therefore 'faster' than turf and this led to an unusually high number of injuries whilst jumping on all-weather surfaces; consequently all-weather jumping was suspended in 1994. The three recognised states of going on all-weather racecourses are: fast; standard; slow.

Considerations in the construction of racecourses and gallops

To move round a curve a horse must generate a centripetal force acting towards the centre of rotation which restrains its tendency to leave the arc. This it does by leaning inwards. When the horse is going left-handed, the left limb is adducted, and the lateral side of the hoof strikes the ground first.

$$\text{Centripetal force} \propto \frac{mv^2}{r}$$

where, m is the mass of the horse, v is its velocity (speed) and r is the radius of the curve around which it is travelling. In other words, the tighter the curve and the faster a horse gallops, the greater the centripetal force which must be generated. The degrees of banking required for travelling at different speeds around bends of different radii to allow the horse's feet to land squarely are known, but courses are still rarely banked. Alternatively, transition curves may be used to reduce the centripetal force.

Treadmills

Both low speed (on which horses walk and trot only) and high speed equine treadmills are available (see Fig. 16.1). Low speed treadmills are used for carrying out controlled exercise (often on an incline) in walk and trot and are owned by many

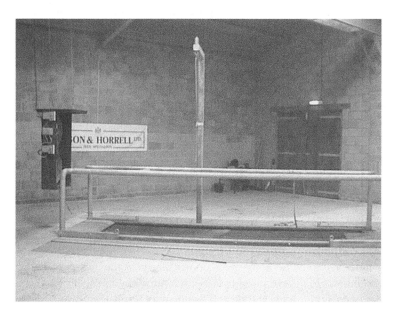

Fig. 16.1 High speed treadmill.

large yards. They cost in the region of £5000 to £10000. High speed treadmills are used mainly by clinicians and researchers and cost between £40000 and £60000. High speed treadmills are capable of inclining to around 10% (6°), which allows the intensity of the work at any given speed to be increased. Treadmills are useful for exercising a horse when you have no suitable rider, for rehabilitation following injury, to control the workload, to progressively load, and to work in a straight line. In this respect they often provide a more suitable mode of exercise than the horsewalker.

The disadvantage of treadmills compared with the horsewalker is that only one horse can go on a treadmill at a time. Treadmill exercise is not a substitute for ridden work but they are very useful to provide hill work, and if a high speed treadmill is available, to provide fast work when ground conditions prohibit working outdoors. However, horses do not compete on treadmills, and therefore it goes against the rules of specificity to do too much of your work on a treadmill. Furthermore, some people believe it can be rather boring for the horse, this is not necessarily true because, unlike us, many horses like to have a very fixed routine.

Quite a large building is needed to accommodate a treadmill, to allow enough room for safe loading and unloading. High speed treadmills are longer than low speed treadmills to accommodate the longer stride of the horse at high speed. High speed treadmills are approximately 6 metres long and 1.2 metres wide. The treadmill consists of a steel plate covered with a rubber belt. The life expectancy of the rubber belt is about 2–3 years if it is in use daily by shod horses. High speed treadmills are very noisy, to the extent that it is difficult to speak to other people in the treadmill room once the horse is galloping. The noise of the horse's hooves hitting the belt often raises concern about the concussion to the horse's limbs whilst running on the treadmill, but injuries on high speed treadmills are quite rare. Concussion is reduced by inclining the treadmill. The high speed treadmill provides an even, level footing, an advantage of the treadmill surface which may outweigh the fact that it is hard. Treadmills used for clinical exercise testing may have a top speed of up to 16m/s (35m.p.h.) and should accelerate to top speed within a matter of seconds. For any canter or gallop work, a safety harness should

be used to support the horse if he stumbles or suddenly loses ground on the treadmill. The harness is linked to an automatic trip switch, so the power to the belt cuts out if the harness takes the horse's full weight; the weight of the horse then very quickly decelerates the belt to a halt. In the event of this happening, the horse does not go flying forward as one might assume. A galloping horse on a treadmill has no momentum, and so the transition from gallop to halt is really quite unspectacular. When working horses on high speed treadmills there should be two handlers at the front of the horse (one each side to keep the horse straight), someone else to operate the treadmill, and possibly a fourth person towards the rear of the treadmill to help move the horse on if he moves too far towards the back. The horse should wear a bridle for control rather than a headcollar. For high speed work the horse will also need a sturdy leather surcingle to which the safety harness is attached. Neoprene boots that cover the fetlock and bell boots (overreach boots) should be worn all round for high speed work. Large fans are placed in front of the treadmill to provide air movement over the horse as in field conditions: the horse would get hot very quickly without these. There should be a buffer bar at the front of the treadmill to prevent the horse getting too far forward; this is normally padded as many horses will gallop right up against it. Horses can still pull quite hard, even on a treadmill. The horse's shoes should be checked before performing any fast work: because the rubber of the belt has a high coefficient of friction and 'grabs' the foot, shoes that would survive outside do not last long on a treadmill at high speed. It is vital to check for studs or road nails, as these literally shred treadmill belts.

Unless absolutely necessary, the handler should not stand directly in front of a horse when it is galloping because it tends to make them back off. It is also unwise to stand directly behind the treadmill because, even though the horse is not moving, if a shoe were to come off it would move with some speed. It is better not to have people coming in and out of the treadmill room when a horse is working at high speed, particularly if the horse is being exercised for research purposes, as higher levels of adrenaline and lactate may result, simply as a result of the horse becoming excited.

A successful protocol for introduction of a horse to treadmill exercise is as follows. The horse should be brought into the treadmill room and the fans switched on, so that it becomes accustomed to the noise. The horse is walked onto the flat treadmill. Before the treadmill belt starts, the horse is made to step backwards and encouraged with verbal commands to walk forwards to the bar a few times. Once the horse has got the right idea, the treadmill should be started just as it is about to step forwards. The horse may be unsteady for a few strides and spread all four legs wide, or even plant its feet, but will normally adapt within a matter of minutes. Horses normally canter in the first session quite happily but only once they are comfortable in trot. The horse should be trotted for at least 5 minutes or however long it takes to relax and start to move in a rhythmical gait. Low speed treadmills are used to produce controlled exercise without the need for a rider. They are very useful in the case of a horse who has had enforced rest, for example due to a tendon injury, as the horse can be made to do a set piece of exercise in a safe environment where it is unable to become too boisterous and risk further injury. As the treadmill can be inclined and it provides a uniform surface, it can be the ideal introduction back to work for the convalescent horse. It is preferable to lungeing or loose schooling because the horse's speed can be regulated and it works in a straight line. Horses can still be worked in tack on a treadmill, i.e. side reins, long reins to maintain straightness, etc.

Swimming pools

Swimming is a very popular addition to the training programmes of many racehorses. It can provide a fairly strenuous yet non-load bearing workout and is therefore is a very useful means of applying a training stimulus to the muscular, cardiovascular and possibly the respiratory system without any stress being applied to the skeletal system. It may be incorporated routinely into the training schedules of competition horses (mostly racehorses) or perhaps only used when work on the gallops is prohibited, for example due to lameness such as bruised soles or due to ground conditions being too soft or too hard. Many yards introduce all their horses to swimming so that it can be easily

incorporated into the programme as and when required.

The first pools for horses started appearing in England in the 1960s. Swimming became very popular in the 1980s, with pools being introduced into yards all over the country, but the cost of maintaining pools has led to a recent decline. Pools may be situated outdoors or indoors and are either circular or straight. Circular pools with separate entry and exit ramps might be considered the most flexible as these often have a 'straight' side with the straight forming one 'side' of the circuit. Horses can then be swam only along the straight side or around the circuit. Circular pools allow the horse to swim continuously. With straight pools the horse must come out, turn around and go back in at the end of each length or they must be tethered so they swim 'on the spot'. All pools should be at least 2.5m deep. A good-sized circular pool should be about 60 metres in circumference. A ramp that is 7m long with a 2.5m drop produces a suitable slope. The flooring of the ramp should be rubber matting and it should have vinyl padded sides. A non-slip metallic walkway around the outside is suitable for handlers. A central island is also provided for the handler, with moveable bridging between the island and the outside of the pool. This is most convenient when swimming continuously in a circular pool as the handler or handlers can be on either the inside or the outside of the pool.

For swimming, the horse should wear a nylon cavesson headcollar, and will need boots on all legs at least until it becomes accustomed to swimming, although horses are more likely to injure themselves getting in and out of the pool than when actually swimming. First-time swimmers may also be fitted with a tail rope to prevent them from somersaulting in the water. The first time the horse swims, it is normal to use only the straight side of a circular pool, the horse going straight in one chute and out the other side, before being walked round into the entry chute and swam for a circuit. This introduces the horse to the entry chute and the water more gradually. When introducing a horse to any new experience, it is better to do a little less than you think it is capable of on the first day, so that it is not unduly fatigued by the exercise. If you attempt to do too much in the first two or three sessions the horse may be reluctant to enter the pool on subsequent occasions. There are very few horses that can not be trained to swim successfully provided they are introduced carefully and slowly. The duration of the swim may be increased by perhaps one or two circuits each session.

Once a horse is introduced to swimming, it may swim 8–10 circuits of a 60 metre circumference pool in 4–5 minutes. Horses can be swam at a fast speed for a short time, e.g. 4–5 minutes, or at a more leisurely pace for 15 minutes, depending on the sport for which they are being prepared. Most horses are capable of building up to an hour of swimming, and National Hunt horses may swim for a longer period, swimming for perhaps two miles, changing direction frequently. The training value of swimming is increased if the horse is encouraged to swim at a reasonably fast pace.

Physiological effects of swimming

Swimming provides a medium to high intensity workout without subjecting the musculoskeletal system to high levels of concussive forces, and so making swimming part of a racehorse training programme (particularly for 2 and 3-year-olds) may reduce the incidence of problems such as bucked shins. Horses normally swim in a trotting gait but individual strategies vary enormously. Swimming is particularly popular as part of the training programmes of trotters and pacers because of the similarity of movements. The back of the horse will be held just under the surface of the water, the head will be raised and the nostrils shut except to inhale. Large thrusts from the hindquarters produce significant lumbosacral flexion in an effort to push forwards through the water. Swimming may improve respiratory muscle strength because, during inspiration, the horse has to expand the chest wall against the pressure of the water.

There are a number of factors that should be considered when interpreting the physiological response of horses to swimming. First, buoyancy. The more body fat a horse has the closer it will be to having neutral buoyancy (Neutral buoyancy is the point at which the tendency to float is exactly matched by a tendency to sink). Body fat is less dense than water and will float. Thus, Thorough-

breds in training with very low body fat will have a low buoyancy and will tend to sink if they do not expend any effort to stay afloat. Because of the buoyancy effect the horse's bodyweight is in effect lower. On land the horse has to work against gravity, and during running on the flat the body may only move as little as 15–30 cm above the ground during each stride. In a pool the effect of gravity is diminished due to buoyancy. On land the horse also has to overcome air resistance and friction through contact with the ground. However, as the horse is able to reach fast speeds it develops significant inertia (Inertia describes the difficulty of making something move, or, if it is moving, the difficulty of making it stop. It also describes the difficulty of changing the direction of a moving object. For example, a tanker has high inertia because of its high mass. It can take several miles to turn a large tanker.). In the pool the situation is, of course, very different. The resistance of the water is high and the horse only travels at slow speeds so it has little inertia. The horse is well adapted to moving through air in that the limbs present a small frontal surface area which reduces resistance. However, most animals that have evolved to be efficient swimmers have limbs adapted to increase the surface area for moving water (flippers, paddle-like feet, etc.), making it easier for them to move through the water. A horse's legs are not so efficient, so it has to work hard in water for only a little forward travel.

On land the horse usually has a respiratory frequency that approaches the stride frequency at walk, trot, canter and gallop, and we have learnt that respiration and stride are linked in a 1:1 ratio during canter and gallop in healthy horses. However, in water the horses stride frequency is reduced. The respiratory cycle also shows a change, with a rapid inspiration and a prolonged, laboured exhalation, compared to their approximately equal duration during running. On land, the timing of limb movements aid respiration and this is absent during swimming. It should therefore not be surprising to learn that the respiratory strategy adopted by horses during swimming is entirely different to that on land. The respiratory rate during swimming is much lower than on land, around 30–40 breaths/min. For a given workload the horse must achieve a certain level of ventilation to maintain oxygen delivery and elimination of carbon dioxide, whether on land or in water. Thus, if the rate is lower we would expect the tidal volume to be increased. Whilst horses clearly do take larger breaths during swimming, to date their ventilatory response to swimming has not been reported in the scientific literature. During maximal exercise on land a 500 kg horse might achieve a maximal minute ventilation of 1800 l/min, from a respiratory frequency (stride frequency) of 120 breaths/min and a tidal volume of 15 litres. If during maximal swimming exercise the respiratory rate was reduced to 40 breaths/min, in order to maintain the same level of minute ventilation the horse would need to achieve a tidal volume of 45 litres, which is close to total lung capacity and therefore not possible. It is therefore likely that horses would be forced to hypoventilate during maximal swimming exercise, leading to increased blood lactate concentrations compared to exercise at a similar intensity on land.

Just as on land, the speed at which the horse swims will determine how hard it works. A leisurely swim at around 1 m/s for 10 minutes may only increase the heart rate to 150 bpm, while swimming at 3 m/s for the same time may raise the heart rate to near maximum. We have learnt that the horse produces a lot of heat during exercise and the harder the horse works the greater the rate of heat production. The horse has a very high sweat rate to attempt to dissipate heat produced by the muscles during exercise, but during maximal exercise the horse diverts blood from the skin to the muscles (at the expense of thermoregulation). Whilst evaporation is a good means of dissipating heat, which occurs when a horse sweats on land, conductive cooling is even more efficient. During swimming a substantial amount of heat can be dissipated by conductive transfer to the surrounding pool water, provided this is lower than the horse's skin temperature, and the horse does not need to sweat. If the horse's skin temperature during swimming is in the region of 35°C and the surrounding water is 15°C, then the capacity for conductive heat transfer from the horse to the water is very high. It is not good for a horse to swim in a pool where the water is at the same temperature as the horse. In this situation no conductive heat transfer can occur,

the horse cannot dissipate heat by sweating and evaporation, so heat loss is restricted to that lost via respiration. This is an ineffective way to dissipate heat. In this situation it would be easy to induce marked hyperthermia in a relatively short period.

Water treadmills

There are currently around ten water treadmills in the UK. The water treadmill consists either of a tank with a ramp down to it and a treadmill in the bottom or a chamber at ground level into which water is pumped once the horse is loaded (see Fig. 16.2). Either design currently costs in the region of £30 000 to £50 000. The disadvantage of water treadmills with approach ramps is the size of the room (about 25 metres long) necessary to accommodate the entry and exit ramps which measure about 17 m altogether. Ground level water treadmills can be accommodated in a room 10 metres by 7 metres, but then the horse usually has to back out of the machine when it has finished exercising. Both designs use tanks of water of approximately 9000–11 000 litres that may be emptied and refilled once a week. The need to change the water is largely dependent upon the degree of use the machine has and the success of the filtration system. Top speeds are usually in the region of 6 m/s. The treadmill belt should have very fine control, starting very slowly and be capable of going up to a trot speed. Fine speed control is vital, as even small adjustments in speed can significantly affect the quality of the gait once the horse is in water. Water treadmills often have water or air jets at the front and sides. The water is usually heated to between about 12 and 19°C. The water treadmill is more versatile if it is also designed to run dry.

Gait adaptations to water treadmill exercise

Water provides buoyancy (which ought to decrease workload at any given speed) and greater resistance than air (which ought to increase the work done when compared to the same speed on a 'dry' treadmill). Both the buoyancy and the resistance

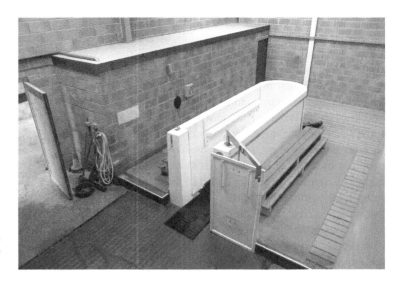

Fig. 16.2 The Aqua-Fit water tread-mill, Equine Therapy Centre, Hartpury College.

effects of the water appear to alter the stride pattern when compared to dry treadmill or overland movement. When horses walk in water of about carpal (knee) depth, they adopt a round action with a good degree of hock flexion in particular. In walk in deeper water (up to the point of shoulder or above) horses tend to choose a combination of low stride frequency and long stride length which probably minimises the effect of the water resistance. In trot, they show a high degree of vertical displacement when compared with overland locomotion.

Application of water treadmills for training and rehabilitation

Heart rates during water treadmill exercise are only slightly higher than those of dry treadmill exercise at the same speed, but vary considerably depending upon the gait of the horse, and the depth and temperature of the water. All horses benefit from around two 10–15 minute introductory sessions to water treadmill exercise for them to become accustomed to the procedure; following this, most reasonably fit horses will work quite happily for up to 30 minutes or more at walk and trot.

Water treadmills are useful for rehabilitation because they provide a mode of exercise in which concussion is reduced, but one in which the horse can be encouraged to work in a 'round' outline, i.e. with the back in flexion rather than extension. Water treadmill exercise has been criticised as it is reported to overdevelop the forelimb muscles. Certainly, horses should be encouraged to work in a desirable outline whilst in water. Horses that do not go forward naturally over ground are likely to go hollow and pull themselves along in the water. It is important that horses are still required to 'drive' from behind, even when working in water. Water walking does not lead to high heart rates and can therefore be safely done with a horse that is at a relatively low level of fitness. However, trotting in water requires considerable coordination and effort from the horse, and can produce heart rates of up to approximately 170 beats/min. It is possible to use the water treadmill for training purposes, but horses would have to be trotted at speeds of around 4 m/s to approach the lactate threshold and for water treadmill work to be a useful substitute for, say, canter work. Water treadmills are a valuable tool in rehabilitation programmes because they provide a form of controlled exercise in a novel environment that is highly appropriate for the rehabilitation of many, but not all, injuries; therefore all water treadmill exercise for rehabilitation purposes should be carried out under the direction of the veterinary surgeon in charge of the case and by an experienced handler.

KEY POINTS

- Some deformation of the surface is required in the early phase of stance to prevent slipping. Firm surfaces allowing little deformation increase the chance of slipping, particularly if the surface is also wet.
- Vertical impact forces are at a maximum in the load-bearing phase of stance, resulting in maximal compression in which the foot of a galloping horse may penetrate the surface by 3–7 cm.
- A material with a low impact resistance makes the horse work harder, as more energy is lost to the surface each time the foot hits the ground. A surface with a high impact resistance is a 'fast' surface, and one with a low impact resistance is a 'slow' surface.
- Gallops are normally situated on rising ground because horses can be worked harder at lower speeds, the vertical impact on the forelimbs is reduced, and it is easier to pull up.
- The 'kickback' of a surface can be reduced by watering, using a surface which is bonded by oil or monofilament fibre, covering with loose sand and rolling, or by using a large particle material, such as wood chips or rubberised fibre, which kicks up but does not go very high.
- For turf racecourses there are seven official states of going: hard; firm; good to firm; good; good to soft; soft; heavy.
- All-weather surfaces are generally firmer and therefore 'faster' than turf. The three recognised states of going on all-weather racecourses are: fast; standard; slow.
- Treadmill exercise is not a substitute for ridden work, but treadmills that can be inclined are very useful to provide hill work, whilst high speed treadmills are useful to provide fast work when ground conditions prohibit working outdoors.
- Swimming provides a non-load-bearing form of rehabilitation work. It is useful work for horses whose injuries, e.g. bruised soles, prevent load-bearing work. It is useful for training youngsters, as it provides a means of aerobic conditioning without subjecting the musculoskeletal system to high levels of concussive forces.
- Water treadmills are useful for rehabilitation because they provide a mode of exercise in which concussion is reduced, but one in which the horse can be encouraged to work in a 'round' outline, i.e. with the back in flexion rather than extension. The heart rates that can be achieved during water treadmill exercise are often much lower than those observed during swimming exercise.

Chapter 17

Practical training

How fit does the horse need to be?

If we exercise an unfit horse and a fit horse we would expect to see a difference not only in performance, but in a number of other areas as well.

Response of a fit horse to exercise

- Good, expected or acceptable performance
- Clinically normal response during exercise and recovery
- Physiologically normal response to exercise
- Rapid recovery
- Normal behaviour
- Normal post-exercise thirst and appetite.

Response of an unfit horse to exercise

- Poor performance
- Abnormal or extreme physiological responses to exercise
- Prolonged recovery post-exercise
- Stiffness/lameness/injury/illness
- Ataxia and weakness
- Reduced or greatly increased thirst and appetite
- Depression.

These are of course extreme examples; in reality for many types of competition, the horse will perform perfectly well without having completed any specific fitness training, having gained enough fitness through hacking, schooling and perhaps even competing regularly. This is probably true to a large extent with sports such as showing and even dressage and showjumping at the lower levels, where the amount of work done as part of skill training

prepares the horse adequately in terms of cardiovascular fitness.

How much fitness training is actually needed will also depend a great deal on the type of horse on which you are competing. Thoroughbreds are naturally athletic, and would not take much preparation to be able to cope with, for example, an affiliated novice level one-day event. For novice one-day events, horses that can easily cover the ground at 520 metres/min should need little more specific fitness preparation than the work done in schooling and skill training. As long as the horse is being exercised for $1\frac{1}{2}$ hours most days and has had some canter preparation, this should be adequate. The only time specific preparation is necessary is if the horse is a native or coldblood type, that really has to be in fifth gear at 520 metres/min, or if the course is particularly taxing. Novice horse trials fitness has been described as equivalent to being 'hunting fit', although this is a rather nebulous term, because it rather depends on with whom you hunt, whether you keep up with the rest of the field, over what country you go and how often!

Sports with a lesser skill component and considerably larger fitness component such as flat racing or endurance riding do need specific fitness training if the horse is to at least complete the competition, or more so for a good performance.

How long will it take?

We are rarely in the position of embarking on a training programme with a horse which is previously untrained or which has no fitness at all. Perhaps the only true example would be a horse that had been kept stabled all its life. People can often underestimate the amount of exercise some horses get from being in the field, and a previous season's training gains may not all be lost. Things might be a lot simpler if we did know that we really did have no existing fitness, because at least then we would know that we were at 0% on the fitness scale and could then start from scratch! It is more likely that we have to start with a horse whose position on a scale from 0 to 100% is unknown (see Fig. 17.1).

So if we are training a horse that we know has been trained before but by someone else, how do we know where we are when it comes to our yard, perhaps in early season or perhaps later in the season? This is always a difficult decision for a trainer as there are no absolute measures of fitness. An unfit horse that has a lot of ability can show very similar responses to exercise as a moderately fit but athletically untalented horse. If we don't know, the best plan is probably to err on the side of caution, try and assess the horse as to how well it copes with exercise of lower intensity, continue with a programme of long, slow distance work, only adding work of higher intensity after the horse has completed some basic 'aerobic training'.

In terms of time-scale, one of the most intensive training programmes is that of an advanced three-day eventer. Traditionally, event horses that have had a complete break following the previous season will complete approximately 16 weeks' training before the major spring three-day event at Badminton. If the mature horse is kept ticking over all year round, it does not need to do pure long, slow, distance (LSD) work at the start of each season. When designing a programme for any horse

you should work backwards from the event and add on at least 7–10 days for unforeseen setbacks, such as unworkable ground conditions or minor injuries.

Probably the longest training programme is that of the 160 km (100 mile) endurance horse. This is the ultimate challenge for the endurance horse. It takes about 3 years to get a novice horse ready but perhaps only 3–4 months to get a mature, previously conditioned horse, fit for a 160 km (100 mile) ride.

Can you bring all the systems to a peak at once?

Even if we had a magic formula which told us exactly what type and amount of work to do with our horses for any give stage in their lives and any given competition, we are still faced with trying to train several systems (muscular, cardiovascular, skeletal) at once, with each system responding to different training stimuli at different rates.

Bringing all these systems to a peak at the same point in time can prove difficult. It would appear that training for maximum increase in bone mass can reduce the shock absorbing capacity of articular cartilage, and training for improvements in aerobic capacity actually reduces the horse's anaerobic capacity. We are unlikely to get all systems and all components of all systems to optimal fitness at once.

How do I construct a training programme?

To design a training programme, imagine a triangle, with the training peak at the top of the triangle. The top of the triangle represents 100% fitness. The higher the peak of your triangle, the wider the base should be; in other words, the fitter you expect the horse to be and the higher the intensity of the work effort required, the greater the preparation required. Also if the base of the triangle represents low intensity work and the peak, high intensity work, the implication is that as intensity of the work increases, the volume (amount) of work should decrease. The training programme of most

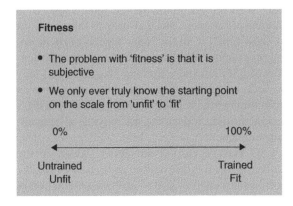

Fig. 17.1   Fitness scale.

competition horses can be divided roughly into three stages as shown in Fig. 17.2.

Successful training depends on progressive loading. This means that the horse is gradually and systematically exposed to increased volume and intensity of work, and in the later stages volume is decreased whilst intensity continues to be increased. The demand of work depends on:

(1) The speed or intensity of the workout
(2) The distance or duration of the workout
(3) The frequency with which the workouts are performed.

Incremental increases in demand should be separated by intervals that allow sufficient time for the horse to adapt. In practical terms, this may mean that you step up demand every week, but then maintain that workload for 1 week, before stepping up demand again.

When complete adaptation to a level has been achieved, no further training response from that level of work can be expected; you need to increase the load to get a further response. At lower levels of training, improvements in aerobic capacity (assessed by measuring $\dot{V}_{O_2\text{max}}$) are seen in a relatively short space of time; as training levels increase, improvements in $\dot{V}_{O_2\text{max}}$ are smaller and take longer to achieve.

The challenge of training is to get the skeletal, muscular and cardiovascular systems to handle the increased demand without straining any to the point of fatigue. Staying in a narrow zone between adaptation and failure gets harder as performance goals increase.

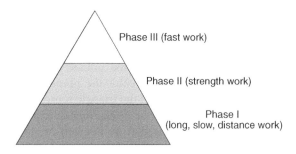

Fig. 17.2   Three stages of a training programme.

Phase I: long, slow distance (LSD)

Cardiovascular and muscular systems respond to incremental increases in work in only a few weeks. Indeed, many of our cardiovascular responses to training such as increased plasma volume and increased heart mass, occur in response to relatively low intensity work. However, an adequate period of long, slow distance work is considered to be useful in training certain musculoskeletal structures and lessens the risk of musculoskeletal injury later in the programme.

As a rough guide, any mature horse which is being brought up from previous fitness should perform about 1 month of LSD before moving onto faster work. For immature horses such as racehorses in their first year of training, LSD should take between 3 and 12 months. This sounds a lot, but the horse will probably not be far off this figure once it has completed a normal programme of sales preparation, backing, early schooling, etc.

How much LSD and how often?

The amount of long, slow, distance work (LSD) is determined by the final level of fitness that is being aimed for (the height of your triangle!). The amount of LSD performed should be proportional to the training goal. LSD may involve walking and trotting for up to about $1\frac{1}{2}$ hours. Regardless of the discipline for which the horse is being prepared, no horse needs to do more than 2 hours' LSD per day, although many horses, such as riding school horses, would be perfectly capable of more than this.

In the early stages, the horse may only be carrying out LSD, and will therefore perform six or seven LSD sessions per week. In the later stages of a training programme, this may drop to three sessions to allow time for all the other aspects of the training programme. We also need to evaluate the benefits of LSD later in a training programme. It may do little or nothing for either increasing or even maintaining fitness, but it may help with the horse's mental attitude, reduce the risk of tying-up or maintain suppleness.

LSD may be carried out under saddle, on the lunge, or on a horsewalker or a treadmill. The horsewalker enables you to exercise several horses at once, but the quality of the walk would not be comparable with ridden exercise. Many trainers of eventers and racehorses have their horses walk for up to an hour a day on a horsewalker. Some people argue that walking on a horsewalker is 'boring' for the horse; however, it is probably preferable for equine athletes to spend a period on a horsewalker if the alternative would be to spend 1 hour in the stable. On a treadmill, horses can be put in tack that enables you to work horses 'in an outline', but it does not save on labour unlike the horsewalker.

Phase II: strength work

In phase II we begin to challenge the horse's body more and undertake exercise of intensities up to and around the anaerobic threshold. The intensity of work done depends on the ultimate goal, but having completed about one month of LSD, our horse should be able to work at canter and gallop for up to $1\frac{1}{2}$ miles by the end of phase II. LSD should not be neglected at this stage, but will be cut back to three times a week. In phase II the cardiovascular system is challenged by working around the anaerobic threshold (at heart rates from 150 to 180 beats/min, depending on the individual horse), for 20–30 minutes at least twice a week.

At this stage, serious biomechanical skill training, such as jumping exercises and schooling are introduced. Now that the horse is asked to work harder, it is all the more important to warm up and warm down correctly. A horse which is sufficiently warmed up will be better able to provide the energy for that work by aerobic means.

Hill work can also be introduced in phase II to strengthen hindquarter muscles. As well as working uphill, the horse can be worked downhill to strengthen the pectorals, shoulder and forearm muscles and also the quadriceps muscles in the hindquarters which have to work against gravity (eccentric contractions) to balance the horse.

Working around the anaerobic or lactate threshold can be expected to bring about a delay in the point at which this threshold is reached, allowing the horse to work harder and for a longer period before lactate appears in the blood. Phase II work can also be expected to bring about changes such as a decrease in fibre size and an increased number of mitochondria within the muscle cells.

Exercising up, down and across gradients is excellent preparation for event and endurance horses as it teaches them to balance and to have better control of their limb placements, whilst placing a diverse loading pattern on the skeleton that mimics the competition situation. Useful alternatives at this stage would be exercises such as swimming or walking in water, both of which will require more muscular effort than walking on a horsewalker if the horse cannot be ridden for some reason. Alternatives to ridden exercise may be needed if the horse has a problem such as bruised soles or a sore back but is not to drop behind in its training programme.

At this stage, endurance horses may also benefit from dressage training to develop their abdominal and hindquarter muscles sufficiently so that they are able to work with a supple, supported back.

Phase III: fast work

A specific phase III may only really be necessary for sports that have a significant anaerobic component. Any horse that has to gallop in competition will require specific speed training. In the final phase of a training programme, true fast work is introduced. Galloping a horse introduces a certain amount of risk. Fast work should be planned and surfaces chosen carefully. Galloping horses is ultimately the best way to prepare them for fast work and to attempt to increase their anaerobic capacity. What if we don't have suitable facilities? How else can we increase the intensity of work in this final stage?

Intensity of work can be increased by working horses up gradients so they are working against gravity (see Fig. 17.3). This is the most commonly used method of increasing intensity without the need to increase speed. Horses' heart rates can easily be elevated by 30–40 beats/min when working at any given speed but on a moderately steep slope, with the added advantage that peak vertical forces through the forelimbs are lower than when working on the flat.

Believe it or not, one of the most effective ways of increasing the intensity of work without working at high speeds is to draught load the horse. This has been done by adding loads to the sulkies pulled by trotters or by draught-loading horses on a treadmill. Weights of up to 100 kg can be added to a rope

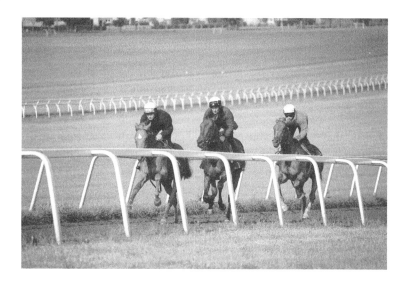

Fig. 17.3   Hill work.

which runs over a pulley, connected horizontally from behind the treadmill to a harness. Horses can work in trot, but produce heart rates of over 200 beats/min and blood lactate levels of 5–16mmol/l, indicating that they are having to work anaerobically. Draught loading is unlikely to become popular with trainers of 2-year-old racehorses, however!

The intensity of work for any given speed can also be increased by working against a resistance, either by riding into the wind or by deep going, e.g. sand. Working in deep going comes with inherent risks of straining muscles, tendons or ligaments, whilst working into the wind cannot always be arranged! It is easy to underestimate how much harder the horse may find a piece of work on a windy day. Think how exhausting it can be simply to walk down the street in a real gale. Running into a strong oncoming wind may explain unusually high heart rates and unusually low performance in an otherwise fit and healthy horse.

At the end of the day, the most effective and most commonly used method of increasing power and speed is to gallop. Fast work can be carried out by continuous (conventional) or interval training.

What is the difference between continuous and interval training?

As an example, let's say we have a horse that needs to be able to gallop at 600m/min for 4 minutes in competition. In preparing the horse by continuous training, we would carry out fast work of longer duration but lower speed, and of shorter duration and higher speed, but would probably avoid exactly reproducing the speed and distance seen in competition. In other words, we may gallop the horse at 700m/min for 1 minute, and canter at 500m/min for 7 minutes. We may carry these out on different days, or simply put our minute of 700m/min on the end of a slower session. One of the biggest drawbacks of this method is finding a suitable place to carry out this work. Ideally you would want a circular all-weather track, so that you could canter for long periods of time.

Interval training a horse can be done with a much shorter gallop than the continuous method. One of the major drives to selection of one or other method depends on the facilities available. If you cannot afford 1600 metres (8 furlongs) of all-weather gallop, but only 800 metres, you have to go up it twice as many times to have done the same amount of fast work! In other words, the training programme used may often be a product of the facilities available, with some riders and trainers actually practising interval training by default. If you have a 500 metre gallop, then you know that once up the gallop is little use and so you probably use two canters on an 'easy' day, one canter and one or two gallops on a 'moderate' day and one canter and three or four gallops on a 'hard' day.

Interval training involves using multiple exercise bouts separated by relatively short rest or recovery periods. This offers the opportunity to increase the volume of exercise and so increase the total training stimulus, whilst providing a method of carrying out all the necessary fast work in a smaller space and/or over a shorter distance. For years, many trainers have considered interval training to be better than continuous training for certain types of horses, particularly event horses, although the scientific evidence for this is still lacking.

The risk of injury is also proposed to be decreased for interval training because, although the total volume of work may be greater, the individual bouts of exercise within an interval workout are shorter. For example, if in a continuous programme on a gallop day the horse was required to gallop 2000 metres (10 furlongs or 1.25 miles) then the interval equivalent may be three gallops of 800 metres each, with 10–20 minutes' walking in between (total of 2400 metres). Thus, in the interval training programme the horse only has to gallop 800 metres in any one 'interval'. Whilst inevitably the horse will become progressively more fatigued (tired) at the end of each successive 800 metre interval, this does appear to be less than would occur for a similar intensity (speed) over a longer distance in one go.

In human athletes, interval training is used specifically to develop anaerobic capacity. So far studies have failed to show significant differences in improvements in anaerobic capacity in interval trained horses compared to those trained continuously. However, studies comparing the two are inherently difficult to perform, as the volumes of work vary between interval training and conventional training programmes. Scientists may choose to set up the experiment so that either (i) two groups of horses perform the same volume of work, (ii) an interval trained group performs the training at the same intensity, but a greater volume than a conventionally trained group. Neither are entirely satisfactory in terms of experimental design to demonstrate which training method is better.

In human athletes interval training is also thought to decrease risk of injury. Whether or not interval training reduces the risk of injury in horses largely depends on how it is used. In an interval programme, horses are less likely to be fatigued than when carrying out a similar total duration of continuous work, and this would certainly be expected to decrease the risk of injury because fatigue increases the risk of musculoskeletal injury. However, because interval training reduces the apparent level of fatigue reached in any one interval, the horse may be asked to go faster for longer periods of which it would otherwise be incapable in a continuous training session, perhaps before the musculoskeletal system is sufficiently prepared, and this could increase the risk of injury.

It may be that interval training does not induce a specific training response by virtue of the nature of the training stimulus applied, it simply enables trainers to carry out a greater volume of work with their horses. Against this is the fact that interval type exercise has been shown in a number of different studies on horses to induce far more extreme metabolic changes than a single bout of maximal exercise to fatigue. For example, one of the first studies demonstrating that the ATP concentration of muscle actually decreases in horses with exercise was carried out using an interval exercise protocol where the horses galloped maximally four times over 620 metres, with around 20 minutes' rest between intervals. Also, whilst blood lactate concentrations as high as 25 mmol/l and perhaps occasionally as high as 30 mmol/l would be seen after a single bout of maximal exercise, blood lactate levels as high as 35 mmol/l (45 mmol/l in plasma) have been reported following four maximal intervals over 700 metres. As the metabolic conditions within muscle during and following exercise play an important role in determining which genes are switched on, the more extreme conditions following interval type work may well be an advantage in terms of training stimulus.

How should interval training be carried out?

Interval training consists of work periods which are built into sessions, varying according to:

- Speed
- Distance
- Time of work
- Duration of rest or recovery periods
- Number of repetitions.

For example, an interval training workout could consist of three periods of galloping at 500 m/min, with 3 minute rest periods in between. Possibly the easiest way to organise an interval training programme is by riding at a set speed for a fixed time, with predefined rest periods.

Alternatively, the horse could be ridden at a predetermined heart rate for a given period of time, or over a known distance. The duration of rest periods does not necessarily have to be predefined, but can vary according to the recovery of the horse's heart rate. For example, you may wish to start the next bout only after the horse's heart rate has dropped to 50% of that of the preceding exercise, so if the horse is worked at 180 beats/min, you would rest until the heart rate is below 90 beats/min.

Interval training provides a certain amount of inbuilt flexibility to the training programme, as there are many ways of progressively loading the horse:

(1) Increasing speed
(2) Increasing distance
(3) Increasing duration of interval
(4) Decreasing duration of rest
(5) Increasing the number of repetitions.

Practicalities of interval training

For an interval training programme to be managed correctly, it should be kept simple. It is not necessary to dismount at the end of each bout to take pulse and respiratory rates, and is indeed highly impractical. At the end of a piece of fast work, the last thing you should do is drag the horse to a halt so that you can take measurements. Decide how you want to run your programme, whether by speed, duration of work bouts, whatever, and then apply the principles of progressive loading, by always increasing distance or duration before speed, and never increase the two together. It is very easy to overdo interval training because horses often appear to cope so well with the work when it is broken down into smaller 'intervals'. Don't be tempted to do an extra interval too early on in a programme. Stick to what you have decided upon in advance and use a heart rate monitor to assess the workload during an interval and recovery between bouts and at the end of a session.

Interval training for three-day eventers may progress to three 8 minute canters at 550–570 metres/min with 5–10 minute recovery intervals. For the purpose of interval training, you can usually be confident that your horse is recovered enough to continue working when the heart rate is below 100 beats/min within 1–2 minutes of finishing an interval. In general terms, if a horse which has coped well with a piece of work, the heart rate should drop markedly in the first 30 seconds as it slows down. If you do not see that initial rapid phase, you have definitely overdone things. Heart rates should be back to warm-up levels (not resting levels) within 5–8 minutes of finishing a bout of interval training. The recovery periods can be relatively short when you have a circular place to gallop in a field or on an all-weather track, but in some cases if you have to use the same stretch of land or all-weather track you may be able to turn around and go back the other way. Of course, if you have a track or gallop on a fairly steep slope then you will not want to gallop downhill. In this case you may be forced to trot and walk back to the start of the track or gallop. This does not really present a problem even though the recovery period between intervals will be longer. For example to walk 800 metres ($\frac{1}{2}$ mile or 4 furlongs) will take around 8 minutes at a reasonably active walk (1.7 m/s or about 110 metres/min).

For the flat racehorse, appropriate interval training may incorporate 20–40 second sprints of 900 m/min. However, the horses which may benefit the most, the 2- and 3-year-old sprinting Thoroughbreds, are often least able physically and mentally to cope with true interval training. Usually, top speed work is done at the end of the work bout, e.g. 600–1600 metres at 800 metres/min and then 200–600 metres at 95–100% maximum speed. One of the dangers of interval training is that repetitions of high intensity work cause rapid depletion of glycogen stores. After fast work, glycogen stores may be depleted by 50% or more. On an adequate diet, it takes about 72 hours for the horse to replenish these fuel stores, and so it would make sense not to perform high intensity interval training workouts more than twice a week to ensure that glycogen stores are not gradually eroded throughout the training programme.

Human athletes often describe continuous training as 'boring', and prefer to perform interval training workouts. There is no doubt that some horses feel the same, but this can also work against you. Interval training is too exciting for some horses, and these horses may work better if trained using continuous periods of fast work. This is particularly the case if you have to use the same field, track or gallop for all interval work.

Learning to ride at a set speed

Riding alongside a car is useful to get a feel for speeds of travel. For fast work it may be easier to simply time yourself over a set distance (which can be measured using the type of measuring wheel used for setting out showjumping and cross-country courses and the start and end marked) and see how effectively you can get to an 'optimum time' when you are performing your fast work. A heart rate monitor can be useful to find out at what speeds the horse travels most efficiently, useful information for both event and endurance riders. In practical terms this is generally only important between trot and canter. Horses, when left to their own devices, select the most energy efficient gait. If the horse is asked by the rider to extend in trot, when it would naturally select canter, it will be found to be working at a higher heart rate. If the horse is then allowed to go at the same speed but to change into canter, the heart rate may well decrease by 5–10 beats/min, even though the horse is travelling at the same speed. Using the heart rate monitor will help the rider establish a feel for the horse's optimum gait for any given speed.

How hard should the horse work and how soon should I increase the intensity?

Even though two horses may run at the same speed, over the same distance, it does not necessarily mean that they have exerted themselves to the same extent. A naturally more talented horse that has a greater cardiovascular capacity and higher maximal oxygen uptake may well perform a piece of work at a heart rate 20 beats/min lower than a less talented individual. For any individual horse, heart rate during exercise is proportional to speed, so the harder the work, the higher the heart rate (until maximum heart rate is reached; see Chapter 10). Heart rate is proportional to speed, but the slope of the line (how much the heart rate increases for increase in speed) varies according to the fitness and ability of the individual.

To find out how hard your horse is working at a particular speed and in any given ground conditions, you should carry out some sort of standardised exercise test over a course of a couple of miles (3000 metres or so). Monitor your horse's heart rate over this course at weekly intervals, noting any change in ground conditions. If you ride at the same speed, you should see a decrease in the mean heart rate over the same course. If there is no further improvement in heart rate with time, you can select a tougher 'test', or ride at greater speed over your set course.

As a horse gets fitter, it can work at the same speed with a relatively lower heart rate, and can therefore work for longer before its maximum heart rate is achieved. Also, in a trained horse, heart rate recovery will be more rapid. By performing tests like these, you should first see a decrease in the horse's submaximal heart rate, and then an increase in the intensity of work the horse can carry out for any given heart rate.

Another factor that will affect how hard a horse is working based on heart rate is its maximal heart rate. Maximal heart rate decreases with age. The intensity of work performed based on heart rate can be described by expressing it as a percentage of maximum heart rate, so if a horse has a maximal heart rate of 200 beats/min and is exercising at 150 beats/min, this is equivalent to an intensity of 75% of maximal heart rate or 75% HR_{max}. (This is the same principle as expressing oxygen uptake at any speed as a percentage of maximal oxygen uptake.) However, imagine the situation where we have a 2-year-old horse with a maximum heart rate of 240 beats/min and an 18-year-old horse with a maximum heart rate of only 180 beats/min. If we work both at a heart rate of 170 beats/min, the younger horse is working at $(170/240) \times 100 = 71\%$ HR_{max} whilst the older horse is working at $(170/180) \times 100 = 94\%$ HR_{max}, so although their heart rates are the same, the older horse is working much harder.

Load carried

Horses that carry weights in competition should be trained with similar weights. In theory, intensity of work done should be proportional to total load carried, whether it is carried as the horses own body mass, the rider's own body mass, a gut full of fluid or lead on the saddle. Studies have shown that the horse's heart rate is no more elevated by carrying a dead weight than by carrying a rider, although it might be argued that, in terms of added effort required by the horse, a dead weight and a decent rider are both preferable to a fatigued, uncoordinated rider. Timeform ratings used in racing in the UK are based on the idea that 'handicapping' a horse with a particular load will reduce its performance by a predictable amount. This would seem to make perfect sense: surely increasing the load reduces performance, and by adding a load of 4.5 kg (10 lb) you would reduce the performance twice as much as by adding a load of 2.25 kg (5 lb). Unfortunately it does not seem to be so simple. You would expect that by increasing the load you would have increased the intensity of the work, and the heart rate would be appropriately elevated for any given speed – not so! It appears that increases in heart rates (measured during exercise on a treadmill lasting several minutes) are not significantly increased until an increase of 10% of the horse's own body mass is added. Whilst in theoretical terms we talk about the heart rate being the same for the same work under the same conditions on different days, even when the work is carried out on a treadmill in a controlled environment, there is day to day variation. Part of this is physiological and part is due to the accuracy of measuring heart rate during exercise. In theory we know there must be a difference, but in practice in scientific terms, we need an increase in load carried of 10% to be able to demonstrate the effect. It doesn't mean that 1% less load carried is not beneficial or that an extra 1% is not detrimental. In racing, there can be no doubt that the handicap system works, and this is based on relatively small weights (loads) being added. For example, a 450 kg horse handicapped with an extra 4.5 kg (10 lb) would only be carrying an extra 1% body mass. However, sports where a minimum load must be carried unfairly penalise smaller horses. For example, if the minimum load that must be carried is set at 75 kg, a 450 kg horse would be carrying 16.7% of its body mass, whilst a horse of 600 kg would be carrying only 12.5% of its body mass and would hence be at an advantage. Therefore a more fair way would be to stipulate that the minimum load carried should be a fixed percentage of the horse's body mass, for example 15%. The drawback of such a system is that it would require each horse to be weighed before a competition and that weighing-in and weighing-out would be more complex.

It is also perhaps surprising that additional load carried does not appear to affect placings of endurance horses, presumably because the horse is normally trained and competed by the same person, and has thus performed all their training carrying such a load. However, if the horse was able to switch to a lighter rider just before the competition, it would perform even better! It may also be that heavier riders naturally tend to select heavier horses.

Ideal body condition

Horses can lose anything from a few kilograms up to 40 kg in the course of competition. Racehorses often tend to have an 'ideal weight' (ideal mass) at which they perform more consistently, and it is often suggested that they should be within plus or minus 10 kg of their ideal mass when they race. A study that looked at the relationship between body condition score and completion rate in a 160 km (100 mile) endurance ride (Garlinghouse & Burrill 1999) found that condition scores had a significant effect on completion rate, with an increase in distance completed of 31.81 km for each incremental increase of one point in condition score. It was concluded that condition score was more important than the mass of the rider or the rider's mass in relation to the mass of the horse. In this study horses were assigned a condition score before the start of the race on a scale of 1–9 as described by Henneke (1985). The results demonstrated that the average condition score amongst all horses (completers and non-completers) was 4.49, whilst those that successfully completed the course had an average body condition score of 4.60. It was suggested that those horses with a slightly higher body condition score had optimal stores of body fat, reflecting a higher energy content of the diet or lesser energy expenditure during training.

A mark of a good horse is often considered to be maintenance of body mass during a competition. Good racehorses tend to lose less body mass in the course of a race than less talented individuals, whether this is down to effort expended, stress or reduced feed and water intake.

Organising the weekly work

As well as having a week-by-week work plan, keep a diary in which you record exactly what work was done, how the horse felt, heart rates (if taken), and all other relevant information. It is a good idea to itemise the horse's ration alongside the workload, so that any diet based problems can be identified. This diary may be of greatest value the *second* time you bring that particular horse to peak fitness, as it may be possible to avoid previous problems.

Many racing yards run on a 3 day cycle, allowing two 3 day cycles per week and one day off. Wednesday and Saturday (and in some yards, Tuesday and Friday) will be phase III days, and Sunday is the day off. Racing would count as a phase III day. Phase I, II and III work is done on successive days, so the horse has an easy, a moderate and a hard work day, in that order. This guards against glycogen depletion and possibly against overtraining.

In a large yard, with lots of horses, there may be three 'lots', with the first lot doing the fastest work, the second lot perhaps doing phase II work, and the third lot doing phase II or LSD work. In a smaller yard, there may only be two lots, in which case the first lot will be cantering and the second lot, LSD. This way, the day is organised in the same way, and horses can be fitted into lots according to their individual needs. The need to ride horses out in different lots is mainly related to labour. You can therefore have 30 horses and 10 riders and three lots, or employ 30 riders to ride one lot each. A weekly work programme might look like this:

- Monday – LSD (60–90 min) or two slow canters
- Tuesday – Medium work, e.g. 2 × 1200 metres (600–800 metres/min)

- Wednesday – Fast work, e.g. one warm-up canter (~600 metres/min) and one gallop over 800–1400 metres (at 900–1000 metres/min)
- Thursday – As Monday
- Friday – As Tuesday
- Saturday – As Wednesday
- Sunday – Rest or 60 minutes' walking.

As preparation for novice horse trials the horse may be doing about 1–1½ hours' work daily, consisting of in 1 week:

- 1–2 fast work days
- 3 LSD days
- 1 skill training day
- 1 day off.

Figure 17.4 shows the work programme in the final 2–3 weeks for a group of six horses being prepared by experienced riders for a one-star level three-day event. For each day the type of exercise is given together with the amount of time the horses spent at different heart rates. For example, on all days by far the most time was spent below heart rates of 120 beats/min and heart rate during training only increased above 160 beats/min on around half the training days and at most for up to 3–4 minutes. Whilst these horses all competed successfully in the three-day event, it is clear that at novice and one-star three-day event level, the training intensity required is relatively low.

How long can you keep a horse at a peak?

Once we think we have the horse at a peak, ready and raring to go, how long is it feasible or wise to keep them there? Most trainers will only bring the horse to peak fitness right before a major competition. The horse will be let down slightly after the competition and then tick over at a level of fitness just below peak. This may mean reducing the intensity and/or volume of all training sessions, or cutting out canter and gallop days. Some flat racehorses are maintained just below competition fitness for weeks on end, racing as often as twice a month. Whilst the horse may be physiologically capable of maintaining peak fitness for weeks or months, you are probably risking musculoskeletal injury by trying to stay at a peak too long. You may also

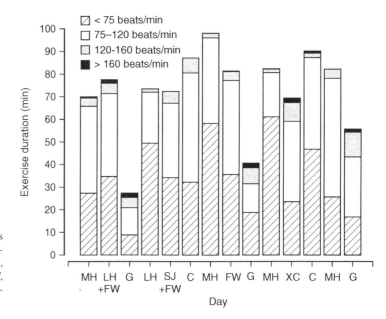

Fig. 17.4 Work programmes of horses being prepared for a one-star level three-day event. Key: LH, light hacking; MH, medium hacking; C, canter; G, gallop; FW, flat work; SJ, showjumping; XC, cross-country jumping.

encounter behavioural problems with the horse becoming 'sour' and losing interest in work. There are many arguments for and against the idea of giving horses a complete holiday at grass for up to 2–3 months at a time. Some trainers believe that it is better to keep the horse in work 12 months of the year, but to reduce the workload for a couple of months of the year.

For many types of competition horse, there will be a long enough break in the competition schedule in which they could have a complete holiday, but this is probably more appropriate for mature horses that are not trying to move up through the grades and may have fewer, but higher quality, competitions to attend. Provided that younger horses are turned out for a period of time each day, and have a varied work programme, there is really no need for them to have a complete holiday. Many trainers worry about the harm that can come to a horse left to its own devices in a field all day, and there is no doubt that a respectable number of tendon and ligament injuries are sustained, not in competition, but whilst careering round a field 'on holiday'. This is really a decision for the individual trainer, as there is no scientific evidence as yet to suggest that a significant decrease in workload is preferable to a complete rest. There may also be a

financial argument for giving more advanced horses a complete break, as this leaves more time to prepare youngsters during the out of season period.

What do you do if the horse has an enforced lay-off?

As a rule of thumb, if the horse is off for 4 weeks, allow 2 weeks to get back to your previous level of work; if it has had 4 months off, take 8 weeks to get back to the previous workload. Horses do maintain their aerobic capacity for several weeks following a lay-off, but it is best to err on the side of caution, particularly if the lay-off was due to injury. In the case of injury a return to work should only be undertaken with the advice of your vet and/or physiotherapist.

Keeping athletes on the road

Back-up team

Always use the best back-up team in terms of vet, farrier and physiotherapist you can find, even if you think you can't afford them; in fact, you probably can't afford not to. Good foot balance is of vital importance to prolong the longevity of the competition horse. Never underestimate the impact poor foot balance can have on performance. If you are very lucky, you may get away with not having your horse shod regularly, but this may significantly reduce its working life. Too many people only worry about their horse's feet when they have a problem, but foot care should always be a priority. The feet of the competition horse should be trimmed and re-shod every 4 weeks. Use an equine vet with experience of dealing with competition horses. Choose a farrier whose work you have seen and if possible is recommended by your vet. It is not a coincidence that a large proportion of horses that end up requiring therapeutic treatment for musculoskeletal injury have to have their foot balance corrected first.

Diagnosis and treatment

Any therapy the horse receives should be carried out under veterinary supervision, and you should be wary of anyone who does not seek veterinary referral before embarking on treatment of a horse. A correct diagnosis of any problem is the first step in successful treatment. Equine sports therapists may not always be qualified physiotherapists, but if they are good, vets will use them. Similarly, many qualified physiotherapists may not necessarily have experience of competition horses.

Record keeping

Keep a diary. This should outline all work done, all feeding programmes, physiotherapy treatments, shoeing, etc. You can only improve on last season's training programme if you know what you did last season. Having a diary may help you to avoid making the same mistake twice, and also helps you reproduce a winning formula when you find it.

Air quality and respiratory health

Let your horse breathe air which is as clean as possible! As a species, the horse is a natural athlete. Horses respond very well to training, and they have an excellent respiratory system which requires nothing more than to be looked after if it is to function to its maximum potential. The rider, however, is often not such a fine physiological specimen, often tending to do things like smoking to deliberately compromise their respiratory function! Keeping your horse in a poorly ventilated stable with dusty food, hay and bedding is the human equivalent of a 20 a day habit. How many top level international human athletes are smokers? Investment in a low dust management regimen for your horse may work out a little more expensive in the short term, but will work out better in terms of performance in the long run.

Even on good management, many competition and racehorses will have significant levels of airway inflammation as a result of other factors such as frequent transport and lower airway infections. In routine surveys of showjumpers, eventers, dressage and endurance horses that are thought to be fit and healthy by their riders, it is not uncommon to find that around two-thirds to three-quarters have airway disease that requires treatment.

KEY POINTS

- Training programmes should be based on the principle of progressive loading, whereby the speed or intensity of the workout, the distance or duration of the workout and the frequency with which the workouts are performed is progressively increased.
- At lower levels of training improvements in aerobic capacity (assessed by measuring $\dot{V}_{O_2max}$)

are seen in a relatively short space of time; as training levels increase, improvements in $\dot{V}_{O_2max}$ are smaller and take longer to achieve.
- Fast work can be performed either as continuous training or interval training. Interval training involves using multiple exercise bouts separated by relatively short rest or recovery periods.

- Interval training allows horses to perform a greater volume of exercise and higher intensity of exercise than can be performed in a single continuous bout because fatigue is avoided.
- High intensity interval training workouts should not be performed more than twice a week in order to ensure glycogen stores are not eroded throughout the training programme.
- Even though two horses may run at the same speed over the same distance, it does not necessarily mean they have exerted themselves to the same extent. Heart rate is proportional to speed but the slope of the heart rate/speed relationship varies according to the fitness and ability of the individual.

- To find out how hard your horse is working at a particular speed you should carry out a 'standardised exercise test'. This can be repeated periodically throughout the training programme. By performing such tests, you should first see a decrease in the horse's submaximal heart rate and then an increase in the intensity of work that can be carried out for any given heart rate.
- Use the best farrier you can find because good foot balance is of vital importance in prolonging the competitive career of the horse.
- Pay attention to the stable ventilation and maintain a dust free environment for your competition horse as this helps guard against airway disease and reduction of performance.

Chapter 18

Exercise testing

Why would you want to use an exercise test?

Trainers have various methods for judging how much work a horse needs to get fit for a competition. Usually, the experienced trainer relies simply on feel. At best, they may listen to the horse's breathing, time the horse over certain distances, compare the performance of one horse with that of older horses with known performance or simply note how keenly the horse goes up the gallops. This is the art of training horses, and it comes with years of experience. The trainer with his stopwatch and the scientists with their treadmills are both conducting exercise tests, but the methods and the circumstances in which they are carried out vary according to the nature of the data required; in other words the test must suit the application.

Exercise tests can be used to assess the fitness of a horse, to compare the fitness of one against another, to monitor changes in fitness throughout a training programme, to assess functional capacity (e.g. maximal oxygen uptake), to characterise horses according to their ability as a spinter type or stayer type, and to verify normal function (e.g. exercising videoendoscopy of the upper airway). Remember that at present there is little or no information regarding the fitness of an individual horse that can be gained from resting measurements.

Exercise tests can also be used to study various training protocols. Despite the popularity and widespread use of methods such as interval training, there is still little scientific evidence regarding the efficacy of different training regimens. Actually scientists are only just starting on the road to determining the effectiveness of different training methods, and it is likely to be a very long road if the experiences of human sports science are anything

to go by! It may seem odd that we have had the benefit of access to high-speed treadmills for over 30 years now, but we are still lacking scientific evidence relating to the effectiveness of different training methods. The main obstacle to training studies has been cost. For example, to compare conventional training and interval training programmes would require somewhere around 20 horses trained in each way, ideally all of the same age, sex and breed, and the clearest response will be seen in previously untrained horses. The training programme would probably last for 16–20 weeks and each horse would have to be managed in the same way and horses in the same training group would have to do the same work. Effectively, we are describing a study that, to carry out, would involve taking over a training yard.

Exercise testing may be necessary to carry out research in areas such as nutrition, biomechanics, endocrinology, drug metabolism and physiology. In such cases, the exercise test is a means to an end. Exercise testing is also used increasingly to try and predict performance potential and to investigate causes of poor performance. Exercise testing large numbers of untrained horses might enable one to pick out the horses with athletic characteristics, such as those with the lowest heart rate for a set piece of work, or identify cardiac or respiratory abnormalities as early as possible. This is dealt with in more detail in Chapter 19.

Standardisation and specificity

The two most important points in any exercise test are standardisation and specificity. Exercise tests can be carried out in the field or on a treadmill. If you are interested in determining the maximal oxygen uptake of a racehorse, it would be ideal to be able to do this under the specific conditions in which the horse normally exercises, usually on grass with a rider on its back. Exercise tests should also be standardised so that comparisons of test results can be made, either comparing results from one horse on two separate occasions, or results from two or more horses carrying out the same test.

Standardisation is difficult in a field situation due to changes in the going (ground conditions), the rider's weight, the wind conditions, and inability to precisely repeat a test in terms of speed and the environmental temperature and humidity. Field tests have the advantage of specificity and treadmill tests have the advantage of standardisation. One of the major disadvantages of field testing is the limitation to the number of variables that can be measured. In the early days of equine exercise research, determined scientists would ride the horses themselves, taking blood samples from indwelling catheters as they raced around the track and throwing the samples to other researchers placed around the track, but this is probably not the easiest way to conduct your research. To make data collection easier, equipment for field testing should be 'on-board', i.e. able to be carried on the horse, or 'telemetric', i.e. wireless and transmit information from the horse to the scientist, so that as little equipment as possible need be carried by the horse and rider. Gradually, the techniques available for field testing are improving. Nowadays, the following pieces of commercial equipment are available for field testing:

- Heart rate monitor
- On-board ECG
- Telemetry ECG
- Telemetric equipment for measuring ventilation and $\dot{V}_{O_2}/\dot{V}_{CO_2}$ (at the time of writing none of these systems for field use have been fully validated)
- Systems for collecting blood samples automatically during exercise.

The price ranges of all but the heart rate monitor mean that the use of such equipment is not commonplace. Besides this, in the UK, any equipment or sampling that is considered to be invasive or cause harm, suffering or distress can only be carried out by vets during the course of a clinical exercise test, or designated scientists or vets who have been granted a licence from the Home Office of the UK Government to do so in the interests of research.

Examples of field exercise tests

Many racehorse trainers use very simple forms of field exercise tests. They need to know when a horse can run a certain distance in a given time or at a certain speed. This may not be the distance or the time over which the horse is supposed to race, but merely gives the trainer some measure of the degree of ability or fitness of the horse. For example, when the horse can run up the gallop at home in 1 minute 20 seconds it is ready to race, or when the horse stops blowing by the time it has walked to the bottom of the hill after the third canter it is ready to race, or when a 2-year-old can keep up with a good 3-year-old on the gallops it is ready to race. These are forms of exercise test, however basic. They provide valuable information to the trainer. But the trainer has to learn by experience because the test is highly specific to his facilities and his way of training. Probably the next step up from simply timing horses on the gallops is to use a heart rate monitor.

Fitting a heart rate monitor

The modern heart rate monitor generally consists of two metal or rubber electrodes which are connected by wires to a transmitter. The wires and transmitter can be held in a saddle cloth or surcingle, or the electrodes can simply be fixed under the girth. The electrodes pick up the electrical activity of the heart and this signal passes through the wires to the transmitter. The rider wears a receiver unit in the form of a watch that picks up the heart rate by telemetry. The signal is in the form of weak radio waves and these are only capable of travelling a short distance, usually less than 1 metre, and so the watch must stay relatively close to the transmitter to pick up a continuous signal.

To ensure that there is a good electrical contact between the electrodes and the skin, either the electrodes are soaked in water before being put on the horse or a gel containing salt is put on, depending on the design. In the case of rubber electrodes it is usually necessary to wet the coat in the area where the electrodes will sit (Fig. 18.1) to obtain a reliable resting heart rate and a heart rate during the early stages of exercise, when the horse starts to sweat this will improve the contact because sweat is a

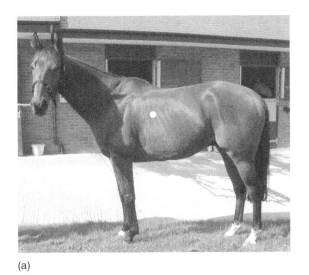

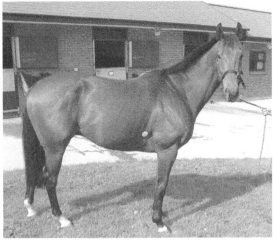

(a)   (b)

Fig. 18.1   Position of electrodes for use with a heart rate monitor.

good electrical conductor due to the presence of electrolytes. Gels such as KY jelly (which is water based but has no salts in it) or special electrode gel (which is also water based but contains electrolytes) can also be used to maintain electrical contact. Oil based gels or creams should not be used because these may insulate the electrodes from the skin.

The electrodes are usually placed under the girth, one between the horse's front legs or slightly to one side of the midline and one on the middle of the thorax on the left hand side. To get the best possible contact, you should make sure that this latter electrode lies directly beneath the girth straps, and not just behind them. When doing fast work, the electrodes should be firmly attached to reduce movement, which is important in maintaining a good contact. If the electrodes are not held firmly against the coat so that they maintain a constant contact, the movement may result in false readings (see Fig. 18.2).

Once tacked up, the watch (receiver) can be fitted to the rider's left wrist, or to a breastplate (provided it is kept close to the transmitter). When the girth is tightened, on most models you should see a flashing black heart on the display of the watch (receiver) that tells you that you have a contact. The heart rate appears a few seconds later.

There are essentially two types of heart rate monitor available: those that store the heart rate data so that they can be played back at a later date

either through the watch or via a computer, or those that simply display the heart rate but have no facility for recalling previous readings. With the latter it can be difficult when working with horses to verify that the system is working correctly. The watch can usually be programmed to display and/or record the heart rate every 5, 15 or 60s, depending on the sort of information you require and for how long you want to record the heart rate. For exercise, the 5s interval is normally chosen, but if you wanted to use the watch to study behaviour or transport or to get a reliable indication of your horse's resting heart rate over a long period of time, a longer interval can be chosen. You can check that your horse is working within preset heart rate limits by setting the alarm on the watch so that it beeps if you go above or below predetermined threshold levels. For example, if you are going to try and ride at a heart rate of 170 beats/min you may set the alarm to 165 and 175 beats/min. When the heart rate is outside this range the alarm will sound and it saves you having to look at the watch to know how hard you are working your horse. On some systems the heart rate display is quite small and can be difficult to read during exercise, especially in wet weather or with a horse that is difficult to ride.

After the heart rate has been recorded, most systems will provide information such as maximum and minimum heart rate and average heart rate. Some systems even allow time markers to be entered. These can be used to mark the start and end of

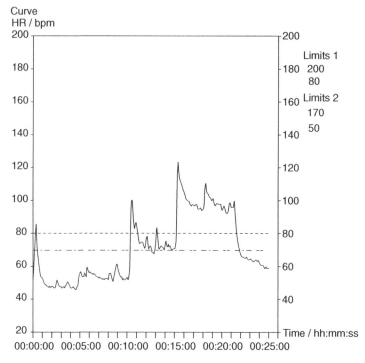

(a) Good heart rate trace

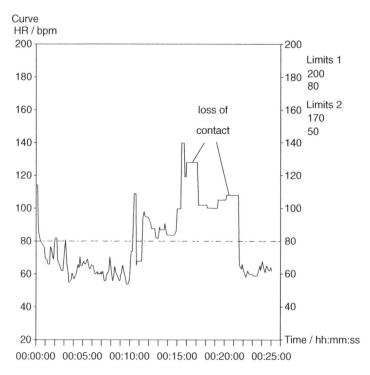

Fig. 18.2   Examples of (a) good and (b) poor heart rate traces of horses undertaking the same exercise test. (Graphs supplied courtesy of Polar Heart Rate Monitors, www.polar.co.uk.)

(b) Poor heart rate trace

a change in pace such as the start and end of a gallop. This allows you not only to see the heart rate but to estimate speed if you know the distance. Markers can also be used in research studies to mark the start of a treatment or part of an experiment.

Troubleshooting

If you have problems getting a black flashing heart on the display, if the flashing heart is not regular, or if it appears to flash twice very close together followed by a pause and then two more flashes close together, or the heart rate tends to stay at a certain value despite variations in work, you can make the following checks:

(1) Are the electrodes/skin of the horse sufficiently wet?
(2) Are the electrodes far enough apart? The closer the electrodes are together the smaller the electrical signal from the heart. The electrodes should be at least 30 cm apart. This can be a problem with some horses when using the human all-in-one electrode and transmitter chest straps.
(3) Tighten the girth again and make sure the electrodes are in place, one directly under the girth, and the other directly under the line of the girth straps.
(4) It is possible that the horse has too thick a coat; it is often difficult to get a contact on an unclipped horse with a long winter coat.
(5) Check that the receiver is not moving beyond the distance necessary to pick up the signal. With some models the receiver can be 'primed' by touching it on the transmitter and the heart rate should appear on the display after having done this.
(6) If you have run through all these checks, and you are still having problems, you may think about changing the battery in the watch: they run out just like any other watch battery.
(7) Check that the wires or electrodes have not been damaged.
(8) The watch relies on the horse producing a regular heartbeat. If you have problems with only one horse, it is possible that that particular horse has an arrhythmia (irregular heartbeat). Many horses may drop beats at rest due to second degree AV block which disappears

once the heart rate is increased above 40–60 beats/min and this is perfectly normal. In fact, if you watch the flashing heart, you should be able to see the dropped beats even if the heart rate is not registered. However, it is very unlikely that the reason the heart rate monitor does not work is because of a heart problem in your horse. If all else fails to get the heart rate monitor which works on other horses working on one horse, find a stethoscope and listen to the heart or palpate an artery whilst looking at the heart rate monitor screen. In nearly 15 years of using heart rate monitors on horses we have only seen three horses in which severe cardiac abnormalities have been the cause of a heart rate monitor not working. Therefore it can occur, but it is very rare.

Simple field tests using a heart rate monitor

Simple exercise tests can be carried out with a stopwatch, a heart rate monitor and a couple of distance markers placed in a straight line at least 400 metres apart, but they can be as far as 1600 metres apart. The exact distance between the markers can be measured with a trundle wheel. Warm the horse up using short periods of walk (10 minutes), trot (5 minutes) and canter (2 minutes). Run the horse between the markers three or four times (at increasing speed each time), and at speeds appropriate to the horse's level of training. Start each run well before each marker so that the horse has reached a steady pace before you pass the marker and start the stopwatch or use the marker on the heart rate monitor. The same applies at the end of each run – stop the watch or mark the heart rate monitor as you pass the marker (many heart rate monitors also have a stopwatch function built in to them and they will even calculate the lap times for you), but don't try and pull up sharply or slow down before reaching the marker. Time the horse between the markers at each speed and record the heart rate throughout each run, and for at least 5 minutes at the end of the last run. Plot a graph of heart rate versus speed for that horse on that day taking the heart rate over the last 10–15 seconds at the end of each run. It is particularly important to ride the horse at a steady speed. Reproduce the test on a regular basis, maybe every 2 weeks, to determine if there is any improvement in submaximal heart rates or recovery rates. This test can also be carried out on a round or oval track or an all-weather track if it is available. The round or oval track has the advantage that you can exercise the horse continuously and go from one step straight into the next.

For a continuous test on a round or oval track, ideally we would want the horse to exercise for 2–3 minutes at each speed. The number of laps that have to be completed may therefore become more as the speed is increased. For example, with a 400 metre loop, if the horse was trotting at 3.5 m/s (210 m/min), the two laps would take 3.8 minutes. However, at 9 m/s (540 m/min), two laps would only take 1.5 minutes, so it would be better to do three laps, which would take 2.2 minutes. If each step is a minimum of 2 minutes then heart rate is more likely to stabilise to reflect the intensity of the exercise. It is also important for the rider to maintain a steady speed on each lap.

The horse starts trotting at a fixed point on the track (usually the middle of a straight side if on an oval track) and the stopwatch is started. Each loop is timed. After the test, the speed on the last lap at each speed is calculated by measuring the distance and dividing by the time. The heart rate is then averaged over the whole lap or over perhaps the last 30s of the same lap. The mean heart rate for each speed is then plotted against mean speed. The point at which speed changes can usually be clearly seen on the heart rate trace. However, for a more refined approach the stopwatch function on the heart rate monitor can be started at the same time as the stopwatch being used to record the lap times. The 'lap' feature on the stopwatch is then used to record the time at the start and end of each lap (rather than stopping and resetting the stopwatch each lap). In this way, the time of the start and end of each lap recorded using the stopwatch corresponds to the times stored in the heart rate monitor. Some heart rate monitors also have a feature that enables markers to be put into the watch by the rider. These can be entered to correspond to the finish/start of each lap, although this can be difficult when riding in a confined space and at speed.

These type of tests can probably be carried out in less than 15 minutes with the advantage that environmental temperature and humidity will have little influence on the heart rate response to exercise. This becomes more of a factor in longer duration tests. Ground conditions will always have an impact on the heart rate response to exercise, whatever the length of test.

To measure heart rate recovery following a test like this you must first:

(1) Pick a 'recovery heart rate'. It is practically impossible to get a horse back to a 'resting' heart rate following exercise if it is tacked up and standing in the middle of a field or at the top of a gallop after exercising, regardless of how long you are prepared to wait. It may well take several hours for the heart rate to return to resting pre-exercise values even when the horse has been taken back to its stable. Instead, you should set a target heart rate of say 60 or 80 beats/min, and time how long it takes for the horse to reach that heart rate when it has been warmed down in a predetermined fashion. An alternative approach is to take the heart rate at a fixed time after exercise. Normally the heart rate early on in the recovery period, around 1–3 minutes from the end of exercise, is the least influenced by excitement and appears the most reliable as an indicator of the preceeding effort.

(2) Standardise the exercise carried out by the horse during its 'recovery'.

When carrying out field exercise tests, the rider should never pull the horse up from a gallop to a standstill. Allow the horse to slow down back into trot and into walk, perhaps over 30–60s and then keep the horse walking. Horses that are pulled up to a dead stop inevitably show an overshoot of heart rate at the end of the piece of fast work, and do not recover so quickly.

A simple exercise test can even be carried out in an outdoor or indoor arena. Using an arena has the advantage that the ground conditions should be more consistent between tests over time. The bigger the school, the faster the horse will be able to canter and so the higher the heart rates that can be achieved. For a school 60 metres by 30 metres, a steady slow to medium speed canter with heart rates of around 140–160 beats/min should be possible. Although it may be possible to speed up on the long sides of a school, a constant pace around the whole school is more important. Place the markers about 2 metres in from the sides of the school and make the corners rounded rather than sharp. As for the field test, a measuring wheel will be needed to measure the distance round the school along the path the horse travels, and a stopwatch will be needed to record lap times to work out speed (Fig. 18.3a). A graph showing heart rate data from such a test is shown in Fig. 18.3(b), together with a plot of heart rate versus speed (Fig. 18.3c).

An exercise test can even be carried out on the lunge which requires less space. There are two ways to approach a lunge test. One is to use a standard lunging test (see Fig. 18.3 a,d,e); for example, 2 minute walk on the left rein, change rein, 2 minute walk on the right rein, transition into trot, 2 minute trot on the right rein, change rein, 2 minute trot on the left rein, transition into canter, 2 minute canter on the left rein, change rein, 2 minute canter on the right rein. The horse is then slowed to walk and the recovery heart rate is taken at 2 minutes from the end of the canter. If a horse is always lunged in the same way then the recovery heart rate at 2 minutes should become lower as the horse gets fitter or increase if the horse develops a problem such as subclinical lameness or respiratory disease. Alternatively, if ten horses that are all of the same fitness (approximates to the same stage of training) are tested, the more athletic horses should have a lower recovery heart rate. This type of test is simple, but will lack some sensitivity. By this, we mean that it may separate out horses of low, moderate and high athletic ability, but that it would probably not differentiate as well between horses of a similar fitness and ability, for example horses competing at four-star three-day event level, unless some had injuries or subclinical disease.

The second type of lunge test is slightly more complicated. It involves counting the number of laps the horse does at each gait and on each rein during the standard 2 minutes. The size and distance of the lunge circle can then be calculated in two ways. The first is to measure the track taken by the horse with a measuring wheel after the test has been completed, but this requires the person lungeing to stay very much on one spot. The other approach is to fix the length of the lunge line to, say, 6 metres between handler and horse. In this way, the distance around the circle can be worked out using the formula $2\pi r$, which for a 12 metre diameter (i.e. radius 6 metre) circle would be about 38 metres. So, for example, if a horse does five laps in

2 minutes at walk on a 38 metre circumference circle, the speed would be equal to the distance travelled divided by the time taken $(5 \times 38\,m)/120\,s$ $= 190\,m/120\,s = 1.6\,m/s$.

The size of the lungeing circle determines how much work the horse does. A 12 metre diameter circle, for example, will make a horse work noticeably harder than a 15 metre circle. This test is essentially the same as the simpler test described above, except that for this test we have the heart rate monitor on the horse and you may like to have an assistant to note the number of laps of the lunge circle on each rein.

All these tests can be used to monitor improvements in fitness during a training programme, provided they are carried out under similar conditions. From each of these tests V_{140}, which describes the speed–heart rate relationship (being the speed at which the heart rate is 140 beats/min), can be estimated. At the end of the day though, the changes in the relationship between heart rate and speed are likely to be greatest early on in the training programme and will be a less sensitive indicator of fitness later on. That is not to say that this type of test may not indicate a medical problem, lameness or viral infection when the horse is at peak fitness.

There is probably little benefit from carrying out a field test in very soft ground conditions and then retesting the horse a month later in dry conditions. Erickson *et al.* (1987) demonstrated that soft going could decrease V_{140} by 1–2 m/s on a muddy track. The tests will be very different because the soft ground will make the horse work harder and so the heart rate will be higher for any given speed. A test carried out in warm or hot conditions may show very different results to one carried out in cool conditions. In general terms, working in the heat results in higher heart rates for the same work in the cool. However, this is also dependent on the duration of exercise. The shorter the test, the less likely that it will be affected by environmental conditions (temperature, humidity, wind and solar radiation). Generally tests under 10–15 minutes will be minimally affected by environmental conditions.

Treadmill testing

Before treadmill testing it is preferable that the horse undergoes a period of training to become

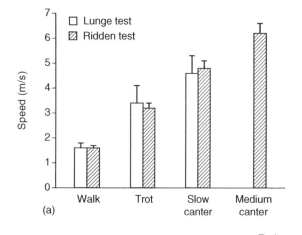

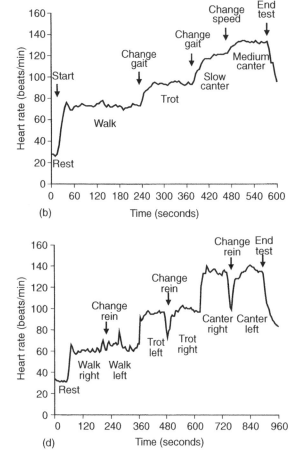

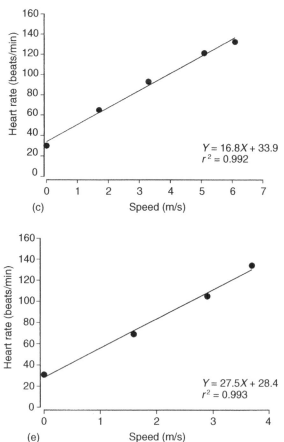

Fig. 18.3 (a) Mean speed for a group of riding school horses in both ridden and lunge tests. (b) Example of heart rate trace from a horse performing a ridden incremental exercise test in an indoor school. (c) Relation between mean heart rate and speed for ridden test. (d) Example of a heart rate trace of a horse during a lunge test consisting of 2 minute periods at each pace and on each rein. (e) Relation between mean heart rate and speed for a lunge test.

accustomed (acclimated) to the treadmill and the other equipment within the laboratory situation, such as masks (see Fig. 18.4), as we would like the horse's behaviour and performance to be as close to that in the field as possible, despite the novelty of the situation. Thoroughbred racehorses have been shown to be able to undertake a standardised exercise test consisting of walk, trot, canter and

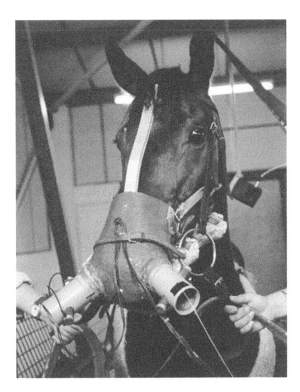

Fig. 18.4 Horse wearing facemask fitted with ultrasonic flow transducers for measurement of ventilation.

gallop during a period of 20 minutes on their first ever treadmill run. However, under these circumstances the horses do not appear comfortable or able to maintain a stable locomotory pattern, and it is likely that most variables of interest will be affected by this, with perhaps the exception of $\dot{V}_{O_2max}$ or speeds eliciting heart rates of above 200 beats/min.

The treadmill environment has the advantage that it allows certain variables to be standardised:

(1) *Speed of running.* The speed of the treadmill can usually be controlled from 1.4 m/s to approximately 16 m/s (35 m.p.h.) and to within ±0.1 m/s.

(2) *Temperature and humidity.* Some laboratories have facilities for controlling air temperature and humidity in the treadmill room. When designing experiments it is important to try and control all variables other than those that you actually wish to manipulate. The effects of en-vironmental temperature and humidity have increasing influence the longer the duration of the exercise.

(3) *Surface conditions.* Treadmill belts are normally rubber, not a surface the horse is used to running on, but it does present an even, stable surface. Because it is firmer than any other surface on which the horse would normally work, many people worry about the degree of concussion on the horse's legs when they are galloping on treadmills. Inclining the treadmill can substantially reduce the concussive forces on the forelimbs, and most high speed exercise tests would be carried out on an inclined treadmill. Although the surface is relatively hard it has the advantage of being even.

(4) *Airflow.* Fans in front of the horse are often used to move air over the body; this is necessary for efficient convective and evaporative heat loss, as would occur in the field. A level of air movement over the horse similar to that of the speed that air would be moving over the horse galloping into still air is required. Thus if the horse is exercising at 12 m/s on the treadmill, the speed of air moving over the horse generated by fans should be similar. However, it is not just velocity but also volume of air that needs to be taken into account. An air velocity of 12 m/s could be generated by a fan only 20 cm across, but the volume of air moved would be very small. Therefore fans at least 50 cm across are normally required. If horses are worked at high speeds with no or inadequate airflow, marked hyperthermia can develop within 1–2 minutes and cause reduced exercise tolerance. A not insignificant proportion of the energy expended in running by the horse is to overcome air resistance, and the fans may help to replace some of the resistance in the treadmill exercise situation.

The inherent disadvantage of treadmill testing is that it is not specific. Horses do not race on moving rubber belts, without riders. Safety regulations in the UK prohibit scientists having horses ridden on high speed treadmills at the gallop, although some locomotion groups around the world have studied horses in this way. The treadmill does, however, allow testing to be carried out on what is effectively a stationary horse, enabling the use of a greater range and sophistication of equipment.

In using any equipment to measure physiological function, such as facemasks for measuring ventilation, or indwelling catheters for taking blood samples or measuring pressures, whether at rest or during exercise, the aim should be to minimise the degree of disruption or alteration in normal physiological responses. Horses can be trained to wear masks during exercise to measure ventilation, uptake of oxygen and output of carbon dioxide, but we cannot take it for granted that the values measured can be directly transposed to field conditions. There is always a chance that the act of putting the facemask on the horse will alter the way the horse breathes or the degree of sympathetic stimulation occurring during exercise. Stress leads to increased adrenaline, which leads to higher submaximal heart rates and higher blood lactates. One way to minimise these inherent differences is to make sure that the horses are fully accustomed to wearing the equipment before any measurements are made. Another way is to measure variables such as heart rate, lactate and blood gases with and without the mask in place to determine if there is any effect of the mask. Even if there is a small effect of the measurement system, provided this is known it may still be considered acceptable to use such equipment, but always bearing in mind the presence of this effect and its implications. The effect is more likely to be a significant hindrance when trying to define absolute values, for example, if we want to describe the $\dot{V}_{O_2max}$ of a population of horses never studied before; if we are using a system that causes $\dot{V}_{O_2max}$ to be overestimated by 20%, then clearly we could draw wrong conclusions about this population in relation to correct absolute measurements made by other scientists using other techniques in other populations. However, if we are trying to investigate the effect of a new feed additive on $\dot{V}_{O_2max}$ we can use an experimental design which would take into account any small errors in measurement of absolute values. For example, in a crossover design, we might study six horses, with each horse's $\dot{V}_{O_2max}$ being measured twice, once without the supplement (control) and once with the supplement (test). At the start three horses would be exercise-tested to determine $\dot{V}_{O_2max}$ with the control (i.e. no supplement) and three would be tested with the supplement. After perhaps a week the tests would be repeated, but the controls

would now get the supplement and the three horses previously supplemented would have no treatment (i.e. become controls). In this situation each horse is said to act as its own control. Because each horse has had its $\dot{V}_{O_2max}$ measured with and without treatment using the same equipment, we can look at the differences (if any) between values of $\dot{V}_{O_2max}$ for the supplemented and non-supplemented horses. In this situation, any absolute error in measuring $\dot{V}_{O_2max}$ has less of an impact on the results because we are looking at differences rather than absolute values.

In probably nearly all circumstances it is better to have horses adequately acclimated to treadmill exercise and any equipment such as masks before carrying out scientific studies. Horses can be adequately acclimated to treadmill exercise for the purpose of conducting a clinical exercise test within 1–2 days; however, you cannot expect these horses to have resting heart rates standing on the treadmill or 'typical' submaximal heart rate responses to exercise. To acclimate horses to the extent that they will stand quietly on the treadmill with heart rates of around 30 beats/min usually means a slower and longer period of acclimation over perhaps 4–6 weeks.

Comparison of overland versus treadmill exercise

After a suitable introduction, running on a treadmill is probably no more unusual to a horse than many of the other things we ask of them. In fact, many racehorses that have been through the starting stalls don't look twice at the treadmill when they are first introduced to it. When first introduced to treadmill exercise, horses tend to move with short, quick strides and are often uncoordinated. They may place both front and rear feet quite wide. After a period of habituation, horses exhibit similar stride kinematics on a treadmill as they do over land. It only takes one or two sessions of 5–10 minutes to get most horses cantering quite happily on a treadmill, able to accelerate and decelerate competently and confidently in response to changes in belt speed. Habituation can be considered to have occurred when the heart rates during treadmill exercise are as would be expected for being ridden at a similar speed and relatively stable, and the gait pattern is stable.

Both the lack of a rider and the fact that the treadmill belt does some of the work for the horse by retracting each limb in the stance phase means that the horse will always find running on a flat treadmill less effort than running at that same speed with a rider over land. For humans running on treadmills, the energy requirements are approximately 10% lower for any given speed. We can compensate for this, however, by carrying out treadmill tests on a slight incline, to bring the energy costs in line with overland running on the flat. It has been estimated that inclining the treadmill to 3.5% produces the same sort of heart rates that would be seen in ridden exercise over land at the same speed with a rider. A different approach would be to load the horse with weights, but to load 60–70 kg of deadweight onto a horse is impractical and can easily cause soft tissue trauma if the weights are not well distributed. Inclining the treadmill is much simpler and more practical.

Where horses are admitted to clinics where exercise testing is carried out, there are many advantages in testing horses as soon as possible: costs to the owner are reduced and the horse does not have to spend quite so long in an unusual environment out of normal training programmes. At the Animal Health Trust, acclimation of clinical cases for poor or loss of performance investigation, or treadmill exercise upper airway endoscopy investigation, usually takes place during 3–5 short training sessions of around 20 minutes each. To keep the number of days that the horse must be in the clinic to a minimum, horses are trained in the morning and afternoon on two consecutive days, with the exercise test itself usually taking place on the morning of the third day. In most cases horses are able to go home on the afternoon of the third day, limiting the time in the clinic to 3–4 days.

Types of treadmill test

Exercise tests, whether they are carried out on a treadmill or a track, in humans or horses, are generally either steady state, intermittent or incremental. Many different types of treadmill test protocol are used depending on the precise nature of the study or clinical investigation. For example, a different type of exercise test may be used to investigate loss of performance syndrome compared with endoscopy of the upper airway as part of an investigation of respiratory noise. An incremental exercise test, a heart rate trace for which is shown in Fig. 18.5, is also the most commonly used exercise protocol to determine maximal oxygen uptake ($\dot{V}_{O_2max}$). This design of test would typically consist of a warm-up at walk (about 10 minutes), a period of trot (about 5 minutes) and then a canter at 6–7 m/s for 1–2 minutes, after which the treadmill speed would be increased by 1 m/s every minute until the horse was unable to maintain its position at the front of the treadmill despite verbal encouragement. Historically these tests have usually been run on inclines of between 3° and 6° and this is still the case today. Whilst most institutes around the world use similar test protocols there is unfortunately no universally agreed standard protocol for determining $\dot{V}_{O_2max}$.

The use of an incline should ensure that the horse will reach $\dot{V}_{O_2max}$ before it reaches the maximum speed of the treadmill. With the older treadmills this was essential as the maximum speed was often only 12 m/s. Today many treadmills can attain speeds of 15–17 m/s and so theoretically a $\dot{V}_{O_2max}$ test could be carried out on a flat treadmill. For clinical cases, the number of steps of this type of incremental test that can be completed is a good indicator of combined fitness and ability. For example, an average fit and healthy racehorse should be able to complete all steps to the end of 11 or 12 m/s, whilst a good racehorse should complete the 13 m/s step (using the protocol described above on a 5° incline). An exceptional performance would be completion of the 14 m/s step, but this happens only rarely for this exercise test protocol. Horses with musculoskeletal problems, or airway or cardiac disease or dysfunction, often reach the point of fatigue at much lower steps.

A steady state test might consist of a warm-up at walk and trot, and possibly even a short (1–2 minutes) slow canter (7–10 m/s), followed by a walk and then a fixed duration single exercise speed. The time of the exercise step may be fixed or can be dependent on when the horse tires, although judging the point of fatigue is somewhat subjective. For example, fatigue might be defined as the first time the horse drops back from the front bar by more than 0.5 metres or it might be when the horse has dropped back but been encouraged back up to the bar three times, or when the horse cannot

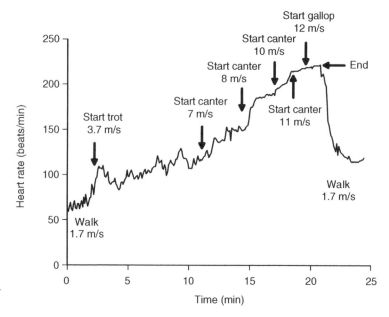

Fig. 18.5 Heart rate trace from an incremental treadmill test.

be encouraged back up to the front bar. In some studies it may be necessary to try and determine if a treatment has an effect on run time to fatigue.

Intermittent exercise protocols can also be used. These may consist of several bouts of canter or gallop at the same speed or increasing speed, interspersed with periods of recovery, much like interval training in the field (see Fig. 18.6). These designs can produce more pronounced metabolic and physiologic changes than seen with single bouts of exercise or incremental protocols. These designs may be particularly useful in studies where a significant degree of glycogen depletion is required to test the effect of different manipulations on the speed of glycogen restoration; they may also be useful in studies of thermoregulation because body temperature will increase over successive bouts of exercise. Higher values of blood and/or plasma lactate can also be reached with intermittent protocols compared with single high intensity bouts. Intermittent exercise can also be useful when the study involves complex instrumentation for measurements during exercise, such as for ventilation, blood gases, blood pressure and gait. Rather than exercise the horse on three separate days at three different speeds, it may be possible to study all three speeds on one day. This is not a suitable design for all studies, but can be applicable pro-

vided the variable being measured returns to baseline between exercise steps. One way around this is to randomise the order of the steps in different horses. So in a study with six horses requiring them each to run for 2 minutes at 8, 10 and 12 m/s, two horses may run the steps in the order 8, 10, 12 m/s, another two may run at 10, 8, 12 m/s and the final two may run in the order 12, 10 and 8 m/s.

A different type of test protocol is one in which the treadmill exercise test is designed specifically to model a form of competition or activity in the field. For example, in studying the response of three-day event horses to different environmental conditions, a treadmill test that was of a similar design to a one-star speed and endurance test was used.

It is probably true that most exercise tests, whether for clinical or research investigations, increase workload by increasing the treadmill speed. This is not, however, exclusive. In certain circumstances it may be desirable or necessary to maintain speed and increase the treadmill inclination. For example, after 10 minutes of walking on the flat the horse may be required to trot at around 3.5–4.0 m/s on a flat treadmill, and after 3 minutes the incline would be increased in steps of 2° every third minute until maximum incline had been reached. The main limitations with this type of test

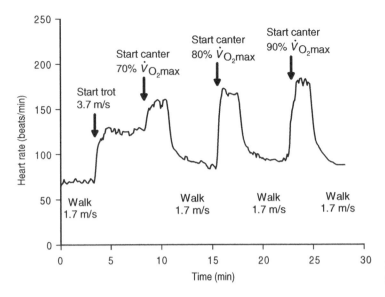

Fig. 18.6 Heart rate trace from an intermittent treadmill test.

are that most horses will not be working anywhere near maximally at the highest incline (7–8°) at trot. Aerobically fit endurance horses, eventers and racehorses may only reach heart rates of 160–170 beats/min at trot on the steepest inclines, and in many cases will not produce plasma lactate concentrations much above 2–3 mmol/l. However, for unfit horses, horses with compromised pulmonary (e.g. horses with RAO) or cardiovascular function (e.g. horses with significant functional heart murmurs), or horses trained for anaerobic type competition (e.g. showjumpers), this type of test is likely to be quite informative. The advantage is that horses can be acclimated to walking and trotting on a treadmill, in most cases, in one day so tests can be carried out either more quickly and/or greater numbers can be processed.

A potential problem with testing horses on steep inclines is that they may not have trained on such slopes during training. If this is the case, then the physiological and metabolic changes during the test may reflect the recruitment and response of the muscle groups needed for steep uphill work rather than the locomotory musculature in general. If these muscle groups are particularly untrained, they may even lead to a falsely poor exercise test performance. Steep inclines may 'unload' the forelimbs, but increase the strain on the tendons and ligaments of the hind limbs. Trotting horses fast uphill on a treadmill at speeds of around 5 m/s on a 5°

incline can produce hind-limb lameness in a large proportion of horses.

What can you measure on a horse exercising on a treadmill?

- Ventilation
- Gas exchange
- Heart rate
- Blood lactic acid (lactate) concentration
- Arterial blood gas analysis
- Mixed venous blood gas analysis
- Airway pressures
- Muscle biopsy
- Blood pressure
- Body temperature
- Sweating rate
- Cardiac output.

Ventilation

Tidal volume, respiratory frequency, minute ventilation and peak and mean inspiratory and expiratory flow rates are the primary ventilatory variables measured during exercise. They can all be derived from measurements of either flow and/or volume. Any device for measuring flow is known as a pneumotachometer (sometimes the shortened term pneumotach or pneumotachograph is used).

Pneumo is derived from the Greek word *pneuma* which means air or breath and tachometer means any device that measures speed or rate. Thus, the output of a pneumotachometer is normally in volume per unit time, e.g. litres/second. The most common design of pneumotachometer works on the principle that any obstruction in the path of airflow will cause a drop of pressure downstream. The obstruction to flow must be great enough for a pressure difference to develop each side of the obstruction but not high enough that it will affect the subject breathing through it. The faster the airflow, the greater the pressure difference. The obstruction normally takes the form of a screen or mesh, or a series of honeycomb tubes (Fig. 18.7). The change in differential pressure with flow rate is also only linear over a limited range. Because of the obstruction, turbulence has the effect of exaggerating the pressure drop across the screen as flow rate increases. Screen pneumotachometers also have the disadvantage that moisture and other respiratory secretions can block the screen and alter the calibration because any further obstruction will, of course, increase the pressure difference and give a falsely elevated flow rate. Some designs can be heated to around 50°C which will prevent condensation of moisture in exhaled breath (which will be around 37–40°C). The other disadvantages of this design of pneumotachometer are that for high flow rates the size must be quite large and therefore they are often heavy. If the correct size is not selected, the resistance of the pneumotachometer may cause the horse to change from its normal ventilatory response to exercise. There are a number of commercially available pneumotachometers that work on the obstruction-induced pressure difference principle.

A different type of device especially suited for use with horses is the ultrasonic pneumotachometer (see Fig. 18.8). Two ultrasonic transducers are mounted diagonally across a tube. Each transducer acts alternately as a transmitter and then a receiver as a burst of ultrasound is sent across the tube and then back again by the second transducer. The phase of the received signal (effectively the time between the signal being sent from one transducer and received by the second transducer) is altered by the speed of the airflow.

The main advantages of the ultrasonic pneumotachometer design are the much lower resistance to

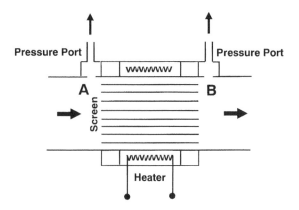

Pressure at A > Pressure at B

Fig. 18.7   The principle of a pneumotachometer.

airflow than the screen or resistance type devices and the fact that the output of voltage with increasing flow is linear. The disadvantage of the ultrasonic pneumotachometer is that the calibration is altered by changes in gas composition and moisture, so if calibration is carried out with room air (21% O_2, 79% N_2 and, for example, 20°C and 50% RH) this will be fine for inspired airflow, but of course expired air has a different composition (e.g. 16% O_2, 5% CO_2, 79% N_2 and 37°C and 100% RH). Fortunately the changes in gas composition, moisture and temperature in expired air approximately cancel each other out and can be ignored for most purposes. As with screen pneumotachometers, moisture build-up can cause problems. However, in the case of the ultrasonic pneumotachometer it is accumulation of moisture on the ultrasonic transducers that changes the calibration. This does not tend to be a significant problem when the period of use is less than approximately 30 minutes. To permit longer periods of use, one system has a facility to flush a low volume of dry air from a cylinder (compressed gases in cylinders usually have close to no moisture, i.e. 0% RH) across each of the transducers to prevent moisture building up. There are only two commercially available systems for horses based on ultrasound technology. The BRDL system has a very low dead space and the facemask only covers the upper face so that a bit and bridle can be used to control the horse (Fig. 18.4). The Spiroson system has a mask which covers the whole face and so has a larger

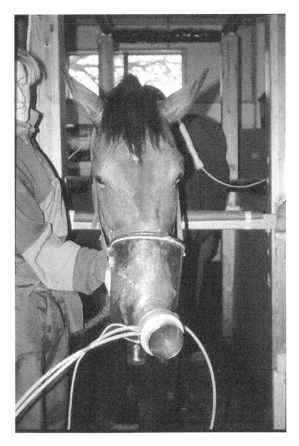

Fig. 18.8 Horse wearing a facemask and pneumotachometer used for measuring ventilation.

dead space, but the inflatable cuff system for sealing the mask to the face appears robust and effective.

One other commercial system for equine use during exercise that incorporates a turbine pneumotachometer is made by Cosmed. To the best of our knowledge there are no published papers describing the validation of this principle in horses during exercise.

A number of different groups have developed their own design of pneumotachometers based on other principles. One of the most well-known systems was that developed by Kimmich and Spaan (1980). This system was based on a flag in a tube that was deflected by the airflow. The flag was connected to a force transducer; the greater the airflow, the greater the deflection of the flag and the greater the force on the transducer. This was the basis for some of the earliest reliable measurements of maximal ventilation in the field (e.g. Hornicke *et al.* 1987). However, the system was difficult to use and

calibrate and was never widely adopted, possibly because the BRDL system was developed commercially at around the same time. Attenburrow (1976) used a thermistor (a type of temperature sensor) positioned in the trachea to measure airflow. This is a relatively more invasive procedure as the thermistor must be inserted into the trachea either by passing it through a nostril and via the larynx which could potentially irritate the airway, or alternatively, the thermistor could be inserted through a small opening in the skin overlying the trachea using a sterile technique and local anaesthesia. Whichever method of positioning the thermistor, the assumption is that a single point measurement of airflow in the trachea will accurately represent flow across the whole cross-section of the trachea. Flow patterns are often complicated in airways and this assumption may not be valid under all conditions.

Irrespective of the method of measuring flow, the equipment must be calibrated before use and preferably also after measurements have been made to verify that no change has occurred. Either flow or volume can be used for calibration of flow measuring devices, although it is desirable to calibrate using values of flow or volume likely to be encountered in the measurement conditions. For example, if inspiratory and expiratory flow rates as high as 50 litres/second are expected to be measured then it would be ideal to calibrate between +50 and −50 litres/second or at least at zero and 50 litres/second. In practice, the linearity of a system is usually determined and then periodic checks are made to ensure this has been maintained, whilst on most occasions a two-point calibration may not span the full range of values for airflow expected.

Flow calibration is usually undertaken using a device known as a rotameter. Air is sucked through the rotameter which in turn is connected to the pneumotachometer and the flow rate can be read from the scale on the rotameter. Rotameters come in different flow ranges and are calibrated for specific conditions (for example, typically the scale may be set for air at 20°C, 0% RH and 760 mmHg (101.3 kPa)). Thus if you used the rotameter with another gas or gas mixture, if the air was a different temperature or moisture content, or if barometric pressure was different, the calibrated scale would not then be accurate. However, if the conditions of the air or gas being drawn from the room through the rotameter are known, a correction to the value read from the scale can be applied.

Volume calibration of pneumotachometers can be carried out using a precision calibrated syringe. Syringes that can deliver volumes of 1–7 litres are available and cover the range of tidal volumes likely to be seen in horses at rest, but during exercise the tidal volume may be double this. Thus, it may be necessary to custom manufacture syringes for calibration of pneumotachometers where exercise measurements are going to be made. A potential drawback to using volume calibration for exercise studies is that the volume will probably be forced through the pneumotachometer quite slowly compared with during exercise. Even by pulling the syringe backwards and forward rapidly it is unlikely that a respiratory frequency of greater than 60 breaths/min could be simulated. During exercise, respiratory frequencies are likely to be double this. Thus, calibrating with volume for exercise at a low 'respiratory' frequency could not verify that the calibration and response of the pneumotachometer would be similar during exercise. However, whilst flow calibration might be preferred, it is not unusual after flow calibration to carry out a volume calibration of a system, just for further verification.

Accurate measurements of volume can also be made using devices known as dry gas meters. These are based on the gas meters installed in homes to measure gas consumption. As they are the basis for charging people for their gas use, these meters are very accurate and reliable. In fact, it is not necessary to buy an expensive dry gas meter if a domestic one can be obtained. However, the commercial systems for physiology do usually have the advantage of a zero button, whilst those for domestic gas consumption cannot be reset to zero. As flow is pushed or pulled through the meter it acts on a set of bellows which turn a dial indicating volume. Dry gas meters are particularly useful for measuring volumes of expired gas collected into Douglas bags over known periods of time. The volume measured might then be used to calculate minute ventilation, oxygen uptake, carbon dioxide production or RER. When used in this way the air is usually drawn through the gas meter by a vacuum source. The dry gas meter is excellent in that its ability to measure volume is not affected by the conditions of the gas, such as temperature, humidity or composition.

However, to make corrections to STPD or body temperature and pressure, saturated (BTPS) it is still necessary to measure the temperature and humidity of the gas in the bag either before or after it has passed through the dry gas meter. If the dry gas meter has a limitation it is probably that gases can only be drawn through them at relatively low flow rates. Exceeding the maximum flow rate damages the delicate bellows mechanism and the meter is likely to be inaccurate or unusable. The small domestic gas meter may have a maximum flow rate of only $5\,m^3$/hour (5000 litres/hour or 83 litres/min). However, larger industrial dry gas meters can have maximum flow rates of $100\,m^3$/hour (100000 litres/hour or 1667 litres/min, close to the maximal minute ventilation of a horse during exercise).

One further consideration which applies to all the different types of pneumotachometer is frequency response. In simple terms this means how quickly the device can respond to changes in the rate of airflow. This is different to the range of airflow rates that could be measured if the flow was constant. A pneumotachometer that can respond to rapid changes in flow rate is said to have a high frequency response, as the changes in rate can be characterised into frequencies. A device that does not respond rapidly would be referred to as having a lower frequency response.

Gas exchange

Measurement of oxygen uptake ($\dot{V}_{O_2}$), carbon dioxide production ($\dot{V}_{CO_2}$) and calculation of the respiratory exchange ratio (RER = $\dot{V}_{CO_2}/\dot{V}_{O_2}$) can be carried out by a number of different approaches and can be divided into those that require a measurement of ventilation and those that do not. Any method for measuring gas exchange will obviously require the analysis of oxygen and carbon dioxide in expired air. Measurements of inspired O_2 and CO_2 can be made, but these can either be assumed ($O_2 = 20.95\%$, $CO_2 = 0.03\%$ but is usually taken to be 0%) or calculated based on barometric pressure, humidity and temperature. The two most common methods of measuring expired O_2 and CO_2 are with electrochemical or paramagnetic oxygen analysers and infrared analysers, respectively.

Electrochemical analysers contain sensors that are commonly referred to as electrodes. These usually consist of either separate or combined measuring and reference electrodes, similar to those used in blood–gas analysers. Paramagnetic analysers work on the principle that oxygen is attracted into a magnetic field and that most other gases are not. The analyser creates a focused magnetic field and any oxygen present in the gas sampled by the analyser is attracted into the strongest part of the magnetic field. Two glass spheres around 2 mm across and filled with nitrogen are mounted on a bar within the magnetic field. Oxygen attracted into the magnetic field displaces the nitrogen-filled spheres and the degree of displacement is related to the oxygen concentration. Oxygen can also be measured using zirconia technology. This has traditionally been used for measuring oxygen in combustion gases, for example in power stations. These gas mixtures are corrosive and would quickly attack normal oxygen measuring equipment. However, zirconia based systems are being used more and more in medicine and physiology because of their fast response times. Measurement is based on the fact that some ceramics, such as zirconia, conduct electricity at high temperature due to movement of charged oxygen ions. The more oxygen in the sample gas, the greater the movement of oxygen ions across a zirconia disk heated to around 800°C.

Carbon dioxide is most commonly measured using a photometric technique based on the fact that some gases absorb a particular wavelength of light. For CO_2 it is a particular wavelength of infrared light. An infrared light source is focused onto a cell through which the sample gas is continuously drawn. The greater the concentration of CO_2, the more infrared radiation it will absorb and the less will reach the detector on the other side of the sample cell.

These analysers are very stable and accurate but have a relatively slow response time. This means that when a gas is sampled by the analyser it may take 1–2 s to give a final, stable reading. This could therefore obviously not be used to follow changes in O_2 and CO_2 in air being breathed out, because the concentrations of O_2 and CO_2 vary throughout the breath.

Respiratory mass spectrometers are able to perform the same analysis but within around 0.002 s. However, they have a lower accuracy and stability than the slow response analysers and usually cost at least six times as much.

Methods for measuring gas exchange requiring measurement of ventilation

1. Non-rebreathing valve and timed collection. This is probably the most simple and robust method. The horse wears a tight fitting mask which is attached to or incorporates a non-rebreathing valve (see Fig. 18.9). In this type of valve the horse breathes in through one valve and out through the other. Therefore the flow of air is always in the same direction. The expired gas is collected into a bag (PVC or similar and commonly known as a Douglas bag) over a timed period. Once the sample has been collected the O_2 and CO_2 content of the expired gas is measured using slow response analysers or a mass spectrometer. This gas is referred to as mixed expired gas because it represents all the gas exhaled by the horse over the collection period. Remember that this will contain both deadspace gas and alveolar gas. The volume of gas in the bag must then be measured to calculate ventilation. This can be carried out by drawing the gas out of the bag through a dry gas meter until the bag is empty.

As an example, if 500 litres of exhaled gas was collected into a Douglas bag over 20 s from a horse exercising on a treadmill at gallop, this would equate to a minute ventilation of $500 \times 60/20 = 1500$ litres/min. If the mixed expired CO_2 was 5% (which could also be expressed as the fractional mixed expired CO_2 $F\overline{E}_{CO_2} = 0.05$) then the rate of production of CO_2 in litres/min is given by 1500 litres/min $\times (5\%/100\%) = 75$ litres/min, i.e. 5% of the volume of expired minute ventilation was accounted for by CO_2. The calculation of CO_2 production is quite simple because we know there was no CO_2 in the inspired air. For calculating oxygen uptake we use a similar approach, but we must allow for the fact that the inspired gas contained 21% oxygen. The easiest way to approach the calculation is to think that the horse breathed in 1500 litres/min $\times$ (21%/100%) litres of oxygen per minute, which is equal to 315 litres O_2 inspired per minute. If the mixed expired oxygen was 17% ($F\overline{E}_{O_2} = 0.17$) then the amount of oxygen in the air breathed out was equal to $1500 \times (17\%/100\%) = 255$ litres/min. Thus, each minute the horse removed $315 - 255 = 60$ litres

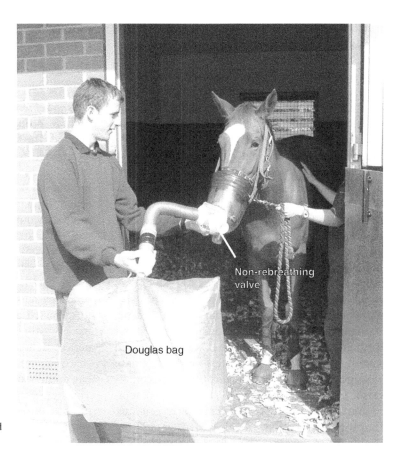

Fig. 18.9 Non-rebreathing valve and Douglas bag.

of oxygen, so $\dot{V}_{O_2}$ (oxygen uptake) = 60 litres/min. A simpler calculation would of course be 1500 litres/min × ((21% − 17%)/100%) = 60 litres/min, but the long approach helps to clarify the concept. The calculation of RER is then 75 (litres/min)/60 (litres/min) ($\dot{V}_{CO_2}/\dot{V}_{O_2}$) = 1.25.

There is one more step that needs to be taken before the calculation of $\dot{V}_{O_2}$ and $\dot{V}_{CO_2}$ is complete. This is to express the volumes of oxygen consumed and carbon dioxide produced at standard conditions. Our calculations of $\dot{V}_{O_2}$ and $\dot{V}_{CO_2}$ are based on the volume of gas we collected. Although this gas would have come out of the horse fully saturated (100% RH) at around 37°C and the volume would also be dependent on the prevailing barometric pressure, after the gas had been in the bag for a while it would have cooled down to room or ambient temperature. A saturated gas is one in which no more water can be introduced without droplets condensing out. The more moisture the air can hold, the less likely it is that codensation will

occur. As the air cooled down it would remain saturated (RH would still be 100%) because the amount of moisture that air can hold decreases with decreasing temperature, i.e. warm air holds more moisture (expressed as grams of water per litre of air) than cold air. That means that our values for $\dot{V}_{O_2}$ and $\dot{V}_{CO_2}$ are currently expressed in terms of the ambient temperature (let's say it was 20°C in the laboratory) and pressure (we'll say it was 780 mmHg (104 kPa)) and saturated with moisture (100% RH @ 20°C). So at this stage our values for $\dot{V}_{O_2}$ and $\dot{V}_{CO_2}$ are by convention referred to as being at ATPS (ambient temperature and pressure, saturated). The problem is, if we carry out a study on another day when conditions are different or we want to compare our data to that published by another group, the precise conditions under which the data were collected will affect the values of $\dot{V}_{O_2}$ and $\dot{V}_{CO_2}$. Therefore, the universally agreed standard for expression of $\dot{V}_{O_2}$ and $\dot{V}_{CO_2}$ is at STPD (standard temperature (0°C or 273 kelvin) and pressure (760 mmHg or 1 atmosphere or 101.3 kPa) and dry (0% RH)).

Tables are published that allow conversion of volumes at ATPS to STPD using a factor (for example, see *Nunn's Applied Respiratory Physiology*, 1993). However, the actual derivation of these factors is based on the application of Charles' law and Boyle's law.

Boyle's law describes the inverse relationship between volume (V) and pressure (P) of an ideal gas at a constant temperature as being a constant (K):

$$P \times V = K$$

Charles' law describes the direct relationship between the volume (V) and temperature (T) of an ideal gas at constant pressure (P):

$$V = K \times T$$

The two equations can be combined to give:

$$P \times V = R \times T$$

where R is the universal gas constant which is the same for all ideal gases.

The formula for converting volumes at ATPS to volumes at STPD based on these gas laws is:

$$\text{Volume (STPD)} = \text{Volume (ATPS)} \times (273/(273 + t)) \times ((P_B - P_{H_2O})/101)$$

Where P_B is barometric pressure in kPa (taken at the time of the study), t is ambient temperature in °C and P_{H_2O} is the saturated water vapour pressure (in kPa) of the gas in the Douglas bag at ambient temperature.

This method of measuring $\dot{V}_{O_2}$, $\dot{V}_{CO_2}$ and RER is relatively easy to perform, requires minimal equipment and is excellent for resting measurements. This method, or slight variations using valves, has been used in some studies during exercise. However, even the resistance imposed by very low resistance valves at the flow rates seen during exercise in the horse appear to significantly affect either the values of $\dot{V}_{O_2}$ and $\dot{V}_{CO_2}$ and/or ventilation and blood gases compared with those measured when using other systems. Other disadvantages include large equipment dead space and weight. The most common effects of valve systems during exercise appear to be a reduced minute ventilation, decreased $\dot{V}_{O_2}$ and $\dot{V}_{CO_2}$ and increased arterial hypercapnia (higher arterial Pa_{CO_2}). Because expired gases are collected and pooled from a number of sequential breaths, usually over 15 seconds or more, valve systems do not provide information on short-term changes in $\dot{V}_{O_2}$ and $\dot{V}_{CO_2}$.

2. Open flow, bias flow, flow by or flow through systems (see Fig. 18.10). All the above terms are often used to refer to the same type of technique for measuring $\dot{V}_{O_2}$ and $\dot{V}_{CO_2}$ in exercising horses. This technique is probably the most commonly used for measuring exercising $\dot{V}_{O_2}$ and $\dot{V}_{CO_2}$ in the horse in different laboratories around the world. The principle of measuring $\dot{V}_{O_2}$ and $\dot{V}_{CO_2}$ with the open flow technique is by dilution. The horse is fitted with a loose fitting mask that allows air to be drawn in around and past the horse's face and the nostrils. The airflow is generated by powerful fans or blowers that are positioned downstream. The airflow rate for any given exercise intensity must always exceed the horse's peak expired flow rates (100 litres/second or 6000 litres/min during intense exercise). This is to ensure that no expired gas escapes from the facemask into the room and that the horse does not rebreathe any expired gas. Gas that escapes or is rebreathed could lead to an underestimation of $\dot{V}_{O_2}$ and $\dot{V}_{CO_2}$, and rebreathing of expired gas higher in CO_2 may stimulate respiration above that due to the exercise intensity. In practice, during high intensity exercise, flow rates of 8000–10 000 litres/min are generally used. The principle of the open flow approach is based on the fact that if all the exhaled gas travels through the system, then if the changes in the oxygen and carbon dioxide levels are measured and the total flow rate is known, $\dot{V}_{O_2}$ and $\dot{V}_{CO_2}$ can be calculated. Because of the high flow rates past the horse's nostrils compared with the actual $\dot{V}_{O_2}$ and $\dot{V}_{CO_2}$, the dilution of the air drawn past the horse by expired gas is small. Therefore the most appropriate analysers for use with open flow systems are the slow-response type.

Taking an example for the calculation of $\dot{V}_{CO_2}$, if the flow rate in the system was measured at 10 000 litres/min and the CO_2 measured downstream from the horse was 0.5%, the $\dot{V}_{CO_2} = (0.5/100) \times 10000$ litres/min = 50 litres/min. For $\dot{V}_{O_2}$, if the oxygen in the downstream air was 20.5%, the calculation would be $\dot{V}_{O_2} = ((20.95 - 20.5)/100) \times 10000$ litres/min = 45 litres/min. RER would be calculated as described above (i.e. RER = 50/45 = 1.11).

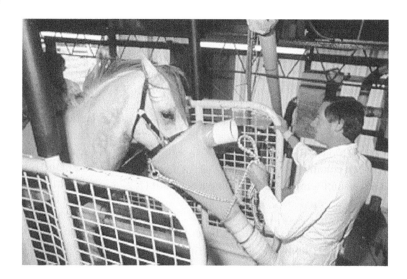

Fig. 18.10   Open flow system.

The open flow technique averages a number of breaths but has been used to study oxygen uptake kinetics in the horse during exercise. The resistance is low, there is essentially no equipment dead-space and rebreathing should not occur provided the airflow rate is high enough.

3. Breath by breath. To calculate $\dot{V}_{O_2}$ and $\dot{V}_{CO_2}$ on a breath by breath basis requires simultaneous, continuous and real time measurements of airflow and respired gas composition. The ultrasonic pneumotachometer is the most suitable flow measuring device, and respired gases must be measured with a respiratory mass spectrometer. The flow and respired gases are integrated to obtain $\dot{V}_{O_2}$ and $\dot{V}_{CO_2}$ throughout each breath. The calculation is usually carried out by either software in the mass spectrometer or by a separate computer taking electrical outputs of both flow and gas signals and using either commercial or custom software, but a good approximation can also be obtained manually working on a chart printout. Examples of flow, CO_2 and O_2 tracings obtained during intense exercise are shown in Fig. 18.11.

The principle of calculation using the breath by breath approach is that instead of calculating $\dot{V}_{O_2}$ and $\dot{V}_{CO_2}$ over a long period of time, such as in the example of the valve and Douglas bag method, $\dot{V}_{O_2}$ and $\dot{V}_{CO_2}$ are calculated over very short periods of time. For example, if at a respiratory rate of 120 breaths/min a single expiration lasts for 0.25 seconds (or 250 ms), if we could sample the flow and

gas signals 250 times during a single expiration, we would have a paired measurement of flow and gas (O_2 and CO_2) every millisecond (one-thousandth of a second). If we look at the first 1 ms of an expiration and, for example, the flow is 50 litres/second, then in that 1 ms, the volume expired would be 50 litres/second or 50/1000 = 0.05 litres/ms, i.e. 0.05 litres. If the CO_2 at the same point in time was 4%, the $\dot{V}_{CO_2}$ for that 1 ms would be (4/100) × 0.05 = 0.002 litres of CO_2 produced in 1 ms. This is of course very small, but we are only looking at one-thousandth of a breath. If the CO_2 produced each 1 ms was the same for the whole of the exhaled breath (lasting 250 ms) the volume of CO_2 exhaled would be 250 × 0.002 litres = 0.5 litres per breath. If the horse was breathing at a respiratory frequency of 120 breaths/min, then the $\dot{V}_{CO_2}$ would be equal to 120 breaths/min × 0.5 litres = 60 litres/min. This is therefore a calculation of CO_2 on a single breath and this can be repeated for each breath; hence, breath by breath.

Of course in reality both flow and exhaled gas O_2 and CO_2 vary throughout the course of each expiration. The software must also be able to accurately determine the start and end of each expiration. One of the most difficult problems encountered when using the breath by breath approach is the fact that whilst the flow signals are occurring in real time (this means that there is no delay between when the flow occurs and its measurement by the ultrasonic pneumotachometer), there is a delay between when expired gas changes occur and when the mass

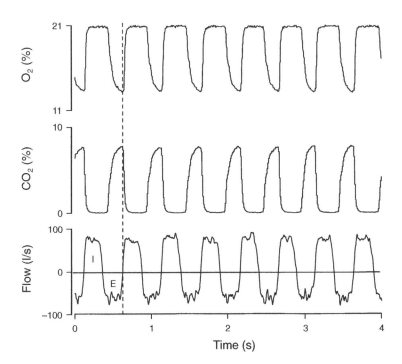

Fig. 18.11 Examples of breath by breath changes in respiratory airflow, CO_2 and O_2 produced by a horse during intense treadmill exercise. Positive flow represents inspiration and is labelled I; negative flow represents expiration and is labelled E. The start of one breath cycle, i.e. the start of inspiration is marked by the vertical dashed line.

spectrometer has made the measurement. This delay is usually quite small (around 250–300 ms) but will cause dramatic errors in the calculation of $\dot{V}_{O_2}$ and $\dot{V}_{CO_2}$ if not taken into account correctly. The delay is not in the actual analysis of the gases but in the time it takes for the sample of expired gas to reach the analysis chamber within the mass spectrometer. This is because the expired gases are sampled continuously by a thin capillary tube placed in the expired flow. The majority of the delay (about 95%) is due to the movement of the expired gases down the capillary and into the mass spectrometer. This means that before the breath by breath analysis can take place, the flow and gas signals must be realigned. This is usually based on determining the points corresponding to the start of inspiration on both the flow and gas traces. On the flow trace the start of inspiration is when the flow crosses the zero flow line and on the gas trace this is most reliably taken as the point when the CO_2 trace falls to zero. The delay in time between the flow and gas traces (O_2 is assumed to be the same delay as CO_2) can then be calculated and the traces aligned by moving the gas traces forward in time so that they are correctly aligned with the flow. Depending on the system or software, the delay may be calculated once at the start of a run of data (as unless the

capillary becomes blocked or damaged the delay should be constant) or on a breath by breath basis, which is probably more accurate.

Methods for measuring gas exchange not requiring measurement of ventilation

Calculation of $\dot{V}_{O_2}$ *and* $\dot{V}_{CO_2}$ *by the Fick principle.* $\dot{V}_{O_2}$ can be calculated using the Fick principle as follows:

$$\dot{V}_{O_2} = \dot{Q} \times (Ca_{O_2} - C\bar{v}_{O_2})$$

Similarly, $\dot{V}_{CO_2}$ can be calculated by $\dot{V}_{CO_2} = \dot{Q} \times (Ca_{CO_2} - C\bar{v}_{CO_2})$. This requires the measurement of cardiac output ($\dot{Q}$) and the arterial and mixed venous oxygen or carbon dioxide contents, as opposed to tensions, in paired samples (i.e. samples taken at the same time). The blood content is the absolute amount of oxygen or carbon dioxide in each millilitre or litre of blood and is expressed either as mmol O_2 or CO_2 per litre or ml O_2 or CO_2 per 100 ml blood. Blood oxygen and/or carbon dioxide contents can be measured in a number of different ways.

- Historically the gold standard for measuring oxygen content has been the Van Slyke method.

This is based essentially on changes in absolute pressure as a result of liberating oxygen as a gas from the blood using a releasing agent such as potassium ferricyanide.

- By the oxygen electrode method which is similar in principle to the Van Slyke technique. A known volume of blood is introduced into an anaerobic chamber (i.e. a chamber with no air present). An oxygen electrode measures the partial pressure of the blood. This initial Pa_{O_2} represents the dissolved oxygen in the plasma and not the oxygen bound to haemoglobin in the RBCs (called 'bound oxygen'). A small volume of potassium ferricyanide is then added which releases all the oxygen bound by haemoglobin. This can now be sensed by the oxygen electrode as it is effectively now dissolved oxygen, and the partial pressure of oxygen is measured again. The change in oxygen partial pressure is equivalent to the oxygen content of the sample.
- With analysers known as oximeters, co-oximeters or haemoximeters which usually measure the absorbance of haemoglobin which changes with the amount of bound oxygen. This can also be seen in the change from bright red (oxygenated) arterial blood to dark-red-blue (deoxygenated) blood.
- From an oxygen dissociation curve. Human blood gas analysers are able to estimate the oxygen saturation and content from a series of equations and formulae describing the oxygen dissociation curve and how it changes with factors such as pH, temperature and carbon dioxide. Equations for horses are available and this technique can be applied, although it is an indirect rather than a direct method.

The oxygen content can also be calculated if percentage saturation of haemoglobin and arterial oxygen tension are known using the equation

$$Ca_{O_2} = [Hb\,(g/dl) \times 1.34\,(ml\,O_2/g\,Hb) \times Sa_{O_2}(\%)]$$
$$+ [Pa_{O_2}\,(mmHg) \times 0.003\,(ml\,O_2/mmHg/100\,ml)]$$

The first part of the equation estimates the bound oxygen as the maximum amount of oxygen that could be bound by 1 gram of haemoglobin to be 1.34 ml. If the haemoglobin concentration was 20 g/dl and the saturation 90%, the oxygen content would be $20 \times 1.34 \times 0.9 = 24.1$ g/dl. The second part of the equation calculates the dissolved oxygen

(oxygen in the plasma) which is much smaller (i.e. 0.003 ml O_2/mmHg arterial O_2 tension per 100 ml of blood). If the Pa_{O_2} was 110 mmHg (14.7 kPa) at a saturation of 90%, the dissolved oxygen content would be equal to $110 \times 0.003 = 0.33$ ml/dl (3.3 ml per 100 ml). Therefore the oxygen content of the blood sample is 24.1 (bound oxygen) + 0.33 (dissolved oxygen) = 24.4 ml/dl.

Mixed venous blood ($\bar{v}$) must be collected from the pulmonary artery and therefore the whole procedure is more invasive than the previous three methods. In practice this approach would rarely be used in order solely to calculate $\dot{V}_{O_2}$, but more commonly by rearranging the original Fick equation to give

$$\dot{Q} = \dot{V}_{O_2}/(Ca_{O_2} - C\bar{v}_{O_2})$$

$\dot{Q}$ would be estimated from measurements of $\dot{V}_{O_2}$ and arterial and mixed venous oxygen contents.

Heart rate

Heart rate is possibly one of the most frequently measured physiological variables in exercise studies. It provides a good estimate of work under most circumstances and is easy to measure and record non-invasively using heart rate monitors or an ECG. Two of the most commonly used variables to describe the relationship between heart rate and speed are V_{140} and V_{200}. These simply describe the speeds at which the heart rate will be 140 and 200 beats/min, respectively. Both V_{140} and V_{200} are calculated from a plot of heart rate against speed. V_{140} and V_{200} will be higher in more athletically gifted horses and will also increase with increasing fitness in an individual horse (see Fig. 18.12). A higher V_{140} (or V_{200}) simply means that a horse can go at a faster speed before reaching a heart rate of 140 beats/min. In general terms, riding school horses might be expected to have V_{140} values of around 4.5–6.5 m/s, whilst fit eventers at the top level should be around 7–8 m/s. Untrained Thoroughbred racehorses in one study were reported to have V_{140} values around 7 m/s and trained Thoroughbreds should have values of around 7–9 m/s. In a study on trained Quarter horses V_{140} was reported to be between 5 and 8 m/s (Erickson *et al.* 1987). Trained endurance horses may also have V_{140} values of around 7–9 m/s.

The speed at which the maximal heart rate is reached ($V_{HR_{max}}$) is also commonly used to describe

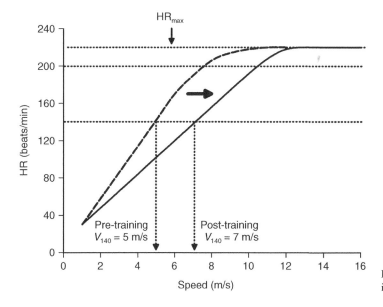

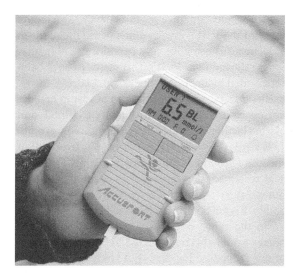

Fig. 18.12 Improvement in V_{140} with increased fitness.

an individual horse's cardiac response to exercise. Idealised graphs showing the relationship between heart rate and speed, for example in an incremental exercise test, often show a clear plateau in heart rate: in reality, this is rarely seen and it is more common to see the increase in heart rate with increasing speed becoming smaller but still increasing slightly with increasing speed.

Blood lactic acid (lactate) concentration

Lactic acid can be measured in blood or plasma. Plasma values are always higher than whole blood values because in any sample the concentration of lactic acid per litre of plasma is much higher than the concentration of lactic acid per litre of RBCs. For example, in one study following single bouts of maximal exercise, the plasma lactic acid concentration was found to be about 2.5 times higher than in RBCs taken at the same time and about 1.5 times higher than the whole blood lactic acid concentration. Lactic acid in plasma can be analysed in many clinical biochemistry laboratories using standard methods on automated analysers. Rapid benchtop dedicated lactic acid analysers which can accept either whole blood or plasma have been around for at least 15 years. More recently, small hand-held analysers about the size of a pack of cigarettes, which can accept either blood or plasma have become available (see Fig. 18.13). These work with

Fig. 18.13   A hand-held rapid lactate analyser.

dry chemistry in the form of a strip onto which the blood or plasma sample is placed. These are very similar to the glucose meters used by some diabetics to check their blood glucose concentrations. Results are obtained within 1 minute. These analysers have been shown to not quite match up to the performance of laboratory analysers but the error may be acceptable, depending on circumstances. For example, the error would probably not be acceptable in a scientific study in which lactic acid was one of the main variables of interest.

Blood samples for lactic acid determination can be taken by syringe and needle, vacutainer or by indwelling catheter. There is little difference between concentrations in venous and arterial blood. It has even been shown that results for a small sample of blood taken from the skin on the shoulder or front of the chest using a lancet are in reasonable agreement with the lactic acid concentration measured in a blood sample collected by venepuncture (i.e. via a needle from a vein). The volume of blood required for lactic acid in blood or plasma analysis is usually small. For the hand held analysers, only a drop of blood is needed (about 10 µl). For laboratory analysis, 1–2 ml may be required. Blood samples for lactic acid should be collected into tubes containing the preservatives fluoride and oxalate to prevent metabolism of glucose to lactic acid by RBCs. In many exercise studies in the 1980s, blood collected for whole blood lactic acid determination was immediately deproteinised (which would denature all the enzymes, including those of the RBCs involved in glucose metabolism to lactic acid) using ice-cold perchloric acid (sometimes referred to as PCA). This seems to have been superseded by the use of fluoride/oxalate.

Blood lactic acid concentration at rest in healthy horses is usually close to 1 mmol/l. Blood and plasma lactic acid tend to increase markedly around 75% $\dot{V}_{O_2max}$ (80–90% HR_{max}) or on the treadmill at speeds of around 8–10 m/s on a 5° incline. The lactic acid response to exercise varies dramatically with fitness, type (sprinter versus stayer), health and ability. V_{LA4} in healthy fit Thoroughbreds is likely to be in the range 6–12 m/s, whilst good endurance horses would also be expected to be at the top end of this range (see Fig. 18.14). A study by Rainger *et al.* (1994) demonstrated that V_{LA4} in a group of fit Thoroughbreds decreased from 9.8 m/s to 5.8 m/s after a period of detraining.

Blood lactic acid concentration after intense or maximal exercise can also be used as a measurement of anaerobic power, with a higher peak blood lactate concentration indicating greater anaerobic capacity which is generally considered to be a good indicator of sprint capacity in horses. In one study of four repeated bouts of intermittent maximal exercise, it was found that the fastest horse on the first 700 metre gallop had the highest plasma lactic acid (32 mmol/l), whilst the slowest horse produced

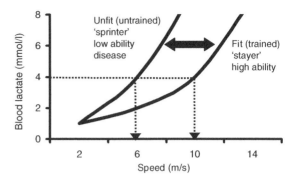

Fig. 18.14 Improvement in V_{LA4} with training.

only 23 mmol/l. However, over the next three gallops the low lactic acid producing horse either equalled or beat the high lactic acid producer for speed. After intense exercise, blood lactic acid concentrations may not peak until 5–10 minutes post-exercise. Thus samples taken immediately at the end of exercise may underestimate the true peak. Similarly, for blood lactic acid concentrations of less than about 12 mmol/l at the end of exercise, the values at 5 and 10 minutes post-exercise will be lower, so a sample collected at this time will also underestimate the true peak value.

Arterial blood gas analysis

Arterial blood can be collected from a catheter inserted into a facial artery, a carotid loop or into the carotid guided by ultrasound, or from a catheter placed in the aorta or left ventricle via a carotid introducer. The difference between arterial blood collected from these different sites is usually minimal and can be ignored in most circumstances. Arterial blood travels rapidly and when sampled will not have passed through tissues or organs; therefore gas exchange and acid–base balance cannot have been dramatically affected. Arterial blood would nearly always be the first choice sample for assessing blood gas and acid–base status either at rest or during exercise. Whilst resting (at 37°C) Pa_{O_2} may be around 90–110 mmHg (12–14.7 kPa); light warm-up walking or trotting exercise may increase Pa_{O_2} by 10–20 mmHg (1.3–2.7 kPa). During intense exercise, many horses develop arterial hypoxaemia (reduced arterial blood oxygen tension). This usually starts at around 60–70% $\dot{V}_{O_2max}$ and becomes progressively more marked with increasing intensity such that in some horses Pa_{O_2} may fall as low as 50 mmHg (6.7 kPa) when measured at 37°C or around 65–70 mmHg (8.7–9.3 kPa) when corrected to true body temperature (see below). When arterial hypoxaemia was first reported to occur in horses, it was thought that these represented poorer quality horses and that this would not occur in the elite horses. If fact, the exact opposite is now known to be true in that in good, aerobic horses, especially Thoroughbreds, the rate of utilisation of oxygen by the mitochondria within the muscles outstrips the maximal rate of oxygen delivery by the cardiovascular system. A horse that does not become hypoxaemic during maximal exercise is likely to have a low $\dot{V}_{O_2,max}$ and/or is an out and out sprinter. A third possibility is that the horse has a cardiovascular system with a huge capacity to deliver oxygen which exceeds the muscles' capacity to use oxygen, although this appears to be rare in good or elite horses competing in primarily aerobic events, and normally it is oxygen usage that exceeds delivery. The same relationship between supply and demand is seen in elite human athletes with the development of arterial hypoxaemia in those competing in disciplines with a very high aerobic component such as cyclists, swimmers, rowers and runners.

Mixed venous blood gas analysis

To look at whole body acid–base and blood gas status, it is necessary to collect mixed venous blood. If a sample of blood is collected from the jugular vein this will show quite marked changes in oxygen, carbon dioxide and pH during exercise, but these changes will mainly reflect what is happening in the head and neck. For arterial blood samples for acid–base and blood gas analysis, the site where the sample is taken doesn't usually make too much difference. This is because all arterial blood comes from the same place, i.e. the left atrium, and we are looking at the blood before any gas exchange has occurred, i.e. before it has passed through any tissues or organs. In contrast, when we sample venous blood we are looking at blood which has passed through an organ or tissue; therefore the oxygen, carbon dioxide and pH in venous blood primarily reflect what was going on in that area. If a large amount of oxygen has been extracted, we might infer that this region is very metabolically (or more specifically, aerobically active at this time).

During exercise, the head and neck muscles, brain and of course other tissues extract oxygen from the incoming arterial blood and produce carbon dioxide and lactate. The major locomotory muscles are at the opposite end of the horse and the venous blood draining this area returns to the heart in the inferior (or caudal) vena cava. Thus, if we could sample this blood during intense exercise we would probably see more extreme changes than in jugular venous blood returning to the heart in the superior (or cranial) vena cava. Whilst this would be of great interest, unfortunately we cannot reliably obtain samples of blood from the inferior vena cava. It is located deep within the body and it is difficult to reliably thread a catheter into it from the jugular vein. What can be achieved reliably is to position the tip of a catheter for sampling blood in either the right atrium, right ventricle or pulmonary artery. The catheter is inserted into the jugular vein and advanced downwards towards the heart following the pressure trace (see Fig. 18.5). The venous blood returning to the heart from the right and left jugular veins and the inferior vena cava meets and mixes in the right atrium. The mixing carries on in the right ventricle and by the time the blood is in the pulmonary artery, it is considered to be fully mixed; hence the term mixed venous blood. This is the most useful sampling site within the body for venous blood for nearly all applications. The downside is that the technique for sampling is relatively invasive.

Not only can blood oxygen and carbon dioxide tensions and contents and pH be measured in mixed venous blood, but blood temperature is often measured in the pulmonary artery. This is sometimes referred to as core temperature (although the same term may also be applied to oesophageal temperature). Again, as for blood gas and acid–base status, the mixed venous blood temperature in the pulmonary artery is particularly useful because it reflects the heat production in all muscles and tissues. Pulmonary artery blood temperature is around 36–37°C at rest and can increase to 44°C during intense exercise. As well as being of primary interest in studies of thermoregulation, the difference between pulmonary artery blood temperature and arterial blood temperature, which will be slightly lower, has been used to calculate respiratory heat loss across the lung.

The most common reason for measuring pulmonary artery mixed venous blood temperature is for the correction of oxygen and carbon dioxide tensions from the temperature at which they are measured to a standard of 37°C. The measuring cell in blood gas analysers is usually warmed to 37°C. Therefore, even after a blood sample has been taken and the sample has cooled down, once inside the analyser it will be heated back up to body temperature, assuming that this was 37°C. This is of course especially important when samples have been kept on ice at around 4°C to reduce the amount of oxygen the WBCs and reticulocytes (immature RBCs) use and to stop the WBCs and RBCs producing lactic acid and changing both pH and carbon dioxide tensions. Storage of blood at room temperature in impermeable glass syringes therefore leads to a decrease in oxygen tension and pH, and increases in carbon dioxide tension.

Temperature also has a marked effect on the oxyhaemoglobin dissociation curve. Increasing body temperature shifts the curve to the right, decreases the affinity of haemoglobin for oxygen and improves oxygen release to the tissues. Decreasing temperature shifts the curve to the left and increases the affinity of haemoglobin for oxygen. This can be a problem when analysing samples taken during exercise on a blood gas analyser set at 37°C because increases in body temperature overestimate both the decrease in oxygen tension and the increase in carbon dioxide tension in arterial and mixed venous blood.

For example, if a horse's blood temperature when an arterial blood gas sample was taken during exercise was 42°C and the Pa_{O_2} measured in a blood gas analyser set at 37°C reads 60 mmHg (8.0 kPa), this will overestimate the true fall in Pa_{O_2}. For Pa_{O_2} and Pa_{CO_2} the error is around 6–7% overestimation per degree Celcius difference between the blood temperature in the horse and the temperature of the blood gas analyser. So although the measured Pa_{O_2} at 37°C (analyser temperature) was 60 mmHg (8.0 kPa), in the horse at 42°C, the true Pa_{O_2} would have been approximately 6% × (42°C – 37°C) = 30% higher = 1.3 × 60 mmHg = 78 mmHg (10.4 kPa). Similarly for a Pa_{CO_2} in the analyser of 70 mmHg (9.3 kPa; 37°C) the true Pa_{CO_2} at the horse's blood temperature would have been 6% × (42°C – 37°C)

= 30% lower = 0.7 × 70 mmHg (9.3 kPa) = 49 mmHg (6.5 kPa). Blood pH is also affected by differences in temperature by around 0.0134 pH units per degree Celcius difference in temperature. Precise correction factors for horse blood have been published by Fedde (1991).

Airway pressures (tracheal/pharyngeal/oesophageal pressures)

Measurements of airway pressure are essential in the calculation of airway resistance and dynamic compliance at rest, and may also be of particular interest when investigating the impact of conditions such as dorsal displacement of the soft palate or laryngeal hemiplegia during exercise. Other examples may include evaluating the effects of a mask or gas collection system, or devices to reduce airway resistance (e.g. equine nasal dilator strips).

The most commonly measured 'airway' pressure is oesophageal pressure. Of course, strictly speaking, oesophageal pressure is measured in the oesophagus and is therefore not an airway pressure. Ideally when investigating lung mechanics we would like to be able to measure pleural pressure. However, this involves inserting a catheter into the pleural space and carries the risk of introducing air which could lead to collapse of the underlying lung (referred to as a pneumothorax), or infection which could lead to pleuro-pneumonia. Even if carried out successfully without either of these adverse effects, this would not be a routine procedure that could be used on a daily basis, for example to follow changes in compliance in a horse with RAO after treatment.

Instead of direct measurements of pleural pressure, oesophageal pressure is usually measured. The thoracic oesophagus lies within the thorax and therefore changes in intrathoracic pressure associated with ventilation are transmitted to the oesophagus. To measure oesophageal pressure, a long stiff catheter with a balloon covering the end (usually a condom for horses) is passed via the left or right nostril. As the larynx is normally open for breathing, it is most common for the catheter to pass into the trachea. The passage into the oesophagus can be aided by flexing the head and neck. The catheter is inserted until the tip is sitting in the pharynx. This is best achieved by offering up the catheter to the outside of the head and placing a mark on the catheter at the distance of the nostril. Once the catheter is in place, it is a case of waiting until the horse swallows and then advancing the catheter rapidly forward by about 20 cm or so. If the catheter has passed into the oesophagus, some resistance will be felt. If it has passed into the trachea little resistance is felt and the horse frequently coughs.

In some cases the horse avoids swallowing when the catheter is in the upper airway. Swallowing can sometimes be induced by moving the catheter slowly backwards and forwards a few centimetres or by squirting 20 ml of water up into the back of the mouth using a syringe. The procedure for inserting an oesophageal catheter is thus essentially the same as passing a stomach tube.

Once the tip of the catheter is in the oesophagus, it must be advanced slowly. Often the oesophagus may initially spasm around the tip of the catheter, and pushing hard may damage the oesophageal surface. The final position of the tip of the catheter determines both the magnitude and the quality of the oesophageal pressure signal. Remember that in a healthy horse the maximal changes in oesophageal pressure may only be about 0.29 kPa (3 cmH$_2$O) during quiet breathing at rest. Because an air filled catheter and external pressure transducer are normally used, any movement (such as head shaking) can greatly affect the signal. An alternative to the air filled catheter and external pressure transducer is to use a catheter-mounted strain gauge, as for blood pressure measurement. These catheters are considerably more expensive and relatively delicate, but they are less prone to movement artefact and can respond to very fast rates of change in pressure, i.e. they have a high frequency response.

There are essentially three ways to determine the final position of the measuring tip of the catheter. The first is to offer the catheter up against the side of the horse and estimate the distance from the nostril to the middle of the thorax. The distance is then marked on the catheter and it is inserted to this length. The second approach is to insert the catheter and once the tip is in the thorax, move it backwards and forwards whilst monitoring the pressure changes. The final position is that which gives the greatest change in pressure between inspiration and expiration (i.e. maximum delta pleural pressure change – maxΔP_{pl}). The third approach is to place the catheter tip using the external approxi-mation and then to take a radiograph (X-ray) of the chest. The catheter is then positioned so the tip lies at a point in the oesophagus just past the back of the heart, which corresponds to mid-thorax (mid-chest) or mid lung. The catheter length inserted is then marked and after the catheter has been withdrawn, the distance is measured. This technique is extremely useful in research studies where measurements may be made in the same horse on a number of different occasions or where the same horse is used in a number of different studies over a period of time.

Whatever method for positioning an oesophageal catheter is used, it is important that the measuring tip is placed to avoid cardiac pressure artefact. This happens when the measuring tip is too close to the heart and small pressure waves are seen on the oesophageal pressure recording as a result of the movement of the heart with each beat.

Large tubes are easier to pass into the oesophagus than thin ones, stiff tubes are easier than soft ones, and a narrow stiff tube will transmit pressure changes the best. However, a large stiff tube is easy to pass into the right position, but may interfere with flow in the upper airway. A soft tube will not damage the upper airway or oesophagus, but will be more difficult to pass and the pressure signal quality may be poor. Soft catheters may even turn around and become bent over during passing. Therefore, a stiff narrow catheter is usually selected, perhaps 3–4 mm in diameter, with 1 mm thick walls. Whilst human oesophageal catheters are available commercially, those for horses must be handmade.

As well as irritating the upper airway or oesophagus from frequent passing, there is always the risk of upper airway haemorrhage due to passing catheters through the delicate nasal turbinates. This can happen to even the most skilled person if the horse happens to shake its head at the wrong time as the catheter is being passed. The bleeding can be quite profuse but reduces with time and often will not recur or seem to have any long-term effect.

Tracheal pressure is measured less commonly. In this case a much thinner catheter without a balloon is passed into the trachea rather than the oesophagus. The presence of the catheter may interfere with laryngeal function and may also cause the horse to cough. To avoid interfering with the function of the larynx, a catheter can be inserted by the trans-tracheal route, i.e. by making a small cut in a small area of anaesthetised skin overlying the mid-cervical (mid-neck) trachea.

Whilst pleural pressure is not commonly measured, it may be required in some circumstances. Techniques for measuring pleural pressure are often more concerned with the actual process of placing the catheter than the process of pressure measurement. Measurements of pleural pressure have the advantage that they are regional, e.g. the pleural pressure changes of the dorsocaudal and cranioventral regions could be compared. Oesophageal pressure can sometimes be limited in that it represents the sum of all pleural pressure changes all over the lung, i.e. pleural surface, and cannot provide information on regional function.

Pharyngeal pressure changes have also been measured at rest and during exercise in horses, using a catheter of similar design to that used for tracheal pressures (see Nielan et al. 1992; Rehder et al. 1995). Pressures in the pharynx can also be measured during videoendoscopy of the upper airway during exercise by attaching a pressure transducer to the biopsy channel of the endoscope. This provides an output of pressure which can be used to calculate respiratory rate, count the incidence of swallowing, and to make measurements of peak and mean inspiratory pressure. The measurements of expiratory pressure obtained using this approach are unfortunately less reliable because during expiration the flow is directly towards the opening of the biopsy channel which, along with the camera lens, is facing almost directly at the larynx. This causes turbulence at the biopsy channel opening and rapid fluctuations and overestimation of expiratory pressure.

Muscle biopsy

Samples of muscle of around 50–200 mg taken using the needle biopsy technique have been used to characterise horses and to determine changes with age, exercise and training, including glycogen usage, lactate production, pH decrease, triglyceride and FFA mobilisation, ATP and PCr decrease, muscle buffering capacity, muscle enzyme activities and histochemistry. The collection of small samples of muscle using the biopsy technique is described in Chapter 3. For exercise studies, a common procedure would be to shave and disinfect an area of skin about 3 cm × 3 cm and to infiltrate local anaesthetic

into two or more areas below the skin. The incisions, approximately 1 cm long, are then made in the skin using a sterile scalpel blade and a pre-exercise sample collected from one site. After exercise a post-exercise biopsy is collected from the second site. It is not usual to introduce further local anaesthetic to collect the second sample.

Blood pressure

Blood pressure can be measured either directly using external pressure transducers or pressure sensors mounted onto the end of catheters. Indirect measurements of blood pressure have been made in the horse at rest using sphygmomanometers, but the accuracy and repeatability are generally poor, and there has not been validation against direct measurements that are considered to be the gold standard.

When making measurements of blood pressure using an external transducer, the distal end (end nearest the horse) of a hollow catheter filled with saline is inserted into a peripheral vein, such as the right or left jugular (or sometimes an artery) and the proximal end of the catheter (the end farthest from and external to the horse) is connected to the pressure transducer. The blood is connected by a continuous 'line' or column of fluid to the transducer and, because fluids are relatively incompressible, the pressure fluctuations in the blood vessel are transmitted to the external transducer. The catheter is positioned by advancing it and observing the pressure waveforms which are characteristic for different regions of the cardiovascular system. The advantages of this type of approach are that the external transducers are relatively inexpensive and robust and because they do not come into direct contact with the horse it is easier to maintain sterility. The main disadvantage is that movement of the fluid within the catheter due to movement and not to true fluctuations in blood pressure is transmitted to the external pressure transducer and sometimes cannot be differentiated from true blood pressure changes. The absolute pressure measured is also dependent on the vertical height of the external transducer. If the transducer is lowered below the height of the tip of the catheter in the horse this will increase the pressure; if it is raised above the height of this point the pressure will fall. The height of external transducers used in horses is therefore usually standardised to the point of the shoulder to correspond with the level of the heart.

With external transducers, the pressure is often measured by a strain gauge that senses the pressure applied to a diaphragm. For intravascular blood pressure measurements the strain gauge is mounted on a catheter. These pressure catheters are often referred to as microtip catheters. The term Millar is synonymous with this design of catheter, after the company in Houston, Texas that makes them, and in fact Mikro-Tip is a registered trademark of Millar. However, in recent years catheters with similar performance and at a more reasonable price have been introduced by companies such as Gaeltech. Furthermore, measurement is not limited to one pressure sensor and it is not unusual to have a catheter with two or three strain gauges mounted at different positions on a single catheter. These may be used, for example, to measure simultaneous pressures along a single vessel, or the sensors may be positioned on the catheter to enable simultaneous measurement of, for example, both left ventricular (distal sensor) and aortic pressure (proximal sensor).

The catheter mounted pressure sensor approach is no more invasive than the fluid filled catheter and external transducer, because of course the open end of a fluid filled catheter must also be inserted into the blood vessel or region where the pressure is to be measured. However, the catheter mounted sensor has great advantages in terms of very high frequency response and reduced noise artefact from movement. On the negative side, these catheters are often four or five times the cost of an external transducer and have a more limited lifespan as they are more delicate. They are also prone to build-up of protein material over the strain gauge surface which can dampen the frequency response and affect the calibration. This can be avoided by thorough cleaning and washing after use. They must also be sterilised each time they are used. The catheters used with external transducers are usually considered disposable and come prepacked as sterile. One other difference between the external and internal measurements is that with the external transducer the pressure measured at the open end of the catheter is referenced to the height of the external transducer (not air), unlike the internal sensor where the pressure measured is the pressure at the sensor with reference to ambient air pressure (independent of height). This can be an advantage if you know exactly where the tip of your catheter is located.

Either internal or external transducer pressure catheters are usually inserted using a special catheter introducer placed in a peripheral vein or artery. For example, pressures in the right atrium, right ventricle and pulmonary artery are measured by placing an introducer in the left or right jugular vein and passing the catheter until the measuring port (fluid filled catheter) or sensor (catheter mounted sensor) is in the correct place. The correct placement is verified by following the blood pressure trace as the catheter is advanced. The typical pressure waveforms seen as a catheter is advanced from the jugular vein to the pulmonary artery are shown in Fig. 18.15. The path that the catheter takes is to a large extent not under the control of the person inserting it. Some catheters, usually for use with external transducers, have a small balloon mounted at the end which is used for making measurements of pulmonary artery wedge pressure, although the balloon can be inflated as the catheter is being positioned and this helps to direct the tip of the catheter with the blood flow, particularly when in the right side of the heart as the catheter is being advanced in the direction of blood flow.

Invasive measurements of arterial blood pressure are complicated by the fact that large arteries lie deeper in the body than veins. A common approach used by groups who are involved in cardiovascular research is to surgically relocate a small section of the carotid artery to a superficial location where it can easily be accessed. This is referred to as a carotid loop. The 'loop' is usually around 5–10 cm in length and can be seen above the jugular vein. An introducer can be inserted into the carotid loop to permit introduction of pressure catheters to measure carotid pressure (which is very close to systemic arterial pressure), or the catheter can be advanced down towards the left side of the heart to measure aortic pressure. Advancing the catheter further into the left ventricle allows measurement of left ventricular pressures. Unfortunately, although left atrial pressure is of great interest and significance for studies of cardiovascular function and especially in many studies of EIPH, because

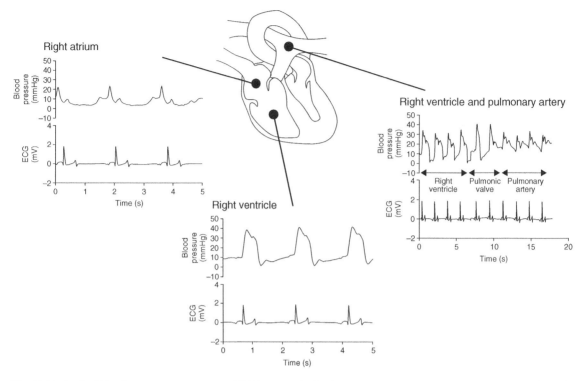

Fig. 18.15 Typical blood pressure waveforms and ECG traces obtained as a catheter is advanced from the jugular vein to the pulmonary artery.

the flow is against the direction of the catheter being advanced (so flow guidance using a balloon is not an option) and because of the configuration of the mitral valve, it is hard to guide the catheter from the left ventricle into the left atrium. However, sometimes when positioning catheters in the left ventricle the tip may occasionally be seen to 'flip' or 'flick' into the atrium, but this cannot be achieved with any consistency. Pressures can be measured in peripheral arteries such as the mandibular artery and the transverse facial artery. These are often used during anaesthesia or for exercise testing where samples of blood are required. Because these arteries are very small (perhaps only 2 mm internal diameter), introducers or catheter tip pressure transducers are generally not suitable for use in these sites and a small catheter (approximately 0.8 mm (21 gauge)) is inserted directly into the vessel. The catheter is connected to an external transducer by a saline filled extension line. However, the signal quality may be poor during exercise due to movement of the extension line.

Body temperature

Body temperatures are often of interest for studies of thermoregulation and for correction of gas volumes or blood gases to standardised body temperature, i.e. 37°C. Many different temperatures have been measured during exercise in the horse, including those of muscle, rectal, venous, arterial, right atrial, pulmonary arterial, airway, oesophageal, guttural pouch and skin. With the exception of skin temperature which can be measured using thermal imaging cameras, measurement is made by a temperature sensor (most often a thermistor or thermocouple) inserted to lie directly at the measuring site. Thermal imaging is an attractive technique as it is non-invasive. However, it only reflects the temperature at the surface. In a horse with a very short coat, skin temperature will be very close to coat surface temperature. In horses with longer coats it may be more accurate to describe temperatures obtained by thermography as coat surface temperatures because they may differ significantly from the temperature of the underlying skin. It is important to recognise that thermography cannot 'penetrate' the skin to give the temperature within a muscle. However, if the muscle is hot, perhaps due to increased blood flow within due to injury, the heat may be conducted to the surface and the effect seen using thermography.

Rectal temperature is probably the body temperature taken most routinely. It is used to correct ventilatory and blood gas data, and in studies of thermoregulation to reflect whole body heat storage. Oesophageal, right atrial and pulmonary artery temperatures may be used for the same reasons. The latter two measurement techniques are more invasive, but the response to changes in heat storage and dissipation is more rapid. Oesophageal temperature changes quite slowly compared to right atrial and pulmonary artery temperature which will both reflect rapid changes in blood temperature, such as occur during external cooling with cold water. Oesophageal temperature is measured with a thermistor or thermocouple on a long (about 2 metres) catheter which is passed via the left or right nostril. The right atrial and pulmonary artery temperatures are measured using catheters with very small thermistors or thermocouples attached inserted into the left or right jugular vein after which the tip with the temperature sensor is advanced until it is in the required location. The placement of the catheter is achieved by following a pressure trace (see Fig. 18.15).

Sweating rate

Sweating rate can be measured either by application of an absorbent material over a known area of skin and recording the change in mass due to sweat absorbed by the material ($1\,g = 1\,ml$). This has the possible disadvantage of insulating the area of skin under the material which may influence local sweating rate. Sweat may also evaporate from the material during the collection period leading to underestimations of sweating rate.

An alternative technique which prevents the loss of sweat by evaporation is the sealed pouch method. A plastic pouch is sealed over a measured area of skin and sweat accumulating in the pouch can be drawn off at known intervals. This technique has the possible disadvantage of both insulating the underlying skin and affecting sweating rates by preventing evaporation. In cool, warm or hot and relatively dry environmental conditions a large proportion of sweat secreted onto the skin would evaporate. With the sealed pouch method sweat is unable to evaporate and the skin can become hyperhydrated, similar to what happens if you stay in the bath too long! Neither of these techniques are particularly suited to looking at the dynamics of sweating (changes over short periods of time) because collection periods of around 10–15 minutes may be needed to obtain a suitable volume of sweat absorbed by the pad or collected in the pouch.

A technique which allows the dynamics of sweating to be studied is the ventilated capsule (Fig. 12.3), the principle being that a capsule of known area is attached to a region of skin, such as the neck, chest or over the gluteal muscles, through which air is either blown or sucked at a known flow rate. If the moisture content of the air entering and leaving the capsule is measured, the sweating rate can be calculated. To measure true sweating rate, the skin inside the capsule must essentially remain dry. If sweat accumulates on the skin surface inside the capsule, evaporation rate rather than sweating rate is measured. The moisture content of air entering and leaving the capsule can be measured using dew point hygrometers or by calculation from measurements of temperature and humidity. Compressed air from cylinders is a good source to use because the humidity is close to zero, although the temperature may also be quite low. Capsules were traditionally made of materials with high thermal conductivity, such as copper, but modern capsules are made in lightweight plastic and can be attached to the coat using straps, skin adhesives, special skin tape (e.g. Blenderm made by 3M) or double sided tape. The limitation of the ventilated capsule is that it is not suited to measurement of sweat composition.

Sweating rate can also be indirectly estimated by measuring body mass change with exercise. However, faecal and urinary losses also need to be accounted for. Even then, the change in mass also includes a component of respiratory water loss.

Cardiac output

Cardiac output is defined as $\dot{Q} = SV \times HR$, where $\dot{Q}$ is in litres/min, stroke volume (SV) is in litres and heart rate (HR) is in beats/min. Of course, HR can be readily measured during exercise, but the direct measurement of SV is generally not possible. One recent study carried out in Japan did attempt to make as near as possible direct measurements of SV during exercise by implanting sensors onto the wall of the left ventricle. However, this is a highly invasive, expensive and technically challenging approach.

1. $\dot{Q}$ by the Fick principle

One of the most common approaches to estimating cardiac output during exercise in the horse is based on the Fick principle, such that $\dot{Q} = \dot{V}_{O_2}/(Ca_{O_2} - C\bar{v}_{O_2})$. The Fick principle is based on the assumption that the whole body consumption of oxygen measured at the mouth $(\dot{V}_{O_2})$ must be a function of oxygen extraction ($Ca_{O_2} - C\bar{v}_{O_2}$ difference) and delivery (cardiac output). Thus, if a horse has an oxygen uptake during maximal exercise of 50 litres/min and the arterial – venous content difference is equivalent to 0.2 litres of oxygen per litre of blood, the cardiac output would be 50 litres/min divided by 0.2 l/l = $\dot{Q}$ = 250 l/min. If the cardiac output (blood flow) remained the same, but the amount of oxygen used by the muscles (i.e. extracted from the arterial blood) doubled, the $\dot{V}_{O_2}$ must have doubled, i.e. 0.4 l/l × 250 litres/min = $\dot{V}_{O_2}$ = 100 litres/min. This approach requires simultaneous measurements of $\dot{V}_{O_2}$ and arterial and mixed venous oxygen content as described earlier.

When $\dot{Q}$ has been estimated using the Fick principle, dividing by the corresponding HR gives an estimate of SV. For example, if $\dot{Q}$ is calculated to be 250 litres/min and HR is 230 beats/min, the SV would be 250 litres/min per 230 beats/min = 1.09 litres (the minutes cancel out).

The accuracy of the Fick principle for estimating $\dot{Q}$ can be affected by a number of different factors, including:

- Errors in measurement of $\dot{V}_{O_2}$ (i.e. primarily flow and respired gases) and arterial and mixed venous oxygen contents.
- Extrapulmonary venous admixture or shunt. This refers to any venous blood which mixes with blood that has passed across the gas exchange surface and which is returning to the left side of the heart. Extrapulmonary refers to this happening outside the lung. Intrapulmonary

shunting (e.g. due to lung disease) is accounted for in the Fick principle. However, the admixture (addition) of venous blood to what is essentially 'arterial' blood reduces both the average arterial blood oxygen content or partial pressure/tension and this is not accounted for when using the Fick principle. Venous blood that effectively by-passes the gas exchange surface without passing through lung itself is primarily of two sources:

- Thebesian veins: a number of small veins draining the cardiac muscle of the left heart drain directly back into the left atrium rather than into the venous circulation or right heart
- Bronchial veins: deep bronchial veins (the veins that return the blood supplying the lung tissue itself with oxygen and nutrients, i.e. the bronchial arterial circulation) drain into the pulmonary venous return to the heart, which is bringing oxygenated blood back to the left atrium.

- The Fick principle does not allow for the oxygen consumption by the lung itself. This may be negligible at rest in healthy lungs, but exercise and disease may increase this error.

2. Indicator dilution techniques

In indicator dilution techniques for estimating cardiac output, a known amount of an indicator solution, e.g. indocyanine green, ice-cold saline or lithium chloride, is injected rapidly as a bolus directly into the right atrium or sometimes into a large vein, such as the jugular vein. The concentration of the indicator is measured continuously downstream, either in the pulmonary artery or somewhere in the arterial circulation. The concentration of the indicator against time is displayed and recorded. There is a delay between injecting the indicator and it being detected downstream. The indicator travels with the blood, mixing as it flows. At the point where the indicator is measured, a rapid rise and a slower disappearance are typically seen. The extent to which the indicator has been diluted reflects the blood flow or cardiac output; the higher the dilution, the higher the cardiac output.

For dye dilution, blood is drawn continuously through a catheter with its tip placed in the pulmonary artery and in turn through an external cell which measures the dye concentration. The more recent lithium dilution method is based on continuously drawing arterial blood through a cell containing a lithium electrode. This approach has the advantage that lithium is not normally present naturally in the blood and that lithium chloride is relatively cheap and innocuous in the concentrations required for this method. Indocyanine dye is expensive, whilst thermodilution is susceptible to errors in both the temperature of the injected saline and measurement of the very small temperature changes that occur in the circulation.

With thermodilution, which uses ice-cold saline as the 'indicator', the blood temperature is measured continuously by a very small temperature sensor with a fast response, i.e. high frequency response, mounted on the end of the catheter. These catheters can be obtained commercially and are referred to as thermodilution catheters or sometimes Swann–Ganz or triple lumen catheters. Whatever design is used, besides the temperature sensor, the catheter must have some means of measuring pressure or a lumen to connect to an external pressure transducer to verify correct positioning of the sensor in the pulmonary artery. When working with large animals such as the horse which have a high cardiac output, relatively large volumes of saline must be injected, usually around 50–100 ml. In man and smaller animals the smaller volumes of saline (about 20 ml) can be injected rapidly by hand, but when working with horses it is normally necessary to use a gas driven pressure injector (driven from a source of compressed air) and a catheter with multiple ports at the end to allow both the injectate to escape rapidly and to prevent a high pressure stream of injectate being directed onto the wall of the right atrium which could result in dysrhythmias.

All indicator dilution methods are considered to be variable over time to the extent that three immediate and sequential determinations should be made and a mean of three similar values should be taken as the true cardiac output.

3. Echocardiography

Pulsed Doppler echocardiography has been used to measure cardiac output in anaesthetised horses. A transducer capable of generating and detecting high frequency sound waves (above 20000 cycles per second, i.e. 20 kHz) is mounted on an endoscope. The endoscope is inserted into the oesophagus via the left or right nostril and advanced until the transducer is lying next to the heart and the aorta can be viewed. The transducer is able to measure both aortic blood velocity and aortic diameter simultaneously. Blood flow past the point of measurement can then be calculated. Because all arterial blood flow must pass through the aorta, this is equal to cardiac output. Currently the size of the probe, the need to be able to manipulate the probe into a position to obtain suitable images and the sensitivity to movement, make it unlikely that this technique could be applied during exercise.

4. Other techniques

Cardiac output has also been measured using radionuclide imaging. A small amount of a gamma emitter such as [99m]technitium pertechnetate is injected into a vein, the right atrium or pulmonary artery. The size of each of the chambers of the heart can then be viewed during each stage of the cardiac cycle using a gamma camera or smaller gamma detectors placed directly onto the subject. This technique has been used to measure cardiac output in human subjects both at rest and during exercise, but does not appear to have been explored in horses.

Another technique that has also been used in human medicine is impedance cardiography. This is a completely non-invasive technique which involves passing a high-frequency current across the chest. The ejection of blood from the left ventricle into the aorta results in a wave of impedance (effectively equivalent to resistance) that can be used to estimate cardiac output. Unfortunately, whilst it is attractive due to being non-invasive, the technique is quite sensitive to motion artefact and again, to date, the use of this technique does not appear to have been reported in horses.

A technique for measuring cardiac output from rest to during maximal exercise in horses has also been recently reported based on the surgical attachment of ultrasonic sonomicrometer crystals to the walls of the left ventricle. The crystals are referred to as transceivers as they both transmit and receive ultrasound signals, which pass easily and rapidly through tissue. Pairs of crystals are used to both transmit and receive a pulse of ultrasound. The time it takes for the signal to travel between crystals is proportional to the distance between them. The nearer they are the shorter the time and vice versa. Therefore by using pairs of crystals placed on opposite sides of the left ventricle, the change in distance as the ventricle expands (filling, i.e. diastole) and contracts (emptying, i.e. systole) can be measured. The change in distance across the ventricle can then be used to estimate changes in ventricular volume. In the only published study to demonstrate this technique in horses (Pascoe *et al.* 1999), out of eight animals only five were reported

to recover sufficiently enough to be able to gallop on the treadmill again. Many complications were also reported following the surgery, including pyrexia (increased body temperature), abcesses, weight loss and lameness and this technique is unlikely to therefore become widely used.

The most common methods employed to measure $\dot{Q}$ during exercise in horses to date have been thermodilution and use of the Fick principle.

KEY POINTS

- Exercise tests can be used to follow changes in fitness that occur with training, to compare the fitness of different horses, to assess functional capacity (e.g. $\dot{V}_{O_2max}$, HR_{max}), to characterise type and to verify normal function.
- Exercise tests are used extensively in research, in areas including nutrition, physiology and biomechanics, to assess the effects of different treatments or manipulations.
- Exercise tests are also used in predicting performance and in the investigation of poor performance.
- Field-based exercise tests may be highly specific (mimic the type of discipline for which the horse is used) but are generally difficult to standardise, whilst treadmill tests have the advantage of being easy to standardise but may lack specificity.
- The range and type of measurements that can be made in the field is almost always more limited than on the treadmill. Equipment available commercially for field testing includes electrocardiograms, heart rate monitors, blood collection devices and ventilation and gas exchange monitors.
- Field based tests may be very simple, such as timing speed over a fixed distance.
- More sophisticated field tests can be carried out with a stopwatch, heart rate monitor and measuring wheel.

- Short duration field tests (less than 15 minutes) are less likely to be affected by environmental temperature and humidity.
- Simple exercise tests to determine the relationship between heart rate and speed can be carried out in fields, on all-weather surfaces, and in outdoor and indoor arenas.
- When carrying out treadmill exercise testing it is desirable to allow an initial period of acclimation to try to ensure reliable data are obtained. This can usually be carried out in as few as three or four training sessions over 2–3 days.
- The treadmill has the advantage that speed, distance, duration, going, temperature and humidity, can all be controlled and reproduced.
- Horses use less energy to run at the same speed on a flat treadmill as over ground on the flat. This is because of absence of the load of a rider and air resistance, retraction of the limbs by the treadmill belt and the difference in the interaction of the feet with the belt.
- It has been estimated that inclining the treadmill to 3.5% produces the same sort of heart rates that would be seen in ridden exercise over land at the same speed with a rider.
- The intensity of treadmill exercise can be increased by increasing speed, incline or both.

Chapter 19

Indicators of performance

What is performance testing?

Performance is what a horse does and can be any test of how good a horse is at a particular discipline; hence the ultimate performance test is the competition itself. In many cases, rather than test a horse in competition we measure some index of physiological function, such as V_{LA4} or maximal oxygen uptake, and try to infer something about performance in different disciplines. Trainers and scientists have many reasons for wishing to test the horse's ability without actually competing it. Performance tests are carried out in order to:

- Try and select individuals that will excel in certain disciplines without actually having to train them and try them in each discipline
- Investigate the reasons for a sudden decline in the performance of a good horse
- Try and ascertain which particular physiological attributes can be used to indicate elite performance
- Establish the impact of various exogenous factors on performance, for example the effect of various diets, supplements, shoes and track surfaces.

The fewer factors which contribute to performance in a particular discipline, the more likely it is that our performance test will provide useful information. Performance indicators are thus more easily applied to some sports than others. Performance in a racehorse could be tested by timing the horse over whatever distance it is expected to race: but what about the dressage horse? Dressage judging is subjective, and that is a simple statement of fact, not a criticism of dressage judges! Objective dressage judging would involve dressage judges analysing large volumes of data relating to the kinematics of the horse and their technical correctness,

with no allowance made for overall impression. The discipline itself is not judged objectively, so the chances of coming up with an objective performance test for a dressage horse have until now been pretty remote. However, recent studies have analysed how dressage horses move and have begun to identify the movement characteristics that are awarded high marks. Thus, it may still be possible to objectively analyse what until now we have always thought of as a subjectively scored equestrian discipline.

It is not much easier to test the performance of a showjumper, or an eventer. Do we set a test to see how high they can jump, or how wide? Neither would be terribly useful because horses are not asked to jump single fences in competition. In this respect the sports in which performance testing is currently likely to be the most accurate are those that are pure tests of athletic ability such as racing and endurance.

A successful performance depends on the optimal interaction of various factors, both internal and external to the horse, all of which must be 'right on the night'! Performance depends upon:

- The genetic make-up of the horse – its inherent physiological and biomechanical make-up and thus its inherent ability (see Fig. 19.1).
- The fitness of the horse or the state of training of the horse – all physiological systems should have been trained appropriately for the competition, so the aerobic capacity of the endurance horse, its thermoregulatory ability and the strength of its musculoskeletal system should have been trained for it to realise its genetic potential (see Fig. 19.2).
- The health status of the horse – a whole range of factors from the actual disease state of the horse through to rather more subtle factors such as the level of hydration and body condition can have a critical influence on performance (see Fig. 19.3).

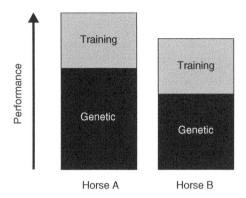

Fig. 19.1 If horse A has more ability than horse B and both receive the same amount of training, horse A will perform better than horse B.

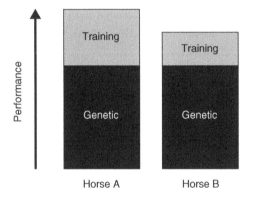

Fig. 19.2 If horse A and horse B have the same ability, but horse A receives more training, horse A will perform better than horse B.

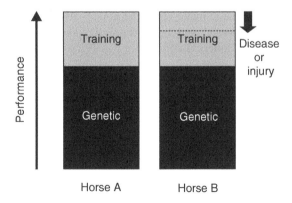

Fig. 19.3 If horse A and horse B have equal ability and are trained to the same extent, but horse B suffers from disease or injury, horse A will perform better than horse B.

- Non-physiological factors, or factors external to the horse – these include all factors other than those related to the horse, such as the track surface, climatic conditions, rider skill or the quality of the competition, and all may influence performance.

Which is best – field tests or treadmill tests?

In our search for a test of performance, the first problem once we have decided on what test we are going to use is to decide where to carry it out. Field testing refers to tests conducted outside, usually under the type of conditions a horse would normally encounter in competition (for examples of field tests see Chapter 18). Knowing that external factors have a real impact on performance, surely we should aim to test performance under the exact competition conditions? The difficulty here is that on any particular day there will be a unique combination of conditions relating to the weather, the state of the going, the size of the rider's hangover, etc., and the chances of being able to reproduce such a test should we want to compare two or more horses are minimal. The alternative is to carry out performance tests in controlled laboratory conditions on treadmills, with the added advantage of the accessibility of so much more equipment for measuring appropriate physiological or biochemical variables. Unfortunately, horses do not run on treadmills in the competition situation. Field tests have the advantage of being specific and realistic, whilst treadmill tests are controllable and reproducible.

Field testing

The track over which the test is to be run should be carefully selected: ideally this should be similar to the competition conditions in terms of surface, gradient and distance. Horses could either be run singly or in groups: generally, horses produce faster times when they are run in groups. The load carried by the horse (including tack and rider) should amount to the same percentage of body mass for each horse. For Thoroughbred racehorses, performance tests could be made up of running horses over anything from 5 furlongs (1000 metres) to $2\frac{1}{2}$ miles (4000 metres), simulating competition conditions. Timing horses over different distances may give an indication of performance, but you will probably find a really good horse stands out in performance tests over several distances.

In a training situation, a simple test of performance may be done as follows: a group of horses are run together (e.g. 2-year-olds and one 3-year-old whose performance has been well characterised over the previous season) over 5 furlongs (1000 metres). The first 4 furlongs (800 metres) may be run at a steady pace, but the horses are then asked to accelerate and compete against each other in the final furlong. If a 2-year-old is capable of keeping up with or passing the 3-year-old whose ability is already known, that may indicate ability.

Even for such a 'pure' sport as flat racing, the tactics used to ride the race may influence the performance the horse produces. Different horses may be suited to running a particular type of tactical race. There may well be a place in Thoroughbred race training for training horses to change pace within the gallop, i.e. accelerate whilst galloping, so that they have a wider repertoire of tactical race types they can run.

Timeform ratings are a subjective measure of how well a horse has performed in the past. Horses are allocated a weight (load) that they must carry in Handicap races depending on past performances. In other words the horses are handicapped according to their ability. The aim of the handicapper is to have all the horses cross the line at the same time by giving more weight to the good horses and less to the poorer horses. This is in order to liven up the betting, as in theory, all horses will have an equal chance of winning. Good horses will have a Timeform rating of over 100 (in lb). If a horse rated 100 ran against a horse rated at 80, then in theory the higher rated horse would carry 20lb more weight (load) than the lower rated horse. Timeform ratings on the flat may range from as low as 30 for really poor horses to over 130 for the elite in each season. There are usually only a small percentage of the total number of horses in training each year that have a Timeform rating of over 100. Over jumps, the Timeform range is slightly shifted upwards from below 60 to over 165. Timeform has been in use in the UK since 1948. The highest ever rated horses at the time of writing are as follows: Flat – Sea Bird II (145); Jumps (Hurdlers) – Night Nurse (182); Jumps (Chasers) – Arkle (212). The Timeform ratings of some other notable horses are Mill Reef (141), Dancing Brave, Shergar and Dubai Millennium (140) on the flat, Istabraq and Monksfield (180) over hurdles and Desert Orchid (187) and Burrough Hill Lad (184) over fences, i.e. chasers. Timeform ratings actually correspond quite well to performance indicators measured during treadmill exercise tests, particularly $\dot{V}_{O_2max}$ and, in one study, V_{LA4}.

In the real world we may be faced with a large group of horses from which we want to select the best for a given discipline. Let's imagine we have the top 12 event horse and rider combinations in the country at the present time. All have performed to a similar level in the present season and all appear free from injury and disease (not like reality!!). We need to pick the six fittest and most athletically gifted horses for a major international competition in 3 weeks' time. Remember that as these horses have all been trained by different people some will be fitter than others and some will be genetically more gifted. A moderately fit athletically gifted horse may be very difficult to differentiate from a very fit but less athletically gifted horse. However, as we are only 2 weeks from the competition, even if we could pick out the gifted horse that could reach a higher level of fitness and therefore perform better, we cannot do much about fitness in 2 weeks. If the horse is not fit enough, that is the rider's loss. What we want are the six horses with the best current combination of athletic ability and fitness. How can we set about picking the six best horses, remembering that we are not looking at dressage and jumping ability as part of our simplified example?

One way would be to send all 12 horses out on a 2 hour hard hack. This would incorporate some long periods of trotting, some galloping and possibly even some jumping: all very similar to the speed and endurance test of the three-day event. All 12 horses would be required to keep together as a group and cover each section in the same time, and at the end of the 2 hour hack we would weigh each horse, perhaps take a blood sample for lactate and measure heart rate recovery. We could then devise a ranking system to score how each horse coped with the work. If one horse finishes the work having only lost 5 kg, with a recovery heart rate of 50 beats/min and a blood lactate of 2 mmol/l, we might suspect this horse is more likely to cope with the rigors of the forthcoming competition than a horse which loses 20 kg, has a recovery heart rate of 90 beats/min and a blood lactate of 20 mmol/l. This is an exaggerated example, but provided the amount of work undertaken is of sufficient intensity and/or duration, it should be possible to separate out those horses that cope with the work well from those that find it more of a struggle.

Testing for performance using a treadmill

When we run a group of horses on a treadmill using a standardised exercise test protocol and all horses complete the full exercise test, unless we see one horse particularly struggling or one horse which looks as though it could have carried on all day, we cannot really speak about performance. Under fixed conditions such as these we set a workload and measure functional changes in response to the exercise. We are measuring physiological or metabolic or some other form of function. Of course, if all the horses complete the exercise test then we might say they all performed the test well, but we won't know anything about the maximum performance that each horse could achieve. We might infer differences between horses if we found one that could run at 10 m/s with a steady heart rate of 140 beats/min compared with another that was already at 220 beats/min at the same speed, but we couldn't be sure.

Exercise tolerance and run time to fatigue

If we want to find out something about performance or exercise capacity using a treadmill, we have to use a different approach in which the 'performance' of different horses can vary. One way of doing this using a treadmill is to use a 'run to fatigue' test. In this type of test, horses are run at near maximal speeds until they cannot keep pace with the treadmill. However, run to fatigue tests are not true tests of performance as such, because there is no equivalent competition where this is required. Exercise tests in which physiological function and metabolic responses are monitored are more often incremental in fashion. After a suitable warm-up in

walk and trot the treadmill speed is increased every minute starting at around 7–8 m/s and continuing to 12–14 m/s. An indication of a horse's ability is the number of steps of the incremental exercise test that it can complete combined with its physiological responses to the exercise. For example, a good Thoroughbred middle distance horse racing over distances of, say, $1\frac{1}{2}$ miles (2400 metres), would be expected to complete at least the 12 m/s step of such a test. However, the performance of such a test would almost certainly be dramatically reduced, i.e. the horse would fatigue at a lower speed, if the horse was unhealthy or unfit. Thus, in investigating performance potential we must take into account both health and fitness. The specificity of the test also comes into play, because whilst the better performing (in competition) healthy and fit middle distance flat horses and National Hunt horses perform well on this type of incremental test, sprinters and showjumpers tend to perform relatively poorly, i.e. the test is loaded in favour of horses that will perform well in disciplines lasting around 2–10 minutes. It would almost certainly not help you identify good showjumpers as these rely on anaerobic power, and it may not help identify elite endurance horses because they need to be able to maintain a high average speed of around 4 m/s over 10 hours rather than 16 m/s for a few minutes.

Aerobic capacity ($\dot{V}_{O_2max}$)

In disciplines such as flat racing over distances of around 1 mile (1600 metres) and upwards and jump racing, i.e. in disciplines where the intensity of exercise is both high and in excess of 1–2 minutes, the better performing horses will be expected to have a high maximal aerobic capacity, as indicated by maximal oxygen uptake ($\dot{V}_{O_2max}$). $\dot{V}_{O_2max}$ can range anywhere between around 110 ml/min/kg in a very poor Thoroughbred up to as high as 210 ml/min/kg in elite horses. Top level, non-Thoroughbred event horses would be expected to be in the region of 140 ml/min/kg. A recent study has shown that there is a strong correlation between $\dot{V}_{O_2max}$ and heart size assessed by ECG (Young *et al.* 2002). Again, good sprinters or showjumpers would not necessarily have or need a high $\dot{V}_{O_2max}$.

Heart rate

The aerobically better horse is capable of running at any given speed with a lower heart rate (HR); to put it another way, a good horse will be able to run faster before reaching any given HR. The point at which HR no longer increases with incremental increases in speed is HR_{max}, and the velocity at which this occurs (V_{HRmax}) is a pretty good indicator of performance in primarily aerobic disciplines. The same theory applies in the measurement of V_{200}, the speed at which the horse has a heart rate of 200 beats/min. V_{200} is estimated by carrying out a stepwise test as described above, and then plotting the relationship between HR and speed on a graph. There is a good correlation between V_{200} and $\dot{V}_{O_2max}$ which is useful because V_{200} can be measured quite easily under field conditions, and since $\dot{V}_{O_2max}$ correlates well with racing ability, so does V_{200}. A similar test for V_{200} could just as easily be performed on a track.

Lactate production

Measurement of the blood lactate response to incremental exercise has also been used as an indicator of performance. V_{LA4} is normally used, i.e. the speed of running at which the horse has a blood lactate of 4 mmol/litre. Evans *et al.* (1993) published a study showing that for Thoroughbred horses racing on the flat there was a negative correlation between lactate produced during a strenuous sub-maximal (10 m/s, 5°) standardised treadmill exercise test and Timeform rating. In simple terms, the horses that had the lower lactate had the higher Timeform rating. This implies that horses with low V_{LA4} are not likely to be good flat racehorses. This is probably true for the races of 8–10 furlongs (1600–2000 metres) or longer. However, there are two possible reasons for horses having particularly low V_{LA4} values: one is that the horse has a low aerobic capacity and is not able to run particularly fast before it has to rely on anaerobic energy production. The other possible explanation is that the horse is naturally a sprinter with a high percentage of large diameter type IIB fibres and relatively lower numbers of mitochondria: such horses are more likely to rely on anaerobic energy production and will reach V_{LA4} first. V_{LA4} is normally between 8 and 10 m/s on a 10% incline for Thoroughbred horses, and may be as high 10–12 m/s for elite endurance horses. Three-day event horses are often intermediate between Thoroughbred and endurance horses, and showjumpers are likely to have very low V_{LA4} values.

The effect of training on indicators of performance

Perhaps with the exception of $\dot{V}_{O_2max}$ which only increases by around 10–15% with training, the other indicators of performance (V_{140} or V_{200}, V_{LA4} and run time to fatigue) are all dependent on fitness. Once a training programme has been started it is hard to say exactly what point any given horse has reached when a test of this type is undertaken. The problem then is one of differentiating between horses on the basis of both combined fitness and ability. The best time to carry out these types of tests to select horses on the basis of their innate (i.e. genetic) ability is therefore before any training has been undertaken. Of course, the trainer, rider or owner can turn around and say that this would be a bad time to undertake such a test because there may be an increased risk of injury due to lack of fitness. The second choice would then be to undertake such tests when all horses have been fully trained, say 6 months down the road. Of course at this point we will have lost some horses through injury and not all horses will have responded physiologically to training the same way. Another problem presents itself in that we want to look at these horses after training, but what training programme are we going to use? We don't want to train all the horses as sprinters, because horses with a naturally high aerobic capacity will respond poorly to such training. On the other hand, we don't want to train all the horses as middle distance or stayers because this will diminish speed in any horses that are genetically sprinters. Usually Thoroughbred horses tend to be trained how they are bred: if the breeding says the horse should sprint, it's trained as a sprinter and vice versa.

Biomechanical indicators of performance

To predict performance using biomechanical indicators, we must have previously studied elite horses in various disciplines, in order to understand what physical and functional characteristics contribute to elite performance. Certain biomechanical indicators may only be possible to detect after the horse has undergone a certain period of ridden work, for example, the ability to collect. However, the race-horse that has a long stride for the length of its legs will have a long stride when untrained and unfit as well as when trained and fit. One of the best indicators of the biomechanical performance of the horse is static conformation. Subjective assessments of the horse's conformation and gait characteristics are currently the most common and succesfully applied indicators of biomechanical attributes in common practice, whilst results from scientific studies are beginning to produce information relating to the significant factors for performance in individual disciplines.

Biomechanical traits associated with elite performance

Thoroughbred racing

The singularly most important contributing factor to the performance of most Thoroughbred race-horses is stride length. A long stride length for a Thoroughbred would be more than 6.5 metres when galloping at racing speed. A long stride length is likely to be associated with high maximum gallop velocity. There is also a relationship between tidal volume and stride length, so the horse with a long stride may have ventilatory advantages as well as biomechanical advantages. A long stride length is achieved by having minimum overlap duration of lead hind and non-lead forelimb stance. In some horses overlap times can decrease to as little as 50 ms with increasing speed.

Three-day eventing

Good eventers tend to give the impression of being slightly rectangular in body shape (the distance from the point of the shoulder to the point of the buttocks is greater than the distance from the point of the croup to the ground) rather than square like dressage horses or showjumpers. This is possibly because long body length is also associated with a longer stride. A long stride length has also been shown to be associated with good marks in the dressage phase as well as ground covering ability in the cross-country phase. Elite event horses often have excellent forelimb conformation and, whilst this may not make any significant contribution to performance, it certainly increases the chance of the horse staying sound long enough to reach the higher levels of the sport.

Showjumping

Good showjumpers are usually very tall. Height is an obvious advantage in the high jumper; after all, we don't see many 5ft high jumpers in human athletics. They are also wide through the shoulders and hips (Langlois *et al.* 1978). Elite showjumpers tend to have larger hock angles than other horses (Holmstrom *et al.* 1990). Showjumping technique has been studied in some depth. A good horse alters its stride very little on the approach to the fence, and only in the stride before take-off are any real adjustments made to the canter stride. Less talented horses appear to have to prepare several strides out from the fence. Good horses also tend to place their limbs closer to the fence on take-off and on landing; in other words they 'get into the bottom of their fences'. For years, trainers of showjumpers have known that the power generated by the hindquarters was all important in take-off, but recently this has been proved using accelerometry. Barrey and Galloux (1997) showed that good jumpers generate the majority of the force for take-off with the hind limbs.

Dressage

Dressage horses are usually tall, 'uphill' horses, with relatively short necks, a long sloping shoulder and a large angle at the elbow joint. One of the critical factors for the dressage horse is the ability to 'collect', that is to transfer and carry weight on the hind limbs. At the top level of the sport the movements required can lead to significant compression of the hock joints, so conformation of the hind limb that confers strength and soundness is paramount. Horses are also required to produce a long stride length in the extended gaits by advancing the hind limbs well underneath the body and this is aided by having a long, forward-sloping femur. Good trot quality is enhanced by a naturally slow stride frequency and a long swing phase. The time elapsed between hind limb contact and diagonal forelimb contact (advanced placement) should be high. According to the FEI definitions, the horse should be able to 'extend the stride by increases in stride length at a constant stride frequency'. In practice this is rarely seen, and even elite horses will increase stride frequency at maximal extension.

Poor performance and loss of performance investigation

Bearing in mind the number and complexity of systems and control mechanisms involved in producing a good performance, investigation of poor performance or loss of performance can require real detective work. Some cases are never really solved, possibly because the horse is not so much suffering from a loss of performance, more a case of 'never really had it to lose'!. The causes of reduced performance either compared to a previous higher level of performance or to expectations, for example based on breeding, may be due to:

- A lack of ability
- A lack of fitness
- Illness or injury in one or more body systems
- Behavioural problems
- Poor riding
- The horse being competed in an inappropriate discipline.

Accurate diagnosis of the causes of poor performance or loss of performance is of great importance both for the client, rider, owner or trainer, but also because continued training and/or competing of a horse with an underlying medical condition or an injury has implications for its welfare.

Many people often use the terms poor performance and loss of performance interchangeably, but in the context of clinical investigation they have important differences. The term poor performance implies a lower level of performance than expected in an individual horse or group of horses (for example a whole stable or single crop of foals) when trained or competed. The comparison may also be made on the basis of what is expected from the breed. For example, any Thoroughbred should be able to canter at 600 m/min and an inability of an individual to do so would be cause alone for a categorisation of poor performance. The expectation of a certain level of performance may often be on the basis of the horse's breeding or appearance, e.g. conformation. A lack of innate athletic ability is therefore a possible cause of poor performance. Loss of performance is different and implies a current lower level of performance in a horse that has previously performed at a higher level. In the case of loss of performance, a lack of innate athletic

ability can, of course, be ruled out as the horse has already demonstrated this to a known extent. An underlying medical condition is more likely to be a cause of loss of performance.

Sadly the most common diagnosis of poor performance is simply a lack of ability, although, even if this is suspected, all other possible medical causes should be thoroughly investigated. An example of a horse with poor performance due to lack of ability would be as follows. A 2-year-old racehorse is referred for poor performance investigation mid-way through the flat racing season. The horse is sound, has completed all its training sessions, but has never been able to maintain pace with other 2-year-olds on the gallops over distances between 4 and 8 furlongs (800 and 1600 metres), i.e. the horse is not particularly inclined to sprinting or staying. Resting examinations do not reveal any abnormalities of the musculoskeletal system, the respiratory system or the cardiovascular system and routine haematology and biochemistry are all within normal ranges. The horse undergoes an incremental treadmill exercise test to fatigue but only just manages to complete the 10 m/s step of the test. At 9 m/s the horse had already reached a maximal heart rate of 230 beats/min. After the test the horse shows a rapid heart rate recovery and is under 100 beats/min within 1 minute from the end of the 10 m/s step. No abnormalities are detected in pulmonary, cardiovascular or musculoskeletal systems. The conclusion is that the horse appears to have no obvious medical conditions, is fit (based on the rapid post-exercise heart rate recovery), but has a poor exercise capacity and the most likely reason is a lack of ability. This is of course only an example; in reality, the diagnosis of poor performance due to a lack of ability may be complicated by less than adequate fitness and subclinical disorders, the likely significance of which for performance must be judged.

'Behavioural' problems may well frequently contribute to loss of performance and poor performance. These may relate to the interaction of the horse and a particular rider. If this is suspected, it is useful to observe the horse when ridden in different surroundings and by a different rider, as well as by the horse's usual rider. Horses can sometimes become bored and lose interest in competing. Sometimes a learned aversion to exercise may result from a previous episode of injury or an unpleasant experience, and this can be difficult to quantify. However, the horse that has, for example, experienced dorsal displacement of the soft palate during exercise may still associate exercise with the unpleasant experience of dyspnoea, and even after successful treatment be reluctant to exercise. We know the condition has been successfully treated but have no way of convincing the horse of this fact.

In investigation of poor performance or loss of performance the main aim is to characterise the functional capacity of the body systems necessary for optimal athletic performance and to determine if these are functioning correctly. This includes determining whether disease, injury or dysfunction of any of these systems is present. The systems in which we are primarily interested are the musculoskeletal system, the respiratory system and the cardiovascular system. The reason we know this is from epidemiological studies of racing and other sports, and from the findings of poor performance or loss of performance in cases referred to clinics.

Poor performance and loss of performance may result from overt (obvious) disease. For example, if a horse races badly and has a marked nasal discharge after the race we might well attribute its loss of performance to the presence of respiratory disease. Similarly, poor performance in a 2-year-old that 'roars' badly when on the gallops is almost certainly due to laryngeal hemiplegia and would not be unexpected. At the level of overt disease the 'diagnosis' may well be made by the owner, rider or trainer. If the disease is more subtle the condition may not be obvious to the owner, rider or trainer, but is likely to be diagnosed by a veterinary surgeon. However, low-grade disease or dysfunction which is only apparent during exercise and is not severe enough to produce clinical signs at rest may often require specialised investigation during treadmill exercise. Low-grade disease may often be impossible to diagnose at rest due to the body's large reserve capacity, and this applies particularly to the respiratory and cardiovascular systems. Low-grade disease without overt clinical signs but sufficient to affect physiological function is termed *subclinical* disease, and diagnosis of such conditions can present the equine clinician without access to a treadmill a very difficult diagnostic challenge. The techniques used for the investigation of poor performance and loss of performance will vary from horse to horse, and may also depend on the sport in which the horse is being used.

Various methods for the objective assessment of racing ability and training state have been used in the horse. Resting haematological variables are not good indicators of fitness state, but certain parameters such as a reduced or elevated WBC count may be useful as indicators of 'unfitness' to race or compete. Various parameters of exercising heart rate and blood lactate such as V_{200} (the speed at which heart rate is 200 beats/min) and V_{LA4} (the speed at which blood lactate concentration is 4 mmol/l) have been used in exercise tests. It has been suggested, for example, that V_{LA4} is higher (meaning that blood lactate starts to accumulate at a faster speed) in Standardbreds that perform well compared to poor performers (Couroucé *et al.* 1997). With increasing fitness, heart rate at submaximal speeds decreases and blood lactate accumulation is delayed; hence V_{200} and V_{LA4} show an increase with training. There are drawbacks, however, to the use of such parameters for fitness testing or comparison of ability between individuals. Firstly, there is the need to standardise testing procedures and conditions, which can be very difficult in the field on different occasions. In addition, because both the heart rate and blood lactate responses to exercise are affected by other factors such as disease, age and excitement, it is difficult to interpret their relevance to fitness in isolation. Finally, the relevance of these variables depends on the horse's use; in sprinting animals, production of high concentrations of blood lactate may represent a desirable high anaerobic potential rather than lack of fitness.

Overtraining is unlikely to be a common cause of poor performance or loss of performance in the horse (see Chapter 15). Whilst there are reports that overtraining in Swedish Standardbred racehorses is associated with an increase in RBC volume (Persson and Osterberg 1999), other workers have generally been unable to demonstrate this.

In cases where poor performance or loss of performance affect a whole stable rather than an individual animal, the approach must be aimed at finding something that could affect many individual animals simultaneously. In this situation, individual animals still need to be examined to characterise the problem, but the cause may include infectious disease, dietary deficiency, imbalance or excess, or some other factor common to all horses, such as pollution of the water supply. To confirm or rule out infectious disease, blood samples can be collected from all animals (or a representative sample of horses if the numbers are very large) and submitted for viral serology and WBC count and differential counts. Nasopharyngeal swabs can also be taken and submitted for virus isolation. Tracheal washing would also be frequently carried out to confirm or rule out respiratory disease, with washes being submitted to a laboratory, most commonly for cytological examination and bacteriology. Beyond this it is often essential to visit the yard and observe all working practices. Rather than simply have samples of feed delivered for analysis, the process of feeding should be observed and samples of the amounts fed actually collected into clean bags for weighing and possibly for analysis. In one case, the cause of poor performance in a large number of horses in a racing yard was identified as excess vitamin C supplementation. The only abnormalities were a low blood bicarbonate and pH, but the disturbance was enough to markedly affect performance. In a another case, poor performance of a whole racing yard was attributed to a switch from oats to naked oats (oats with the outer fibrous husk removed). The trainer had decided to switch to naked oats, but half way through the season many horses were performing poorly both on the gallops and when racing; they appeared to be carrying much more 'condition' (i.e. they were fat) than would be expected and following exercise 'blew' for much longer than expected. Treadmill exercise testing of three horses from the yard confirmed the trainer's observations, but no common abnormality was detected. A visit to the yard and observation of the feeding process identified the problem as overfeeding of naked oats. When the change had been introduced, the person responsible for overseeing the feeding of the horses had failed to understand the difference between naked oats and ordinary oats and had continued to feed the same volume (i.e. number of 'scoops') of naked oats as ordinary oats. Because naked oats have had the fibrous husk removed, one scoop of naked oats would contain less fibre and a lot more starch (i.e. carbohydrate = energy) than a scoop of ordinary oats: the horses

were therefore being overfed. A return to feeding ordinary oats resolved the problem within 1–2 months.

Water samples should also be collected. It has not been uncommon for individual yards to have large numbers of horses showing increased muscle enzymes in plasma as a result of pollution of water supplies with nitrate fertiliser washed from fields.

A full and detailed history is also an important part of investigating poor performance and loss of performance. The owner, trainer or rider who keeps good records will usually be able to provide an accurate and detailed history of treatments, feed deliveries, changes in feeding practices, vaccinations, worming and training programmes.

In investigating poor performance or loss of performance it is important to recognise that most cases are likely to have more than one underlying reason. A study of horses referred to the Tufts University for poor or loss of performance investigation suggested that as many as 84% had more than one abnormality detected (Morris & Seeherman 1991). Of course, the finding of an abnormality does not mean that it is the current cause of poor or loss of performance, especially if the condition has been present for some time. However, it is possible that an abnormality present for some time combined with a more recent problem may be enough to produce a noticeable reduction in performance when each alone would not.

Orthopaedic disorders and respiratory diseases have been identified as the two most common causes of lost training time and wastage in racehorses in training (Jeffcott *et al.* 1982; Rossdale *et al.* 1985; Evans 1988). Injury and dysfunction affecting the musculoskeletal and respiratory systems are also the most frequent causes of loss of performance in both racehorses and sports horses. Although the frequency of lameness or other orthopaedic conditions is recognised to be high in racehorses and it is known that this can limit performance, the impact is often underestimated, particularly by trainers. Treadmill exercise testing both without and with analgesia (pain relief) can be used to evaluate the effect of a known orthopaedic condition on exercise tolerance (Roberts & Wright 1999). Musculoskeletal disorders may also occur in large numbers of animals in association with a disease outbreak. In one case an outbreak of equine rhabdomyolysis syndrome (tying-up) associated with muscle stiffness and poor performance was attributed to a recent equine herpesvirus infection (Harris 1990).

The prevalence of lower respiratory tract disease due to both infectious and non-infectious causes is high in the horse. In the younger horse (less than 3–4 years of age) the prevalence of infectious respiratory tract disease generally appears to be greater than non-infectious, e.g. allergic, disease. In the older horse, both infectious and non-infectious disease are common. Lower respiratory tract disease in young racehorses in training has generally been considered to be due to some, often unidentified, viral disease; hence the term 'the virus', often used by those in the racing world. However, it is clear that viral induced respiratory disease in the horse is not always caused by one single virus, but most commonly by equine influenza virus, equine herpesviruses or rhinoviruses. It is not possible to differentiate respiratory disease caused by these different viruses simply on the basis of clinical signs, and identification must be based on measuring either the level of antibodies to each specific virus circulating in the blood (viral serology; a high antibody titre to a particular virus suggests it is likely that an animal has been exposed to that virus or vaccinated against it recently) or isolation and identification of virus in a swab taken from the upper airway (nasopharyngeal swab).

It has also become apparent that whilst the term 'the virus' has been used, in fact it is much more likely that respiratory disease in young racehorses in training will be due to bacterial rather than viral infection. Wood *et al.* (1999) studied horses in training in the UK in a number of different racing yards over several seasons; they reported that around 14% of racehorses could be expected to have lower airway disease at any one time and that this was most frequently associated with bacterial infection of the airways rather than viral infection. A number of other studies on racehorses and sports horses have come to the similar conclusion that airway inflammation is more likely to be associated with the presence of bacteria than viruses. The most common bacterial species associated with airway inflammation appear to be *Streptococcus zooepidemicus*, *Actinobacillus/Pasteurella* spp. and *Streptococcus pneumoniae* (Wood *et al.* 1993; Burrell *et al.* 1996).

The stable environment and in particular the air quality may also frequently be involved in respiratory problems in racehorses and other performance horses. One study reported that horses bedded on straw in loose boxes were twice as likely to suffer from lower airway disease as animals bedded on shavings in barns (Burrell *et al.* 1996). More recently, stabling has been shown to be associated with airway inflammation in young Arabian horses (Holcombe *et al.* 2001). The single most commonly occurring medical condition affecting adult horses in the UK is almost certainly recurrent airway obstruction (RAO) which was previously known as chronic obstructive pulmonary disease (COPD). This is the condition also referred to, particularly in the USA, as 'heaves'. 'Heaves' describes the exaggerated respiratory efforts affected horses make to breathe; the resulting overdevelopment of the abdominal muscles results in the formation of a 'heave' line. The reason for the recent change in name is that human medicine also uses the term COPD. However, human COPD is most commonly the result of prolonged smoking and is quite dissimilar to equine COPD. This has led to much confusion in the literature and when human and equine groups have interacted. The term RAO describes the intermittent changes in lung function that are a key feature of the disease.

Some estimates suggest that around 12–15% of horses may have a severe form of RAO producing overt disease. Many more horses are thought to suffer from subclinical RAO. RAO is a respiratory hypersensitivity or allergy with some similarities to asthma in man. In most cases RAO is caused by mould spores commonly found in the stable environment, either from the forage, the bedding or both. RAO can cause significant reduction in lung function, but surprisingly it is often overlooked in the evaluation of respiratory disease in racehorses. A condition with similar clinical signs and features is summer pasture associated obstructive pulmonary disease (SPAOPD). This is also a respiratory hypersensitivity, but in this condition the inciting agent is likely to be some form of pollen, which is in higher concentration outdoors. In general, horses with RAO due to a hypersensitivity to moulds improve when kept at grass, whilst horses with SPAOPD are less affected when stabled.

The prevalence of subclinical respiratory disease in all types of competition horses is high. For example, Herholz *et al.* (1994) examined 112 Warm-blood horses, 60 showjumpers and 52 dressage horses, all judged by their owners to be free of respiratory disease. Pulmonary disease was detected by clinical examination in 53% of the horses. At the Animal Health Trust, Dr Colin Roberts and one of the authors (David Marlin) have commonly found an incidence of airway inflammation of over 75% in elite endurance and three-day event horses 1 month before major competitions.

Detection of disease is complicated by the frequent absence of clinical signs of airway disease such as cough and/or nasal discharge. For example, in a study by Burrell *et al.* (1996) where horses were routinely monitored by endoscopic examination of the respiratory tract, only 38% of horses with lower airway inflammation were reported to have been coughing. Thus, the absence of cough does not imply the horse is healthy (cough has a low sensitivity for detecting respiratory disease). However, in the same study cough was found to have a specificity of 84%. Translated, this means that if a horse is coughing there is an 84% chance that it has respiratory disease (cough has a high specificity for respiratory disease). Given that respiratory disease is common, all horses being investigated for poor or loss of performance should probably have respiratory endoscopy and a tracheal wash.

EIPH is now considered to occur to some extent in all horses working at more than a medium canter. A number of studies have tried to establish if the presence of endoscopic evidence of EIPH, i.e. blood visible in the trachea, relates to reduced performance. However, to date, only one survey (Mason *et al.* 1983) has found a relationship between EIPH and finishing position. In a group of horses subjected to post-racing endoscopic examination following poor racecourse performance, the prevalence of EIPH has been found to be no greater than that of a random sample of racehorses (Roberts & Marlin 2001). Severe EIPH that is graded as 4 or 5 or that results in blood visible at the nostrils would be expected to be more likely to negatively affect performance.

Abnormalities affecting the heart occur frequently in the horse but are often not considered to be of clinical consequence. A prevalence of heart murmurs of 81.8% was reported by Kriz *et al.* (2000) in Thoroughbred racehorses, and Young & Wood (2000) reported that murmurs due to mitral

(bicuspid) and tricuspid valvular regurgitation (leakage from the ventricle back into the atrium during systole) increased in 2-year-old Thoroughbred horses after 9 months of race training. Severe, high grade murmurs, implying greater leakage of blood are likely to significantly affect performance because cardiac output is reduced.

Many horses may also show abnormalities in cardiac rhythm at rest, but many dysrhythmias are not of clinical significance in terms of reducing exercise tolerance. (The term dysrhythmia is a more accurate term than arrhythmia in this context.) An important and not uncommon exception is atrial fibrillation. Atrial fibrillation is a condition where the atria contract rapidly (fibrillate) and out of phase with the ventricles. The contractions are less powerful but do not greatly affect ventricular filling at rest. However, during exercise atrial contraction contributes more to ventricular filling and can markedly reduce cardiac output and exercise tolerance. Atrial fibrillation can be easily diagnosed by taking an ECG. This is most easily seen at rest. The use of colour flow Doppler echocardiography, which permits imaging of blood flow through the heart and recording of the ECG combined with exercise testing to assess the cardiac response to exercise are powerful aids to determine in which cases cardiac function is likely to be limiting to performance.

A not uncommon presentation of loss of performance is the horse in which the only signs are a history of reduced exercise tolerance and/or lethargy. Affected animals may show no other signs of disease, but some are reported with symptoms that may include periodic inappetance or muscle stiffness. Blood samples obtained from affected animals sometimes show alterations in the numbers of WBCs, with low total WBC counts and/or reductions in the number of neutrophils being the most frequently reported of such changes. Diagnosis in these cases is not always possible and when signs are very vague it may be difficult to determine whether the patient really is abnormal. It must be remembered that a small number of individuals will normally have WBC values that lie outside the reference range. A wide range of possible causes of this syndrome have been suggested. A common term used for the condition is 'post-viral fatigue', although few cases have detectable evidence of an initial viral infection. Ricketts *et al.* (1992) reported evidence of enterovirus infection in a number of affected horses, whilst others have suggested that a bacterial infection may be involved in some cases. In mild cases in which a full investigation fails to reveal a definitive cause, some horses respond to the implementation of a carefully graded exercise plan involving bringing the horse into full work over an extended period.

The use of exercise testing for the investigation of exercise-related disorders began around 15 years ago in the UK and has increased markedly as more treadmills have come into use in UK veterinary schools and other institutes. Research into exercise physiology has also allowed a clearer definition and understanding of the normal response to exercise. Before the introduction of the high speed treadmill, clinicians were restricted to resting and post-exercise examination and measurement, and observation of the horse during actual exercise.

Field exercise testing can be useful in some cases, although the sophistication of measurements is less. Modern telemetry ECG systems are able to provide the ECG, from which rate and rhythm can be obtained, and also respiratory rate and rhythm can be measured simultaneously using the same electrodes as the ECG by the technique of im-pedance plethysmography. A further difficulty in field testing is the lack of control over environmental and ground conditions, and the inability to reproduce any kind of standardised test. High speed treadmills permit control of speed, distance, duration, incline, running surface, temperature and humidity. The ability to exactly reproduce an exercise session weeks or months later following diagnosis and treatment should permit even small improvements in function to be quantified.

Treadmill exercise testing can be used to measure exercise tolerance, in terms of run time to fatigue, providing a measure of exercise capacity, as well as facilitating measurement of physiological function during exercise. Rose *et al.* (1995) suggested that there is likely to be a relationship between treadmill run time and racing performance, noting that at the University of Sydney, the best racehorses generally had the longest run time to fatigue on the treadmill. A similar relationship has been evident in patients tested at the Animal Health Trust. Treadmill exercise testing also allows many measurements of physiological function to be made, as

described in Chapter 18. The most common and useful variables measured include heart rate, blood or plasma lactate, blood gases, ventilation and oxygen uptake.

The prevalence of obstructive disorders of the upper airway is relatively high in racehorses, and in many cases the disorder only occurs during exercise. These are referred to as dynamic conditions. Therefore a particularly useful and widely used treadmill diagnostic procedure is videoendoscopy of the upper airway during treadmill exercise. A number of conditions of the upper airway in their severest form can be diagnosed on the basis of a resting endoscopic examination. This is the case for horses affected by severe recurrent laryngeal paralysis (also referred to as laryngeal hemiplegia or 'roaring') (see Fig. 19.4) and permanent epiglottic entrapment which can both be diagnosed by endoscopic examination at rest without the need for exercising videoendoscopy.

Horses less severely affected by recurrent laryngeal paralysis may demonstrate normal laryngeal function at rest, but during exercise left laryngeal dysfunction is apparent, with the collapse of the left arytenoid cartilage into the airway. Recurrent laryngeal paralysis and the associated dynamic collapse of the larynx into the airway results mainly in limitation of inspiratory airflow. Laryngeal dysfunction is usually graded from 1 to 5, with 1 being mild and 5 being complete paralysis. A horse graded 3 at rest will invariably exhibit dynamic laryngeal collapse during exercise, whilst some horses showing a mild degree of paralysis at rest manage to abduct the larynx normally during exercise.

It has become apparent in the last 10 years that disorders such as dorsal displacement of the soft palate (DDSP), which may also be referred to as 'soft palate disease' or 'gurgling', or erroneously called 'tongue swallowing', and dynamic laryngeal collapse in animals with partial dysfunction of the laryngeal muscles, are absent at rest and only occur during intense and sometimes relatively prolonged exercise. This is because for the condition to occur requires either the changes in upper airway pressures that are seen only at the very high flow rates reached during near-maximal exercise, or when fatigue occurs in respiratory as well as locomotor muscles, or a combination of both. DDSP occurs

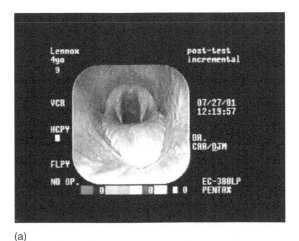

(a)

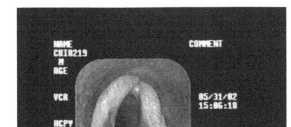

(b)

Fig. 19.4 (a) Endoscopic view of a normal larynx and (b) endoscopic view of horse showing left-sided recurrent laryngeal paralysis.

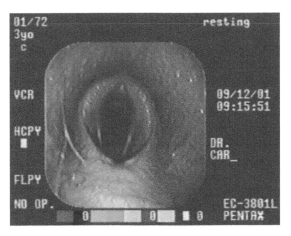

Fig. 19.5 Dorsal displacement of the soft palate.

when the airtight seal between the larynx and the soft palate is lost and the soft palate obstructs the airway (see Fig. 19.5). Before the soft palate actually displaces it is usually seen to billow upwards into the airway, and the horse may swallow repeatedly in attempts to equalise pressure above and below the palate and prevent displacement. Thus, there is a dramatic change in the function of the upper airway during exercise that cannot be inferred solely on the basis of a resting examination. It is often, but not always, associated with a 'gurgling' sound during exercise, and the horse will usually be forced to slow down once the palate has displaced. DDSP is a condition that affects expira-

tion more than inspiration. DDSP has been suggested to be more likely to occur if the horse has had a particularly difficult race, perhaps in heavy going, and this may relate to the degree of fatigue experienced in the upper airway muscles.

An indication to carry out exercising videoendoscopy of the upper airway is when an abnormal respiratory noise is heard during exercise which cannot be diagnosed during a resting endoscopic examination, or when there is some doubt on the basis of a resting examination alone. Exercising videoendoscopy is also indicated in the investigation of poor performance because a significant number of cases which are subsequently diagnosed as DDSP present as having no history of abnormal noise. At the Animal Health Trust around 30% of horses that are subsequently found to have DDSP on the basis of treadmill videoendoscopy have no history of abnormal respiratory noise during exercise. Correct diagnosis is essential if a horse is to receive appropriate treatment. In some cases this may mean receiving the most appropriate surgery, whilst for other cases it may mean avoiding unnecessary surgery, which at best may have no effect on the upper airway and at worst may worsen the condition or cause further abnormalities in function. It may be surprising to learn that not all cases of dynamic airway obstruction require surgical correction, and some horses may respond to rest or treatment for upper airway inflammation.

The importance of exercising videoendoscopy is illustrated by the findings of Kannegieter and Dore (1995) who reported that a complete and correct endoscopic diagnosis was made at rest in only 25% of a group of horses referred to the University of Sydney for treadmill investigation. A resting examination of the upper airway is frequently carried out as part of a poor performance investigation before treadmill endoscopy, and it is not unusual to see horses which have transient or even permanent DDSP at rest which never show the condition during exercise and vice versa.

A typical investigation for poor performance or loss of performance might begin with a routine orthopaedic evaluation to determine whether there are any musculoskeletal conditions present that might either be contributing to poor performance and/or be likely to be worsened by treadmill exercise. This examination would then be followed by a short period of treadmill acclimation. By far the majority of horses would only require two or three acclimation sessions, and the process appears to be best when the runs are over a short period of time. This may consist of morning, afternoon and morning runs over a 2 day period with exercise testing on the second or third day. A small percentage of horses require a longer period of acclimation, and complete failure due to a horse that is dangerous to itself, to staff, or fails to acclimate to a level where it can canter and gallop comfortably, occurs only in around 1–2% of cases.

In some centres, measurements of heart rate and lactate or other physiological variables are made during the videoendoscopy protocol, and the horse is only tested the once. Other centres run physiological and endoscopic protocols on different days or at different times on the same day. At the Animal Health Trust, the protocol used involves carrying out a standardised incremental exercise test during which ventilation, oxygen uptake, carbon dioxide production, lactate and heart rate are measured. At the end of this phase of the exercise test the horse is taken back into walk, the mask is removed and the videoendoscope inserted into the upper airway. The horse is then given a short warm-up and taken up to gallop where speed and/or incline may be increased until the horse fatigues or until a diagnosis can be made. The collection of the physiological

data in the first phase of the exercise test protocol has the advantage of providing detailed information for a standardised test and also gives an indication of exercise capacity. It also serves to tire the horse which can be important for videoendoscopy because many upper airway dynamic conditions can require a component of fatigue of the respiratory muscles in the upper airway.

The protocol used for physiological exercise testing varies with the type of horse being tested. For racehorses and higher level eventers the exercise protocol given in Table 19.1 is used for physiological testing at the Animal Health Trust. Such an incremental test permits exercise capacity to be investigated, and if oxygen consumption at the end of each step is plotted, $\dot{V}_{O_2max}$ may be calculated. In an average Thoroughbred horse in full training, $\dot{V}_{O_2max}$ is around 150–160 ml/min/kg, whilst elite animals of championship status have been found to have values for $\dot{V}_{O_2max}$ in excess of 200 ml/min/kg. For less athletic animals or horses involved in less strenuous activities, protocols involving a lower workload, produced by exercise at a lower incline and/or speed are used.

For exercise endoscopy, incremental exercise test protocols are also used with the starting point, duration and rate of increase of steps again depending on the type of animal being tested. Since conditions such as DDSP frequently occur only

Table 19.1 Incremental exercise test protocol used for physiological exercise testing at the Animal Health Trust, Newmarket

Speed (m/s)	Gait	Duration (minutes)	Incline (degrees)
1.7	Walk	5	0
4.0	Trot	3	5
7.0	Canter	2	5
8.0	Canter	1	5
10.0[a]	Canter	1	5
11.0[a]	Gallop	1	5
12.0[a]	Gallop	1	5
13.0[a]	Gallop	1	5
1.7	Walk	10	0

[a] Test concluded when the patient has difficulty maintaining treadmill speed.

towards the end of a race or event when the animal is fatigued, it is important when racehorses and eventers in full training are investigated that the exercise test continues until either a diagnosis of upper airway obstruction is made or the horse shows signs of fatigue. Table 19.2 shows a summary of the relative incidence of dynamic upper airway disorders in horses presented for exercise endoscopy at the Animal Health Trust over a 2 year period.

Accurate diagnosis of poor performance or loss of performance is particularly challenging, and requires a clear and accurate history; it may involve the expertise of orthopaedic clinicians, cardiologists, respiratory specialists and the facilities of a good laboratory for cytological, haematological, clinical biochemical, serological and bacteriological analysis. It is likely that a number of different subclinical abnormalities may be identified and the skill is often in interpreting the significance that each has to the reduced athletic capacity. At

Table 19.2 Prevalence of dynamic upper airway obstructive disorders in 152 horses referred for treadmill videoendoscopy (courtesy of Dr Colin Roberts)

Condition	Prevalence (%)
Dorsal displacement of the soft palate	37.5
Soft palatal instability	20.4
Dynamic laryngeal collapse	10.6
Axial deviation/vibration of the aryepiglottic folds	10.5
Pharyngeal collapse	9.9
Epiglottal entrapment	0.7
Epiglottal retroversion	0.7

present, detailed investigation of poor or loss of performance cases can only effectively be carried out during treadmill exercise, but with constant changes in technology it may soon be possible to carry out investigations of a similar level of sophistication in the field.

KEY POINTS

- Performance is what a horse actually does, and the ultimate test of performance is usually some form of competition.
- Tests of performance other than in competition may be carried out to select talented horses at a young age, to investigate loss of performance, to study which physiological attributes indicate elite performance, and to study the effect of exogenous factors such as diet on performance.
- Performance testing is likely to be most accurate in sports or disciplines that are tests of pure athletic ability such as racing or endurance, rather than skill.
- Successful performance depends on optimal interaction of factors such as genetic make-up, fitness, health, climate, going and rider skill.
- Performance tests can be carried out in the field or on a treadmill. In the field it is easier to measure maximum performance, whilst on the treadmill it is more usual to study function in

relation to a fixed task. The exception is when exercise tolerance tests or run time to fatigue are used.
- Maximal oxygen uptake tends to be highest in elite racehorses competing on the flat or over jumps.
- $\dot{V}_{O_2max}$ or V_{200} values are usually good indicators of performance in primarily aerobic disciplines because they reflect heart size and cardiovascular capacity.
- V_{LA4} is generally higher in better performing Thoroughbred racehorses competing over 8–10 furlongs (1600–2000 metres) or more, and in good endurance horses. V_{LA4} may be low in Thoroughbred sprinters, Quarter horses, showjumpers and polo ponies which participate in disciplines where short bursts of speed or power are required.
- Biomechanical characteristics can also be used as indicators of performance potential, such as a long stride length in Thoroughbred racehorses.

- Investigation of poor performance and loss of performance requires a thorough understanding of normal function and the attributes required for success in different disciplines.
- Poor performance is often due to a lack of ability, lack of fitness, poor riding, poor management, or the horse being competed in an inappropriate discipline.
- Loss of performance is more likely to result from disease, illness, injury, dysfunction or behavioural problems.

Chapter 20

Feeding performance horses

What do we want from a feed ration?

The diet of the competition horse should supply enough energy both for maintenance and for work. In certain circumstances there may be two primary goals, e.g. young racehorses needing to be fed both for growth and for work, or an eventer which is underweight being fed for work and for weight gain, i.e. to increase its body mass. We need to ensure that the horse's requirements for any given circumstance are met as effectively as possible. The primary drive for most people in finding the optimal diet is usually financial, as the feed bill is usually the greatest single expenditure for a competition yard, greater than bedding and veterinary costs. The feed industry is very competitive, and thus feed manufacturers use very persuasive advertising and marketing to get us to buy a particular type of feed or supplement. Knowing what we want out of a ration can help us to ask the right questions of the feed manufacturers and protect ourselves from unwittingly paying too much for a feed we do not really need.

There are one or two versions of a method of ration formulation available which enable us to calculate what we ought to be feeding, but most competition yards do not use ration formulations to decide what to feed. Most diets are formulated over time on a trial and error basis: if the horse loses body mass, the feed is increased; if the horse gains body mass or becomes too boisterous, the feed ration is decreased. This method using only 'the eye of the master' may actually be more sensitive and responsive than a calculated ration formulation, as the ration formulation is unlikely to take account of all variables such as climate, temperament,

whether the horse is clipped or non-clipped, health status of the horse, frequency of competition, etc. However, a useful exercise is to work out exactly what your current diet provides in terms of energy, and the contribution of both the concentrates and forage within the diet to the total energy provision. If you later encounter any problems with the diet not performing as well as you might expect, knowing exactly what your current diet provides may enable you and/or a nutritionist to come up with a simple solution.

Water – the most important ingredient

Approximately 65–75% of an adult horse's body mass is water. Loss of body water poses an immediate threat to the performance of the competition horse. A loss of water amounting to just 2% of body mass (10 kg in a 500 kg horse) may affect performance. In man, it is as little as 1%, which is a very good reason not to indulge in too much alcohol at the pre-event party! Many of the old horse masters knew the importance of adequate water provision because water withdrawal can actually have a 'quieting effect' on a difficult or dangerous horse, a technique that has been used by unscrupulous dealers and competitors.

Water balance within the body is carefully regulated. A certain amount of water is lost from the body every day in the form of urine, water in faeces and evaporative losses associated with sweating and breathing. Even when the horse is not sweating there is a continual slow loss of water because of the permeability of the skin, known as insensible water loss. These losses must be replaced in the diet and by drinking to maintain the total body water pool. Daily water intake is dependent on:

(1) *Body size*. The amount drunk by a horse each day depends fundamentally on its body size, with large horses drinking more than small horses, so it is useful to talk about daily intakes in terms of ml/kg body mass to compare horses of different sizes. On the same diet, same grazing, the same workload, and in the same climate, horses with free access to water will drink similar amounts of water to within 5–10 ml/kg body mass.

(2) *Ambient temperature*. The next most important factor determining water intake is ambient temperature. Intakes vary from 30 ml/kg body mass to 70 ml/kg body mass over a winter/summer period. This equates to between 15 and 30 litres of water in a 12 hour period for an average sized horse, or between one and three bucketfuls.

(3) *Diet*. The amount of water drunk decreases with increasing moisture content of food. Food containing 30–40% moisture provides the minimum amount of water to meet the needs of the non-working horse. Fresh forage and haylages can contain 60–80% water, so a horse out at grass may not drink at all. Water intake is also influenced by the nature of the diet. As diet digestibility increases, faecal losses are less, so water intake decreases. Water requirement and intake will increase with the level of protein and salt in the diet. In stabled horses around two-thirds of the total water intake occurs in association with feed intake. When stabled horses are fed they can frequently be observed moving between the hay net or manger and water bucket. Again, this probably relates closely to the dry matter content of the diet.

(4) *Workload*. Moderate work increases the water intake about 40% over resting values in cool conditions, and up to 80% over resting values in hot conditions, as sweat losses increase.

(5) *Availability*. To ensure that the horse's needs are met, good quality water should be available at all times. The horse will often consume more than is needed if palatable water is readily available. The increase in intake in this situation seems to occur due to an increase in drinking frequency, not to increased drinking duration or increased drinks during a single drinking bout. This suggests that horses may drink more in a stabled situation simply because the water is freely available. It is not uncommon to hear of horses that consume in excess of 60–70 litres per day. In these cases, measurement of urine creatinine concentration can be used to rule out the existence of kidney disease. If the creatinine is very low this implies a high water intake and a necessarily high urine output. This is known as psychogenic polydypsia and may commonly be related to boredom. Intake is reduced to a minimum if water is unpalatable or even if water has a novel taste, which may occur if horses change yards or are stabled at an event.

The measurement of the total dissolved solids (TDS) within a water sample is the most basic measurement of water quality. A TDS limit of 6500 mg/l has been given as the upper safe limit for horses, although it is likely that intake is reduced due to unpalatability at levels of TDS well below this figure. Highly chlorinated water may be unpalatable due to its strong smell. Some of the chlorine will vapourise, reducing the odour, if the water is stood for a few hours before being presented to the horse.

Water and electrolytes

Body fluids can be described in terms of their solute concentrations, but for physiological purposes are more usually described in terms of their osmolarity. This describes the osmotic pressure of a solution and thus to what extent a solution tends to draw water to itself. Body fluids, both intracellular (that within cells) and extracellular (that outside cells), have an osmolarity in the region of 300 mosm/l (milliosmoles per litre). Any solution that has the same osmolarity as this is described as being isotonic regardless of its actual composition. Thus a 300 mosm/l solution could be made entirely of sodium chloride (NaCl), or potassium chloride (KCl), or even glucose. If a horse loses body water, the osmolarity of its body fluids increase and are said to be hypertonic (osmolarity greater than 300 mosm/l). If a horse loses, for example, sodium only, or gains water only, the osmolarity of its body fluids will decrease and they are then described as being hypotonic (osmolarity less than 300 mosm/l). The major electrolytes that contribute to the osmolarity of extracellular fluid are sodium and chlorine, so extracellular fluid is very similar to a solution of ordinary table salt, equivalent to 9 g NaCl in one litre of water or 0.9% NaCl. A 0.9% NaCl solution is often used as a substitute for extracellular fluid in both clinical and research environments. The major electrolyte within intracellular fluid is potassium. Fluid losses usually occur from the extracellular fluid, but in times of dehydration, intracellular volume will also be depleted in an attempt to minimise the impact of the water loss across both intra- and extracellular fluid compartments.

An increase in osmolarity of body fluids is recognised by sensory cells called osmoreceptors in the hypothalamus that trigger the posterior pituitary gland to increase the secretion of antidiuretic hormone (ADH). ADH increases the permeability of the kidney tubules to water and allows more water to be reabsorbed, thus producing more concentrated urine. ADH levels are decreased if the horse is fully hydrated. For information on how to best replace lost fluid and electrolytes, see Chapter 12.

Meeting total daily energy requirements

A typical daily intake of food is often 2–2.5% of the horse's total body mass; thus if a horse weighs 500 kg it might be receiving 10–12.5 kg of feed per day. Next to water, the most critical component in the diet of the performance horse is energy, in the form of carbohydrate and fat. Probably less than 10% of the total energy requirement comes from the oxidation of protein and therefore requirements for protein do not increase significantly with increased work. For many years people believed that hard working horses needed better 'quality' food and that 'quality' was synonymous with protein. The protein requirements of the exercising horse will only be higher than those for maintenance of body tissues if the horse is also growing, for example 2-year-old racehorses.

For low levels of work you may simply be able to increase the mass of diet currently being fed. Most horses are fed a combination of forage and cereals to meet daily requirements for work. It is recommended that the daily forage provision should be at least 1% of body mass (on an 'as fed' basis): thus a 500 kg horse should receive a minimum of 5 kg of hay per day. In many racing yards each horse receives only 3.5 kg per day, i.e. well below recommended levels. Forage has a lower energy content per kilogram of dry matter than cereals and it may not be possible to meet the horse's daily energy requirement by feeding forage only, as the quantities that need to be fed may exceed the horse's daily capacity for food (approximately 2.5% of body mass) and hence its appetite. In this situation the only way to meet the energy requirements within the horse's capacity is to feed foods that are more energy-dense than forage.

Feedstuffs

Fibre

Fibre sources include hay, haylage, grass, silage, fibre cubes and chaff. Hay can be meadow hay, seed hay or legume hay with an average energy content of 9 MJ DE/kg DM (megajoules of digestible energy per kilogram of dry matter). The digestible energy of the feed is the gross energy minus the energy content of the faeces attributable to it. Meadow hay is made from permanent pastures containing many grass varieties and often some herbs. Seed hay is made from pastures with one or two grass species, most commonly rye or timothy. Alfalfa hay is excellent quality hay which is very useful for feeding competition horses, and is very popular with racing yards in particular. Silage is semidried forage with a dry matter (DM) content of less than 40%. Haylage has a DM content of between 50 and 75%. Silage for feeding to horses must be very carefully produced because clostridial activity can cause botulism, which is usually fatal. Bacterial activity can be controlled by having low pH (approximately 4.5) and relatively high dry matter (more than 25%). Haylage is becoming increasingly used as a result of the difficulty in obtaining good quality hay in the UK. Hay is more likely to produce a respiratory allergy than haylage and is one of the reasons that haylage is often preferred to hay. Haylage has a higher water content than ordinary hay, and whilst many people believe that haylage does not need to be fed in such large quantities as hay because it is usually more energy-dense than hay, it should actually be fed in similar quantities because it contains more water on a weight for weight basis. To reduce the risk of dust and fungal spores in hay being inhaled, hay is often soaked. Perhaps the best method is to keep a water trough or large bin into which the hay net is placed for between 10 and 30 minutes, as even short periods such as this can significantly reduce the numbers of respirable particles released into the surrounding atmosphere. Longer periods of soaking are not recommended because the water-soluble carbohydrate content, nitrogen content and mineral content of the hay are significantly reduced by soaking.

Fibre can also be fed as chaff, and there are a number of different types of chaff commercially available: molassed chaff (highly palatable), those made with unmolassed hay or straw (more suitable for ponies on low calorie diets) and alfalfa ones, the latter being an excellent source of fibre and calcium for horses on high concentrate diets. Chaff is often added to the feed at a rate of about 0.5 kg per feed.

One of the best forms of fibre for horses is grass. The quality of pasture varies enormously from region to region and also throughout the year. In the UK, pasture can provide a significant proportion of the dietary intake during the months between late April and early September. Throughout the rest of the year, certain types of horses and ponies (such as native types) can do very well on a diet based largely on grazing.

Concentrate feeds

These are so called because they provide a more concentrated source of energy than forage, at between 12 and 16 MJ DE/kg DM. Concentrated feed can be provided either as grains or 'straights', or as specially manufactured compound feeds.

'Straights': the most commonly fed straight is oats, but increasingly, competition horses are fed naked oats. These are oats no true husk and therefore they have a much higher starch content than ordinary oats. As a result of their higher starch content

naked oats only need to be fed at 25–50% of the normal amount of oats by weight. Barley is often fed as extruded barley, or as micronised flakes. Both extrusion and micronising are types of cooking process aimed at gelatinising the starch, thereby increasing digestibility of the grain. Extrusion is used to produce various sorts of 'Supabarley', a more digestible form of barley, whilst micronising produces a type of cooked flake which stands up well throughout the mixing process involved in producing a compound feed. Some feed mills also produce steam cooked grains, a process which not only increases digestibility but is claimed to increase palatability. Fewer yards these days rely solely on oats and bran as a basic diet. Wheat bran is deficient in both essential amino acids and calcium and high in phosphate, and thus is less commonly used these days.

Many people use sugar beet pulp because it is a highly palatable, high fibre and high energy feed which is fed soaked. Sugar beet pulp comes in the form of pellets and shreds. Pellets take quite a long time to soak (24 hours) in 1 part sugar beet to 3 parts water, but the shredded sugar beet is soaked in less time (approximately 12 hours) in 1 part sugar beet to 2 parts water. The water that is drained from the sugar beet following soaking may be added to feeds to increase palatability or for endurance horses as a 'high energy sports drink'!

Compound feeds: a wealth of compound feeds are available, largely either pelleted, extruded or in coarse mixes. Feed companies tend to make all their standard rations available in either pelleted or coarse mix form, with the same energy (in terms of MJ DE/kg): the pelleted diet often contains slightly more fibre than the coarse mix but is also often slightly cheaper to buy. Coarse mixes contain grass pellets and a wide range of cooked grains. Whether or not it makes any difference to the horse, owners often like to feed coarse mixes as they can see what is in the feed, even if they are unable to identify all the individual components! The appearance of the feed is all-important because consumers do not want to buy bags of feed that appear dusty. The problem of dust may be reduced by adding molasses to a feed or chaff as it binds fine particles that might otherwise be inhaled. Coarse mixes with additives such as herbs are often popular with owners as they smell good. It is incredible how many owners still feel the need to add a feed supplement to a compound feed, often having already paid a premium price for a good quality compound feed. This really should not be necessary when there are a wealth of diets readily available designed to meet the needs of everything from the broodmare to the veteran to the 'poor doer'.

Quick release and slow release of energy

The main fuels for exercise are carbohydrate and fat. The extent to which each is used depends largely upon the intensity and duration of the exercise, diet and the horse's stage of training. The total daily energy requirement of horses in endurance type events is actually far greater than that of racehorses, because the daily duration of exercise for the endurance horse is usually so much more. The racehorse has a higher *rate* of energy consumption, but a lesser daily energy requirement. If you only consider the intensity of work and not the duration, it is easy to underestimate the amount of energy required by horses doing prolonged submaximal work, e.g. riding school horses.

Carbohydrate can be provided by feeding forage, cereals or a combination of both. The rate at which the horse requires the energy determines what type of carbohydrate ought to be fed. Horses undertaking endurance type work require a prolonged slow release of energy throughout the day, whereas the racehorse needs a quick burst of energy for a short period of time. Endurance horses can be fed higher levels of structural carbohydrate in the form of forage that takes a long time to be digested, absorbed and utilised, providing slow release of energy. Racehorses are fed diets higher in starch, i.e. cereals (concentrate feed), as these are rapidly digested and absorbed and provide a quick release type of energy source. The horse's hay net is our baked potato; his concentrate feed is our chocolate bar, providing a quick burst of energy that does not sustain us throughout the day.

Fuels for slow work

For slow work, horses use a combination of fat and carbohydrate as fuel. The best diet to give horses performing slow work of moderate duration is fibre based, providing a slow release of energy. It is important to understand that the production of volatile fatty acids from the digestion of fibre does provide useful energy for work, as many people think of fibre as just a filler. For slow work of long duration, an appropriate fuel source is fat. Muscles obtain their free fatty acids (FFAs) either from stores within the muscle itself or from adipose. In response to exercise and increased levels of adrenaline, FFAs are mobilised from triglyceride stores in adipose tissue. Fat in the form of oil such as vegetable oil can be used to replace some of the forage in the diet as a means of increasing its energy density. Think of energy density as the difference between eating a kilogram of carrots or a kilogram of chocolate. The mass is the same but there may be 100 times the calories in the chocolate as in the carrots. Fat is more energy-dense than grains and so a combination of fat, fibre and grain may enable the owner to meet the horse's energy requirements, whilst feeding 50% of the ration as hay, more easily than if the ration consisted of grains and fibre alone. The endurance-trained horse will be better able to utilise fat, probably because of their increased number of mitochondria and aerobic enzymes, and hence the necessary means of breaking down fat. Fuel usage on the whole becomes more efficient with the switch to fat utilisation as there is less aerobic breakdown of glycogen and glycogen stores are spared. If glycogen can be spared, the onset of fatigue can be delayed.

Normal horse diets will contain approximately 3% fat (in terms of percentage of the total energy intake). As much as 20% of the total calories in the diet (forage + cereal + added oil) of an endurance horse could come from fat. If fat is so good, why not feed even more? High fat supplementation is fine in theory, but above approximately 20% of the total energy intake, fat tends to upset the hind gut and lead to the production of loose droppings. Remember that we give paraffin oil when we want to help movement through the gastrointestinal tract and dietary fat can have the same effect. When substituting fat for fibre at high levels, care must be taken that the vitamin and mineral requirements are still met by the remainder of the ration, as fat contains no minerals or vitamins.

Fuels for fast work

Fat cannot be used for fast work because it cannot be broken down anaerobically and has a slow rate of ATP regeneration. The primary fuel source for high intensity exercise is muscle glycogen. Relatively little ATP is produced for each unit of glycogen used up anaerobically and so muscle stores of glycogen are quickly depleted in high intensity exercise. In fast work the rate of ATP turnover is high; consequently the rate of glycogen utilisation is high.

When the horse is required to do any cantering or galloping as part of its daily work, the total daily energy requirements may well exceed those that can be met by a forage diet alone. For this reason, a 'concentrate' feedstuff made up of cereals will be needed to replace some of the forage within the diet to provide a more energy-dense ration. The harder the horse works, the greater the need to replace forage with concentrates. Also, a high forage diet may increase gut fill and hence body mass, which may reduce performance. However, adequate levels of forage must be fed for healthy gut function and prevention of certain types of colic.

Feeding minimum amounts of forage to stabled horses often leads to boredom as the horse is left without anything to eat for most of the day. Also, low fibre diets reduce the capacity of the bowel to act as a reservoir for water and electrolytes (particularly important for endurance horses). Low fibre may also lead to carbohydrate 'overload' where the digestive capacity of the small intestine is overloaded, with the result that excess soluble carbohydrate reaches the large intestine causing rapid fermentation. This leads to excess production of gas and lactic acid, leading to colic, diarrhoea and laminitis. Feeding very low levels of fibre very often forces horses to resort to eating their bedding with increased risk of impaction colic. It has also been associated with an increase in incidence of certain types of stereotypical behaviour.

Time of feeding

Following a large hay meal, large volumes of saliva and digestive juices are produced which can decrease plasma volume by up to 24% (Clarke et al. 1990). When a grain meal is fed, horses only produce about half as much saliva. Due to the large influx of fluid into the digestive tract during a hay meal, a grain meal fed at the same time as the hay or shortly after tends to travel through the small intestine faster, thereby reducing grain digestibility. Feeding grain + hay in the morning before a simulated three-day event speed and endurance test conducted on a treadmill resulted in higher heart rates during the treadmill test (Pagan & Harris 1999). This was thought to be due to the increased body mass and reduced plasma volume associated with the hay intake. Feeding grain either with or without hay 2 hours before exercise produces an increase in insulin levels, a reduction in FFA availability, and increases the rate of blood glucose disappearance that is not desirable for prolonged exercise. Feeding only forage before a competition has no adverse effects other than possibly reducing plasma volume and increasing body mass. It is probably wise to feed your eventer small quantities of hay only during the night before the cross-country phase of a three-day event, but grain should be withheld. Frape (1998) suggests that there is a justification for giving a small grain meal to a sprinter between 3 and 7 hours before competitive exercise, and a meal containing more fibre than grain can be given to the endurance horse 5–8 hours before competitive exercise.

Monitoring body mass and condition

It is a good idea to monitor the horse's body mass and condition, and to keep a record of this together with training records. The simplest way to do this is by visual assessment of body condition score, with 1 being very poor with prominent vertebrae, and 9 being extremely fat to the point that there is a crease down the horse's back and bulges of fat over the ribs. Other systems rate condition from 0 to 5; the 1–9 method is that published by Hennecke et al. (1981). Increases or decreases in body condition are often less apparent to someone who sees the horse every single day, as changes are usually very gradual. A safeguard is to make some sort of objective assessment of the horse's body condition, in other words its body mass.

Estimations of the horse's body mass can be made by measuring the horse's heart girth (taken immediately behind the elbow) and the length from the point of shoulder to the point of buttocks (see Fig. 20.1). The following equation (Carroll & Huntington 1988) provides an estimate of body mass using these measurements:

$$\text{Body mass (kg)} = \frac{\text{Heart girth (cm)}^2 \times \text{Length (cm)}}{11\,877}$$

Body mass can then simply be monitored by measuring heart girth because length will not change in a mature horse. 'Weightapes' providing estimates of body mass directly can be purchased, but for the purpose of simply monitoring change in heart girth, a simple tapemeasure will suffice. The best methods to discover the body mass of the horse is of course, to weigh it (see Fig. 20.2) and many racing yards and professional riders now own weighbridges and use them on a regular basis.

The optimal mass of a Thoroughbred racehorse is reported to be within a 7.3 kg range (Lim 1981). If the horse is below optimum mass its energy stores, including muscle glycogen, are likely to be reduced and the risk of fatigue is increased. Better performing horses tend to lose less mass following racing than ones that perform less well; this probably reflects the degree of dehydration suffered by the horse during both the competition and travelling to and from it.

Vitamins for health and performance

Vitamins are complex molecules involved in essential bodily functions. We know that many vitamins have an important role to play in the production and utilisation of energy for exercise, and therefore it pays to avoid deficiencies of these vitamins when feeding performance horses. Plants can synthesise all the vitamins they require for metabolism, but animals cannot and are therefore dependent upon an external supply. There are two main groups of vitamins:

- Fat soluble
- Water soluble.

Fat soluble vitamins are stored in the body; therefore it is not necessary to supply these on a daily basis. Vitamin deficiencies may arise due to poor dietary content, or provision of a balanced diet in insufficient quantities, particularly in situations where the requirement for vitamins is increased for example, increased physical activity and rapid growth. Whilst the levels needed to prevent the onset of clinical signs of vitamin deficiency are known, the optimum levels for performance horses

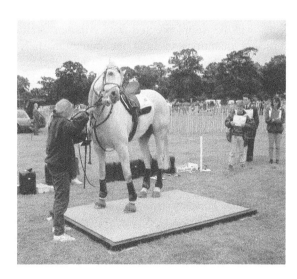

Fig. 20.2   A weighbridge.

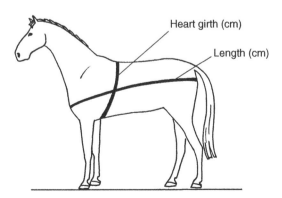

Fig. 20.1   A method for estimating body mass.

are not all clearly established. Taking this into account, vitamin supplementation may be necessary for horses in hard training, particularly those on low forage diets where the provision of vitamins in the diet may be limited.

The fat soluble vitamins (A, D, E and K)

Vitamin A

Vitamin A is necessary for the regeneration of rhodopsin, a photopigment found in the retina. The splitting of rhodopsin using light energy produces nervous transmissions that are sent via the optic nerve to the brain to cause visual sensations. Although the splitting of rhodopsin is reversible, a fresh supply of vitamin A is required to reform the visual pigment completely and so allow the process to continue; thus vitamin A is important, particularly in night vision. Vitamin A is also necessary for the integrity of epithelial tissues and the normal growth of bone. Vitamin A (retinol) is derived from the carotenoid pigments found in herbage, the main pigment being β-carotene. β-Carotene is converted to vitamin A in the wall of the small intestine, but this process is relatively inefficient in the horse.

Fresh pasture and legume hay contain adequate levels of β-carotene, but there are low levels in hay (particularly the hay used in the UK), especially if it has been stored for a few months. There is little β-carotene in grains; in fact most grains (except corn) are devoid of β-carotene. Most compound feeds will be supplemented with vitamin A in sufficient quantities to fulfil the minimum daily requirement. Signs of vitamin A deficiency include anorexia, poor growth, night blindness, a rough, dry coat and increased susceptibility to respiratory infections. Since the liver can store sufficient vitamin A to meet all the horse's needs for up to 6 months, a horse would need to continually consume a diet providing inadequate vitamin A for many months before its stores became depleted. Vitamin A deficiencies are unlikely to be common amongst performance horses.

Vitamin D

Under the influence of parathyroid hormone, vitamin D is converted to its active form from a pre-cursor that is either ingested or produced in skin. It is then converted to 25-OH-vitamin D in the liver and transported to the kidney where further hydroxylation to the most active form, 1,25-$(OH)_2$-vitamin D occurs. Vitamin D is often called the 'bone vitamin' as its most clearly established function is to maintain the plasma calcium and phosphorus levels to those required for the normal function of various mechanisms involving calcium, including muscle contraction, blood clotting and hormone and enzyme action. In the small intestine, vitamin D stimulates the absorption of calcium and phosphorus and is also involved in the mobilisation of calcium from bone to maintain a constant, normal plasma calcium concentration. Vitamin D conversion to its active form is triggered by a fall in plasma calcium. The requirement for vitamin D is closely linked to the dietary concentrations of calcium and phosphorus.

Because vitamin D is involved in the absorption of calcium, it is most crucial during the growth and development of bone, i.e. in the young growing animal. As most mammals can form vitamin D_3 from lipid compounds in the skin in the presence of UV light, it is likely that adult animals need little if any dietary supply of this vitamin. If the horse spends any time outside it is unlikely to suffer from a vitamin D deficiency; similarly if it eats sun dried hay. If hay is stored over a long period, the vitamin D content drops over the season.

Vitamin E (α-tocopherol)

Vitamin E activity is possessed by several tocopherol compounds, but the primary one found in equine tissues is α-tocopherol. Vitamin E acts as an antioxidant, thereby protecting substances in food from oxidation. Vitamin E itself can be destroyed by oxidation, which is accelerated by poor feed storage resulting in development of moulds. Crushing of oats leads to the gradual degeneration of vitamin E by oxidation unless the oats are then formed into a pellet. Vitamin E plays a role in maintaining the stability of cell membranes and works with selenium in this capacity. The requirements for vitamin E are unclear. They are probably increased with exercise, and vitamin E supplementation may improve immune function. One study (Aikawa *et al.* 1984) suggested that vitamin E deficiency is associated with decreased endurance capacity in rodents and another that supplementation with vitamin E increases endurance capacity (Novelli *et al.* 1990).

The requirement for vitamin E depends on the level of polyunsaturated fatty acids (PUFAs) in the diet because oxidation of these fats increases during exercise. Increased PUFA levels in the diet as a result of its supplementation with maize oil, soyabean oil or cod liver oil increases the vitamin E requirement because vitamin E protects PUFAs from oxidation. Vitamin E and selenium deficiencies have been associated with azoturia (tying-up) in horses.

Vitamin K

In normal healthy animals a vitamin K deficiency is very rare because most, if not all, of the daily requirement is synthesised by micro-organisms within the gut. It is also available in green leafy material and so a horse receiving some grazing would be unlikely to be deficient. Vitamin K is essential for blood clotting, but there is no reason why the horse's vitamin K requirement would increase due to increased levels of work.

Water soluble vitamins

B vitamins

B vitamins are normally synthesised in adequate quantities by gut micro-organisms, as well as being provided within dietary intake so deficiency is unlikely. Riboflavin, niacin, pyridoxine, pantothenic acid and biotin are all involved in various aspects of oxidative phosphorylation. Horses on low forage, high grain, diets may not synthesise adequate levels of B vitamins. Because many B vitamins are involved in energy metabolism, requirements for them may be increased during exercise.

Thiamin (vitamin B1)

Thiamin is involved in energy metabolism as a cofactor in enzyme reactions. Thiamin deficiency has been associated with bradycardia (low heart rate), ataxia (loss of coordination) and weight loss. Thiamin deficiency may be a problem in racehorses which use a great amount of energy and may thus be more susceptible to marginal thiamin deficiency because thiamin is required for energy utilisation. Low levels of blood thiamin have been reported in some racing Standardbreds (Loew & Bettany 1973).

Vitamin B_{12} (cyanocobalamin)

Vitamin B_{12} contains cobalt. Horses can synthesise this vitamin in their gut provided the diet contains minimum levels of cobalt. It is required for cell replication, and thus a deficiency may result in decreased RBC number and anaemia. Mature horses on high grain diets and in hard training may need supplementation of vitamin B_{12}.

Folic acid

There is a lack of information on the requirements for folic acid (folate) in the horse. Folic acid is associated with vitamin B_{12}, and so deficiency of folic acid may cause anaemia. Pasture is a good source of folic acid: horses with limited access to pasture, such as stabled racehorses, may require a folate supplement. It is possible that horses in hard work receiving more concentrate feed and less green forage may need higher levels of folic acid than horses at rest.

Biotin

Biotin is available from grass and clover foliage. Whilst it is present in many cereal grains, it is only in a form that is available to the horse in maize, yeast and soyabean. The biotin in wheat and barley is largely unavailable to the horse. Biotin supplementation at a rate of 15 mg/day leads to improvements in hoof wall problems such as weak hoof horn, misshapen hoof wall, cracked feet and crumbly hoof wall.

Biotin supplementation should be used for up to a year in order to allow time for the whole hoof capsule to be replaced by healthier horn, bearing in mind that hoof wall grows at a rate of 8–10 mm per month. After this period of time, a maintenance dose of 2–5 mg/day can be used.

For best effects, the calcium content of the diet should be checked, as a lack of calcium will detrimentally affect hoof horn growth despite biotin supplementation.

Vitamin C

Vitamin C is synthesised in the tissues of horses from glucose and has antioxidant properties. It is also a cofactor involved in the synthesis of carnitine. Thus it has been suggested that animals involved in endurance exercise may benefit from vitamin C supplementation. Vitamin C is depleted by stress, of which chronic exercise may be considered to be a form. Low plasma ascorbic acid levels have been found in racehorses. Vitamin C can be supplemented in the form of ascorbyl palmitate, as L-ascorbic acid is poorly absorbed by horses.

Minerals for performance horses

Major minerals

Calcium (Ca) is essential for enzyme action, hormone action, and for normal nerve and muscle function. Phosphorus (P) is required for the action of various enzymes, and both Ca and P are important structural components of bone. Bone acts as a huge reservoir for these minerals which should be supplied in the diet in the ratio 2:1. Ca may well need supplementing if the horse is receiving a high grain–low forage diet (forage and/or pasture plants, especially legumes, are good sources of calcium) particularly as cereal grains supply higher levels of P than Ca. High levels of P compared with Ca can lead to a decreased availability of Ca. Insufficient Ca in the diet can lead to resorption and increased porosity and weakening of bone. Ca and P should be provided at levels of 2 g/kg of diet and 1 g/kg of diet, respectively, to meet requirements. Many trainers add limestone flour or calcium gluconate (a more bioavailable source of calcium) to the diets of competition horses as a supplementary Ca source.

Ca levels in plasma are affected by acid–base balance. Metabolic alkalosis causes blood Ca levels to fall. Low plasma Ca levels may be seen in horses performing prolonged submaximal exercise due to the calcium losses in sweat and the respiratory alkalosis that can occur as a result of this sort of exercise.

Magnesium (Mg) is an essential component of body fluids, required at a level of 2 g/kg diet. Good sources are forage and sugar beet.

Potassium (K) is an important intracellular ion found in high levels in forage, but is low in cereal diets. It should be provided at a level of 46 mg/kg body mass per day for horses at rest. Prolonged sweating increases requirements.

Sodium (Na) and chloride (Cl) are important components of extracellular fluid involved in the regulation of blood volume. Provision of table salt at a level of between 5 and 10 g/kg diet would provide adequate Na and Cl for a horse in winter without great sweat losses. More may be required in hot weather or when the horse undergoes prolonged, submaximal exercise, in which case it may be necessary to provide additional electrolytes in feed or in drinking water (see Chapter 12).

Trace elements

These are required in smaller quantities than the major minerals, i.e. at levels of mg/kg diet. Copper (Cu), manganese (Mn), iodine (I) and selenium (Se) are all important for normal growth and development. Zinc (Zn) deficiency may reduce appetite and growth rate. Iron (Fe) deficiency causes anaemia, but there are no proven benefits from supplementing iron in horses that are not anaemic with a view to increasing haemoglobin content or packed cell volume. Selenium is part of the enzyme glutathione peroxidase which works closely with vitamin E to protect cell membranes from peroxidation. It has been suggested that the activity of this enzyme increases with training, which may mean that the requirement for Se is increased with exercise. Low levels of serum Se have been associated with poor racing performance in Thoroughbreds.

Probiotics

Performance horses may be exposed to high levels of stress, either in terms of workload, or due to competition or travel, which has a detrimental effect on the health of the hind gut microbial population. Probiotics contain live organisms and their products that are beneficial for intestinal microbial health. Probiotic cultures may include fungi, bacteria, and bacterial and fungal enzymes. Adding probiotics or live yeast cultures to the diet for horses being used for athletic performance may be beneficial.

Herbal supplements

Herbs are often included within compound feeds or are available as supplements aimed at a specific medical or behavioural problem. Owners may be keen to try feeding herbal supplements to their horses for their medicinal properties, thinking that natural must also mean 'safe', but they should be aware that this is not necessarily the case in all circumstances. In trying out herbal blends aimed at a particular problem, say, excitability, it would make sense to change no other aspect of the horse's management or feeding regime in order to judge whether or not the herbal supplement appears to have had a positive effect. Often people try nutritional and management changes all at once, and are then left not knowing which of the changes were responsible for the improvement in the horse's demeanour, but continue to feed the supplement 'just in case'. This area of nutrition would benefit from controlled trials to establish whether or not a particular herbal supplement is beneficial in large numbers of horses with similar conditions.

Perhaps the most important thing to bear in mind for trainers is that not all of these herbal supplements are safe to use under Jockey Club or FEI regulations regarding prohibited substances, so they should be used with caution for competition horses.

Miscellaneous supplements

Carnitine is a non-essential amino acid which may spare glycogen by enhancing FFA metabolism, for which it is necessary. Carnitine is a carrier used for transporting long-chain fatty acids into the mitochondria. It has been used as a nutritional supplement for human athletes in the hope of reducing lactate accumulation and delaying fatigue. When added to the horse's diet, it had no effect on the muscle concentrations of carnitine.

Sodium bicarbonate (baking soda) administration before maximum exertion (i.e. sprint activity lasting a few minutes or less) may be beneficial but is not allowed under Jockey Club rules. 0.4–0.6 g/kg body mass of sodium bicarbonate dissolved in several litres of water is administered by stomach tube, 3–6 hours before an event requiring anaerobic performance. The sodium bicarbonate buffers the high amount of lactic acid produced, thereby increasing the production of muscle lactate and muscle glycogen usage but decreases the extent to which muscle pH falls. Buffering lactic acid delays fatigue and thus may enhance performance. Peak blood buffering capacity does not occur until 2–6 hours after administration of sodium bicarbonate. You should not give a sodium bicarbonate supplement to an endurance horse as these tend to get hypochloraemic alkalosis due to heavy sweating in hot climates.

Methylsulfonylmethane (MSM) a derivative of dimethyl sulphoxide has been shown to reduce degenerative joint changes in animals and is often fed to horses with arthritis.

Oral creatine supplementation has been used successfully in human athletes to increase muscle creatine stores, and thus boost phosphocreatine concentrations. However, creatine in very poorly absorbed by horses.

Drugs and performance

Any factor which enhances performance is known as an ergogenic aid. Ergogenic aids include those which are permitted in competition and those which are not. 'Legal' ergogenic aids would include, for example, the use of electrolytes or even something as simple as verbal encouragement from the rider. Illegal ergogenic aids would include all drugs given with a view to unfairly increasing performance. The use of drugs in equine sport is as old as the sport itself, but the idea of trying to unfairly improve the chances of one's own horse winning is a twentieth century phenomenon, the earliest abuse of drugs having been largely directed towards decreasing the performance of competitors' horses. Because many of the early efforts were directed towards 'nobbling' or 'doping', the term 'doping' seems to have stuck and refers to all attempts to influence performance whether it be performance enhancement, reduction or restoration, i.e. using medication to mask a condition which would otherwise lead to poor performance.

The first reported case of doping related to the common practice in the early 1800s of 'nobbling' horses with arsenic. One such infamous doper was Daniel Dawson, who was alleged to have administered arsenic to horses' drinking water before a race with the intention of backing them to lose, but his crime was uncovered when the horses actually died from arsenic poisoning.

'Doping to win' came to England in 1897, resulting from a spectacularly successful partnership between Gates, an American businessman and an English trainer called Wishart. Gates supplied the cocaine to Wishart who then seemingly carried out extensive 'home trials' with the drug to establish how much to give to each horse and when. The pair made a fortune by running nondescript horses first without the drug and then with the drug (and very good odds!), afterwards selling them on at a tidy profit, only for them never to perform so successfully again. This was obviously not in the spirit of the game, but was completely legal at the time because no-one knew anything about the effects of cocaine on horses. Their scam was finally exposed when another trainer, George Lambton brought the effects of cocaine to the attention of the Jockey Club by openly running his horses on cocaine with considerable success. As a result of this, doping was banned in 1903.

Despite the ban, doping continued, with many cases being brought to trial between the 1930s and the 1960s involving opiates (for performance restoration), caffeine (for performance enhancement) and phenobarbitone (for performance reduction). In 1963, following a spate of drug abuse cases, the Horseracing Forensic Laboratory was set up for the purpose of carrying out routine drug testing and research into both drug metabolism and methods of detection.

All the organisations regulating equestrian sport publish lists of 'prohibited substances' which the Jockey Club defines as follows:

> *'A substance originating externally whether or not it is endogenous to the horse which falls in any one of the categories contained in the list of prohibited substances published from time to time in the Racing Calendar.'*

Most horses that win a race are drug tested. Also, any horse which has performed unusually badly or well may also be tested at the stewards' discretion. Samples (usually of urine) are taken on the course, by field vets. They are sealed in the presence of the trainer and the specimens then taken to the Horseracing Forensic Laboratory in Newmarket. Trainers are held responsible if their horse has a positive drug test, regardless of whether the administration of the substance was intentional or not, and so trainers have to be vigilant regarding the use of feedstuffs and also the application of topical skin and hoof treatments which may be absorbed through the skin.

Drugs for performance enhancement

Performance in a racehorse could be enhanced by either increasing speed, delaying the onset of fatigue, or both. The drugs which fit into this category include the amphetamines, caffeine, cocaine and anabolic steroids.

Amphetamines produce brain stimulatory effects by mimicking the sympathetic nervous system. They bring about the release of noradrenaline and adrenaline into the circulation. In humans, amphetamines lead to mood elevation, euphoria and a decreased sense of fatigue, resulting in their extensive use as a recreational drug. They also cause an increase in basal metabolic rate (BMR) and increased plasma FFA concentration. Sympathomimetic amines, such as clenbuterol (Ventipulmin; also known as a β_2-adrenergic agonist), are commonly given to horses to treat bronchospasm associated with RAO. However, there does not appear to be any real performance advantage in giving these drugs to clinically normal horses. They may improve running speed in horses, but this has not been scientifically proven. Amphetamines can cause cardiac arrhythmias in both humans and horses, and cause an elevation in submaximal heart rate.

Caffeine is found in tea, coffee, cocoa beans (and hence chocolate) and belongs to a group of chemicals called xanthine alkaloids, which are often found in animal feed. Similar substances are theobromine (a metabolite of caffeine) and theophylline. If horses are given feed which is contaminated with small traces of other animal feeds, it is likely that they will test positive for these substances. Caffeine is a central nervous system stimulant with similar (but less powerful) effects to amphetamine. In horses, caffeine may improve running times, but it also increases submaximal heart rates, stimulates FFA mobilisation and the nervous system and causes diuresis.

Cocaine is a potent sympathetic and central nervous system stimulant, and also a local anaesthetic. In humans it induces intense euphoria and an increased self-confidence and alertness. In horses and humans it tends to bring about an increase in heart rate and blood pressure during exercise and a lowering of V_{LA4}. It may increase performance during short term intense exercise but not during prolonged, submaximal exercise.

Anabolic (muscle enhancing) steroids are very similar to the male sex hormone, testosterone. They are synthetically produced hormones which tend to have less masculinising properties than testosterone whilst retaining the anabolic (muscle enhancing) properties. Some human athletes use anabolic steroids in the belief that they not only increase muscle mass, but bring about an increase in aggression and 'will-to-win'. The use of anabolic steroids to increase muscle mass in horses would be likely to have more of an effect in developing youngsters than in mature horses.

Erythropoietin (EPO) is produced naturally by the body and stimulates the production of red blood cells (RBCs). EPO abuse has been widespread in certain human sports, such as cycling. EPO elevates the number of RBCs, which increases oxygen-carrying capacity and, in turn, increases $\dot{V}_{O_2max}$ and exercise capacity. Administration of EPO to horses is known to result in anaemia and death. Even if there is an increase in RBCs in horses, it is doubtful if this would be beneficial as the increase in oxygen-carrying capacity would likely to be offset by a reduction in cardiac output due to increased blood viscosity and increased peripheral vascular resistance.

Drugs to decrease performance

Agents that decrease performance are known as ergolytic agents, and these include sedatives and tranquilisers. A sedative will induce narcosis (sleep) if given in high doses, e.g. romifidine, detomidine, and valium. A tranquiliser (for example, valium and acetylpromazine) are anti-anxiety drugs that

decrease awareness and produce a mentally relaxed state, but will not induce narcosis. Whether or not a drug is ergolytic or ergogenic depends to some extent on the temperament of the horse and the nature of the sport in which it is partaking. A mild sedative may have a beneficial effect on a particularly excitable dressage horse for example! An example of a sedative would be a beta blocker, e.g. propranolol, which causes decreased performance and increased perception of fatigue, with decreased resting, submaximal and maximal heart rate. Promazine, chloropromazine and acetylpromazine, are all phenothiazine derivatives which act as catecholamine blockers, in other words they tend to prevent sympathetic stimulation in response to stimuli. They decrease spontaneous motor activity, decrease blood pressure and decrease athletic performance. Valium (diazepam) is a tranquiliser which can also be used to decrease muscle spasm, while α_2-adrenergic agonists such as xylazine, detomidine and romifidine all decrease the release of noradrenaline and dopamine, and reduce athletic activity.

Drugs to restore performance

The most common drug offences in equestrian sport are those in which drugs such as anti-inflammatories are used to allow a sick or sore horse to compete. These would include the non-steroidal anti-inflammatory drugs (NSAIDs) which inhibit prostaglandin (PG) synthesis. PGs are produced in large amounts in inflamed tissues and are responsible for the increased sensitivity of inflamed tissues. One such NSAID is phenylbutazone (bute), a potent anti-inflammatory and analgesic. The analgesic effect of bute is via its anti-inflammatory property; it does not block pain as an anaesthetic would and therefore does not influence proprioception (awareness of limb position) as an anaesthetic would. In this respect it is 'safer' then a local anaesthetic. Bute administered orally takes 12 hours to take effect, compared with an intravenous injection which starts to act in 30 minutes but will not reduce PG levels for 3–4 hours. Traces of bute can be detected in urine 9 days after administration, with 2 mg taking a fortnight to clear.

Corticosteroids are often injected into joints in order to treat pain and inflammation. Repeated intra-articular corticosteroid injections have been found to cause undesirable side-effects such as cartilage damage, suppression of immune function and possibly suppression of the horse's own glucocorticoid secretion from the adrenal cortex. To minimise these effects hyaluronen is often injected at the same time. Corticosteroids are classified according to duration of activity: less than 12 hours is short acting, e.g. hydrocortisone; 12–36 hours is intermediate, e.g. prednisolone; over 48 hours is long acting, e.g. dexamethasone. They have potent effects on joint pain and should therefore be used with caution, because they can allow a horse to work quite happily on a damaged joint that can ultimately lead to a far more serious joint injury.

A diuretic is something that causes the production of large quantities of dilute urine; therefore they tend to make the horse dehydrated. Despite the fact that they dehydrate the horse, some people think they have an effect in restoring the performance of horses that bleed from the lung during exercise (EIPH) and even that they improve the performance of non-sufferers. An example of a diuretic is frusemide (the US name is furosemide; it is also known as Lasix or Dimazon), a drug which has been used for many years for horses known to bleed, and one which is permitted in racing in certain states in the USA. As a diuretic, the ultimate effect of frusemide is a decrease in plasma volume. This results in a decreased pulmonary arterial pressure, a fact that is thought to prevent or reduce the effects of EIPH. It is also a bronchodilator, and decreases airway resistance in horses with obstructed airways. Interestingly, although frusemide effectively causes dehydration, it has been shown to function as an ergogenic aid. It appears that the loss of 20–30 litres of total body water does not negatively affect performance in short term high intensity exercise. In fact, the reduction in mass carried appears to be positively beneficial because $\dot{V}_{O_2max}$ is not affected.

Advice for trainers

There is much that trainers can do to ensure that they do not inadvertently 'dope' their horses. The most important is to buy horse feeds only from manufacturers and merchants who operate a clean-mill policy. This will guarantee that the feed has not come into contact either directly or indirectly with feeds manufactured for other animals, which may contain stimulants such as caffeine and theobromine. Ask for a written guarantee of the

Table 20.1 Examples of approximate detection periods for various drugs as published by the European Horserace Scientific Liaison Committee (EHSLC)

Drug	Action	Dose	Formulation	Route	Number of horses studied	Observed detection time[a]	Date of issue
Romifidine	Sedative	100 µg/kg	10 mg/ml solution	Intravenous	2	72 h	5/8/97
Acepromazine	Sedative	152 µg/kg	1% granules	Oral	1	96 h	5/8/97
Clenbuterol hydrochloride	Bronchodilator	0.8 µg/kg twice daily for 4.5 days	30 µg/ml solution 16 µg/g granules	First dose intravenous, then oral	2	156 h	3/2/00
Lidocaine hydrochloride	Local anaesthetic	440 µg/kg	20 mg/ml solution	Subcutaneous	2	60 h	3/2/00
Methylprednisolone	Steroid	400 µg/kg	40 mg/ml suspension	Intramuscular	2	>44 days	5/2/97
Phenylbutazone	NSAID	2.2 mg/kg	200 mg/ml solution	Intravenous	1	144 h	5/2/97
Frusemide	Diuretic	1.0 mg/kg	50 mg/ml solution	Intramuscular	2	72 h	5/2/97
Frusemide	Diuretic	1.0 mg/kg	50 mg/ml solution	Intravenous	2	60 h	3/2/00

[a] The observed detection times include both detection of the drug and/or its metabolites. These data are based on limited numbers of observations in Thoroughbred horses which were not in full training. The detection times published by the EHSLC are based on very low numbers of horses studied. The detection times may vary markedly between individuals and with factors such as age, sex, breed, training status, health, concurrent medication or any other factors which may increase or shorten the detection times. The authors cannot except any responsibility for the use of these figures in any way whatsoever.

clean-mill policy. Even with a written guarantee it is wise to keep a sample of all feeds (and supplements) fed in the month before a competition, along with the batch number of the feed, so that the source of any prohibited substance may be discovered in the unfortunate event of a positive drug test. Always extend clearance times for prescribed drugs (see Table 20.1). Tell your vet when you intend to compete so that you can discuss adequate withdrawal times in any given situation.

Topically applied substances can end up in blood by passing through skin or being licked. A common practice is to put Vick up the nostrils of colts travelling with fillies to prevent then smelling them, particularly if one is in season. Even this can lead to traces of camphor being found in a urine sample. Most of the recent positive tests in racing have arisen from substances in common use in stables, such as leg washes, tack cleaning products and disinfectants. Feed additives such as probiotics and electrolytes are usually perfectly safe to use.

KEY POINTS

- A loss of water amounting to just 2% of body mass (10 kg in a 500 kg horse) may affect performance. Horses can be encouraged to drink when they are away at competitions by flavouring the water with apple juice or squash if they have previously been introduced to this novel flavour.
- Body fluids, both intracellular (that within cells) and extracellular (that outside cells), have an osmolarity in the region of 300 mosm/l (milliosmoles per litre). Any solution that has the same osmolarity as this is described as being isotonic; it does not imply anything regarding the actual composition of the solution.
- A typical daily intake of food is 2–2.5% of the horses total body mass; thus a horse weighing 500 kg might be receiving 10–12.5 kg of food per day.
- The most critical component in the diet of the performance horse is energy. Most of the horse's daily requirement for energy is met by the breakdown of carbohydrate and fat. Probably less than 1% of the total energy requirement comes from the oxidation of protein.
- Forage has a lower energy content per kilogram of dry matter than cereals, and it may not be possible to meet the horse's daily energy requirement by feeding forage only because the quantities that need to be fed may exceeed the horse's daily capacity for food and hence its appetite.

- Fibre sources include hay, haylage, grass, silage, fibre cubes and chaff. The average energy range for hay on an 'as fed' basis is 6–11 MJ/kg.
- Concentrated feeds have an energy content of 12–16 MJ DE/kg DM.
- Horses undertaking endurance type work require a prolonged, slow release of energy throughout the day and are therefore usually fed higher levels of forage than horses doing shorter duration faster work.
- Average diets for horses contain approximately 3% fat (in terms of the percentage of the total energy intake), but as much as 20% of the total calories in the diet (forage + cereal + added oil) of an endurance horse could come from fat.
- Racehorses are fed diets higher in starch such as cereals (concentrate feed) because these are rapidly digested and absorbed and provide a rapidly available energy source.
- All horses will have an optimal competition mass. If the horse is below its optimum mass its energy stores are likely to be reduced and the risk of fatigue is increased.
- Most positive drug tests in equine sport these days are due to owners/trainers having unwittingly administered their horse a prohibited substance either via a feed or feed supplement, or by not giving sufficient time for clearance of a prescribed medicine. Even some topically applied products can lead to a false positive result.

Chapter 21

Transport

To compete in nearly all sport at whatever level it is almost always necessary to transport horses. Even the horse kept at home and only ever hacked out probably had to arrive in some form of transport, and occasionally may have to be transported to a vet or farrier. Many thousands of miles are clocked up by horses being transported each year. If only half the horses in the country travelled 100 miles each in a year then that would be 30 million horse transport miles per year. Of these high number of miles, probably 99.9% pass without incident. Of course, accidents do happen. We probably can't do much about a blow-out on the motorway, the horse that puts its foot through the floor or the horse that falls and becomes wedged under a partition. These sorts of problem are fortunately quite rare. However, transport can have effects on health, welfare and on performance, and we may be able to eliminate or reduce the impact of some factors associated with transport and their possible adverse effects. The main effects of transport are usually considered to be increased stress responses, adverse effects on the respiratory and gastrointestinal systems, increased energy expenditure, and adverse effects on performance. These do not occur in all horses or even in the same horse on different journeys, and adverse effects may only be seen in a small number of horses all transported under the same conditions.

Horses are predominantly transported by road and to a much lesser extent by air and sea (Fig. 21.1). It is now quite rare to hear of horses transported by rail, although it was very popular to take horses to races by rail in the 1930s. Of course, before mechanised transport, racehorses would have to be ridden to the races. In general, most of the factors that affect horses during transport are similar whether this is by road, by air or by sea. There are some differences or problems particular to each form of transport which will be highlighted.

What happens to a horse during transport?

It is often assumed that all a horse being transported has to do is stand up. The horse would be standing if it was in its stable or in the field, so what's the difference? Quite a lot. Some studies have shown that heart rates of most horses are higher during transport than if they were standing in their stable. This was originally interpreted as being due to mild anxiety and was almost dismissed as being of any significance. However, more recently it has been shown that for many horses the effort they expend in simply standing in the back of a lorry or in an aeroplane during transport is similar to walking for the same period. Another estimate is that the energy expenditure during transport is twice that at rest in the stable. So imagine you live 50 miles outside London and the day before you are going to run in the annual London marathon, you set off from home and walk for 10 hours, have a night in a hotel and then run the next day! Then think about your horse. This might be over emphasising the potential effects of transport, but in the past transport has often been neglected as an area that could affect both health and performance.

Of course, many of the effects of transport are likely to be related to the duration of the journey. Transporting your horse for under 1 hour is likely to carry a very low risk of health problems or effects on performance. In fact, the current view is that transport for under 3h has negligible or immeasurable effects on the health and performance of horses that are healthy at the start of transport (i.e. not horses that have RAO (COPD), viral infection, etc.). But at the other end of the spectrum there are flights to the other side of the world lasting 18–20 hours flying time, not to mention the time for refuelling, quarantine checks,

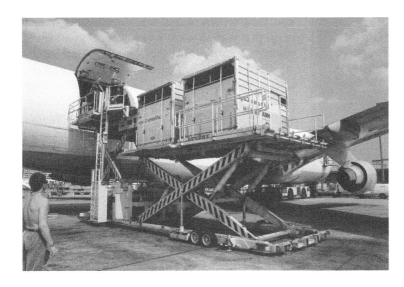

Fig. 21.1 Flight crates containing horses being loaded onto an aircraft.

getting to and from airports, etc. And long journeys are, of course, not just restricted to flying. For competitions held in countries such as Italy, the drive from the UK would be of the order of 3 days. Even allowing for overnight stops and stabling, the actual travel time in the lorry would be near to 24 h. Whilst naturally we would perhaps think that longer travel is always worse, some studies of flying have shown that stress responses for shorter and longer flights, as measured by changes in WBC counts and the ratio of neutrophils to lymphocytes, are not that different. This may mean that the horses are anxious in the early stages of a flight but relax more in the later stages. However, whilst anxiety may be of concern to owners, grooms, riders and trainers, it does not necessarily have immediate implications for health. Leaving out injuries, the main body systems affected by transport are the respiratory tract and the gastrointestinal tract.

Weight loss during transport

One of the most common consequences of transporting horses is dehydration. On the basis of a number of studies of horses transported by either road or air, loss of mass is often in the region of 0.4–0.5% body mass per hour of transport or around 2 kg/h in a 500 kg horse. This figure is an average for horses with previous experience of transport, transported in 'ideal' conditions. For example, if horses do not have enough space, are driven badly, if the tem-perature and/or humidity are high, or if horses are anxious, then losses may increase to as much as 1.5% body mass per hour.

Increased loss of mass during transport can occur as a result of

- Decreased water intake
- Increased sweating
- Increases in the water content of faeces
- Increased insensible water loss.

Decreased water intake

Horses may not drink as much if they are not fed. Around two-thirds of a horse's daily water intake is associated with eating. If the horse is eating less, it will almost certainly be drinking less. If you have taken water in plastic containers, the plastic can taint the smell and taste of the water and this puts some horses off. However, this can often be overcome by adding a small amount (50–100 ml per 15 litre bucket) of apple juice or molasses to the water. Remember though, you must introduce your horse to this at home so that you know if your horse likes flavoured water. If you are travelling for 8 hours and you offer your horse water before the journey starts and during a 30 minute stop after 4 hours' driving, you are effectively allowing access to water for only 30 minutes in an 8 hour day. It's not always the case that the horse will take the opportunity to catch up on its daily water intake. If it is still on the lorry it may be more interested in food, and if you

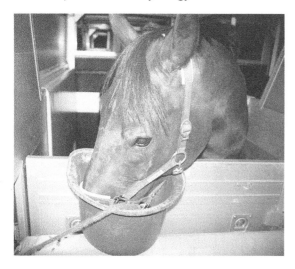

Fig. 21.2   Allow horses to eat and drink when they want to.

unload the horse there may be too many distractions. We might hope that horses will drink and eat normally after transport, but unfamiliar surroundings, separation from stable mates and changes in water may all mean that water intake remains below average. A better approach is to provide feed and water throughout the journey. A soaked hay net or haylage and a bucket suspended in front of the horse allow it to eat and drink when it wants to, not when you decide it's time it should (Fig. 21.2). Again, many people will travel horses with a hay net, but without water available. To prevent water spilling, an old tyre can be placed over the top of the bucket. Horses travelled with feed and water continuously available may be more relaxed and definitely lose less body mass. This approach is unlikely to be needed for journeys under 4–5 h except in hot conditions.

Increased sweating

If a horse is nervous or if the conditions are warm, hot, or hot and humid, then sweat losses may be increased. Sweat contains both water and electrolytes. If you are travelling horses in the summer, make sure that there is good ventilation through the lorry. Don't be tempted to over-rug horses. It would be better for them to be slightly on the cool side than on the warm side. Ideally, this should mean that there is some air movement at all levels within the partition. If there is a lot of air movement across the top of the trailer or lorry (i.e. at the level of the head) but none at the body level then the horse may still get warm and sweat. Good ventilation will also help with air quality. In summer you could, of course, start journeys in the early morning or late in the day to avoid the hottest times. This also means that you are less likely to get stuck in heavy traffic. Being stationary on a hot day is ideal for doubling or even trebling the amount of fluid loss.

Increases in water content of faeces

When the horse is anxious, this upsets the gut and the horse is less able to digest its diet properly; droppings may be passed more frequently and become more watery.

Increased insensible water loss

Although we tend to think of the skin as 'waterproof', in fact it is permeable to water. In dry, and especially warm and dry, conditions, moisture is lost through the skin. This is not the same as sweating. Therefore, even if a horse does not appear to be sweating, in warm or hot and very dry conditions a significant amount of water can still be lost. Insensible water loss is often not a major route of water loss in horses in temperate climates. For example, in the UK the relative humidity rarely falls below 30%. However, in desert conditions with temperatures as high as 40°C, relative humidity may be as low as 5%. Of course, at 40°C, the horse may well need to sweat to keep its body temperature down. However, there is one situation in which insensible losses are greatly increased at relatively low temperatures because of very low moisture content of the air, and that is during flying. Therefore, when horses are flown, even if the cabin temperature is kept around 15–17°C (an ideal temperature range), the very dry air will cause water to be drawn from the skin. This is not just confined to horse flights. The same happens on passenger flights. However, there is little that can be done to reduce or eliminate insensible losses other than to try and ensure the horse remains hydrated by drinking.

Effects of dehydration on health and performance

Dehydration is likely to affect primarily the gastrointestinal tract and the respiratory tract. Reduced fluid in the large intestine may interfere with the bacterial flora and, in turn, with digestion. The risk of colic may also be increased. Dehydration can affect the respiratory tract by causing drying of the airways. This may interfere with the lungs' normal defence mechanisms for dealing with bacteria and potential allergens (e.g. moulds, pollen) or irritants (e.g. dusts). Drying of the airways may affect mucus production and also mucus clearance from the lower airways. Dehydration can therefore potentially induce mild airway inflammation in horses with no history of respiratory disease, lead to a dramatic worsening of inflammation and lung function in horses with pre-existing respiratory conditions such as RAO or a lower airway infection. Mild to moderate dehydration may well have little effect on the performance of healthy horses, except if it induces airway inflammation. However, the level at which dehydration impacts on performance is still poorly understood. One study from the USA showed no difference in time trials for horses transported for 15 minutes compared with when they were transported for 120–150 minutes. There is an anecdotal report that horses losing less than 10 kg after long distance air transport raced better than those losing more than 20 kg. A safe approach is therefore to try and take steps that will reduce dehydration as much as possible during transport and/or to allow sufficient time for recovery following transport.

Recovery following transport

Recovery in body mass following transport does not appear to be the same as following exercise or competition. For example, we know that losses of 5% body mass can easily be restored overnight in eventers following the speed and endurance test. However, a loss of 5% body mass following transport may take 3–4 days to restore fully. This suggests that the loss of mass may be related to something other than simply dehydration following

transport. Certainly, total protein returns to normal fairly quickly following transport, suggesting that the horse actually rehydrates fairly quickly. However, it may be that the effect is related to loss of ingesta and water from the large intestine and caecum.

To assess and manage mass loss associated with transport, the starting point is to actually measure the change in mass. In research studies, a set of portable scales is often used. This approach is most likely to produce accurate results as all measurements will be taken using the same scales, although the scales should still be calibrated each time they have been moved. Differences of 10–20 kg would not be uncommon for different sets of scales, especially if they are not regularly calibrated. If a set of scales are 20 kg out in 500 kg, this doesn't really matter if you use them to calculate amounts of wormers or drugs, to assess mass loss after exercise or to follow your horse's mass throughout the season. However, if your scales show your horse's mass to be 500 kg before transport and a second set of scales after transport show it to be 490 kg, but the second set over-reads by 20 kg, you will think that your horse has lost 10 kg and is OK, when it has actually lost 30 kg and may need fluids. One way around this is to check the mass of your horse on any set of scales before transport and then check the reading of that set of scales with bags of feed. You can then do the same following transport when you are checking the mass of your horse on a different set of scales. Following losses of around 5% body mass, it may take 3–4 days for a horse to come back to its pre-transport mass. If the journey has been long (1–2 days by road or a flight of over 6 hours), if there has been a change of more than 3–4 time-zones, if the feed has changed, and if the climate is much warmer or colder, it may take the horse up to a week to regain the mass lost. Therefore, with journeys such as this, if you have access to scales and trust them, until your horse has shown a reasonable recovery in mass (say 50% of loss restored) it would be unwise to do more than hand walking and riding at walk. If you don't have scales, its better to proceed with caution and incorporate into travel plans some very light days. Remember that horses lose fitness very very slowly and that a week of light work in the later stages of a training programme will have little impact. For horses prone to tying-up it would be wise to reduce the amount of hard feed during a period of recovery from transport when horses are only in light work.

Effect of transport on the respiratory tract

The respiratory tract may be affected by dehydration, which in turn may decrease mucus production and/or mucus clearance. If ventilation is inadequate the horse may also be exposed to a higher concentration of allergens which may originate from hay or bedding. In addition, ammonia from urine acts as an irritant to the respiratory tract. The horse's high head position during transport can also affect clearance of mucus from the airways and cause bacteria that normally colonise the upper respiratory tract to spread to the lower airways. There are many bacteria that live in the airways of normal healthy horses that, given changes in conditions, could multiply rapidly and induce disease or an infection. Several studies have shown that tying horse's heads up for 24h caused marked accumulation of mucopus in the trachea, increased numbers of bacteria and decreased ability to clear mucus from the respiratory tract. However, it has also been found that bacterial counts increase after only 6 hours of head up restraint. Interestingly, it has also been reported that allowing horses to lower their heads for 30min every 6h does not prevent the increase in bacteria in the trachea.

It is probably still important to try and encourage horses to lower their heads occasionally during travelling, for example by feeding them small pieces of carrot or apple low down, as this may assist clearance of accumulated mucus from the airways. This is also why it is important to have rest breaks during road journeys and to take the horses off the lorry (Fig. 21.3).

The air quality during road transport can be improved by ensuring good ventilation, using a low dust bedding material such as paper or cardboard, and feeding fully soaked hay or haylage. In addition, to counteract the irritant effects of ammonia produced from urea in urine by bacteria, there are compounds called zeolites which can be used to absorb and neutralise ammonia. These come as a

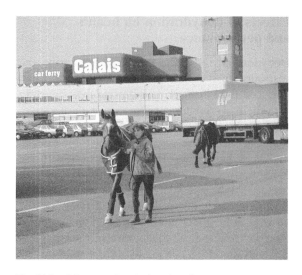

Fig. 21.3 Allow rest breaks in a long journey.

powder which is sprinkled onto the floor before the bedding is laid on top.

Taking steps to ensure air quality is as good as possible are even more important during air transport where the amount of fresh air ventilation is relatively low, air is recirculated, there are frequently large numbers of horses, and it is not possible to take the horses out of the environment and remove urine and faeces.

For healthy horses, transport and poor air quality may only produce mild airway inflammation which, on arrival, resolves rapidly without treatment. For horses with pre-existing RAO, even if mild, consequences may range from a slight increase in airway inflammation which is not apparent, i.e. no clinical signs, to clinical signs including nasal discharge, cough, increased lung sounds, dyspnoea and/or poor exercise tolerance.

All horses are at risk to some extent of developing 'shipping fever' (essentially pneumonia, i.e. bacterial infection of the lung) after extended periods of transport. This is the most common illness affecting transported horses. The signs of shipping fever include depression, decreased feed intake, increased body temperature, cough, nasal discharge and increased respiratory rate. Shipping fever may develop during transport or any time up to around 3 days after arrival. A study of road transport in Japan (Ishida *et al.* 1999) reported that 12% of horses transported for over 24h developed shipping fever and another study reported that 6.3% of horses flown from the UK to Australia developed shipping fever. Perhaps not surprisingly, the risk of shipping fever developing also increases with the duration of transport. The most common bacterium associated with the development of shipping fever has been reported to be *Streptococcus zooepidemicus*. Whilst it is not clear why some horses will develop shipping fever following either road or air transport, whilst all others remain apparently healthy, factors such as air quality, duration, health before transport and how carefully the horses are transported (head position, frequency of breaks, driving, etc.) are all likely to play a part. Shipping fever can often be treated successfully but can also be fatal. For this reason it is always a good idea to take a horse's temperature before transporting it. If your horse has a temperature you are obviously not going to transport it. However, if you don't take its temperature before transport, arrive at a competition after an 8 hour drive and then find that your horse has a temperature, this may put your horse at an increased risk of developing shipping fever. The last thing you want to do with a horse in this state is to turn around and drive home. So you are stuck 8 hours from home with a sick horse on which you can't compete. It has happened!! A pre-transport temperature takes 1 minute to do. Consider making it part of your travel routine, especially for longer journeys.

Orientation during transport

There is some scientific evidence to suggest that horses generally travel better when they are rear facing as opposed to forward facing (see, for example, Waran *et al.* 1996). Rear facing horses tend to have fewer impacts on the trailer sides, fewer total impacts and fewer losses of balance. Rear facing horses also tend to have lower heart rates during the first 15 seconds of travel than the forward facing horses. This is probably because horses have an inherent ability to respond more easily to forces acting caudally (towards the hindquarters), rather than cranially. When travelling rearward, it is more likely that the horse will have room to lower its head and neck to aid balance. Also, if sharp decelerations are made

(more likely than sharp accelerations!), the horse will impact on the trailer/horsebox with its bottom, not its head. Current evidence based on a number of different scientific studies suggests that around two-thirds of horses when travelled loose will adopt a rearwards facing position.

Recommendations for preparation, transport and acclimatisation for the 1996 Atlanta Olympic Games

Our knowledge of how the stressors of heat and humidity impact on a horses health, welfare and performance was revolutionised in the run-up to the Atlanta Olympics as a result of an integrated, international research effort. As well as directly benefiting horses and competitors of all nations competing in the heat and humidity of the Atlanta Olympics, much of the research can now be applied to maximise the health, welfare and performance of horses competing in less demanding competition environments and for the health and welfare of working animals in extreme climates. The International Research Group published detailed recommendations for competitors for the Atlanta Olympics in terms of preparation for travel, management during travel and acclimatisation on arrival in Atlanta. Competitors were advised to treat the recovery from transport and the acclimatisation as two separate 'stressors' and recommended to fly out at least 21 days before their competition, which would ensure that horses were able to fully recover from their long flights before embarking on acclimatisation. The following section gives an insight into the 'work behind the scenes' at Atlanta, being the culmination of four years of research across around ten different countries.

For major competitions such as the Olympics or the World Equestrian Games, preparations should begin several months before travel. These preparations include:

- Diet: any changes required for competition should be introduced at least 4 weeks in advance of the competition. The decision must be made early on as to whether to use feed exported from home to the country of competition or to import feed from the host country and use the same feeds on arrival. If it is the latter, food from the host country can be imported before competition so the horse can become used to the new source. This is especially important with sources of fibre, abrupt changes in which can cause marked disturbance to the gastrointestinal tract. Disturbances in hindgut microflora can be minimised by feeding probiotics (under veterinary guidance) 2–3 days before and up to 5 days after transport, especially for poor travellers.

- Hydration: travel to and competing in a humid and hot climate results in loss of fluid and electrolytes. It is essential that horses are 'trained' to drink electrolytes prior to transport and competition so that they do not refuse them at critical times. This can be done by building up to the required level of electroytes over time, or by getting the horses accustomed to drinking flavoured water in order to mask the electrolytes. The use of flavoured water is good but be aware of any additives in the flavouring that may constitute 'prohibited substances'.

- Veterinary testing: prior to travel, the horse should undergo a thorough veterinary investigation, paying particular attention to any known predispositions to certain conditions. For example, recurrent airway obstruction (equine COPD or 'heaves') can be aggravated by travel, and rhabdomyolysis indirectly by heat and humidity as a consequence of increased electrolyte loss. A horse should not travel unwell or unfit, even if sufficient time has been built into the acclimatisation period. An ill or unfit horse is unlikely to travel or acclimatise well.

- Cooling: in a hot environment, horses should be cooled during training exercise and competition. However, horses from cooler climates may not be used to this and must therefore be introduced to the practice before travel (Fig. 21.4). You may even need to practise at home with warm water.

- Pre-acclimatisation: it may be beneficial to arrange some pre-competition training in a climate similar to that found in the country where the competition will take place.

- Training: horses should be travelled fit for competition. Once the horse sets off for an international competition the priorities are to minimise the stresses of transport and to acclimatise accordingly to the new climate. You can not expect to 'train' the horse as well during this period of time and therefore all the normal fitness training should be complete before travel. In addition, it is useful to actually reduce or 'taper' the training intensity in the 2–3 days prior to travel to ensure that horses are fully hydrated and physically recovered prior to travelling.

- Bodyweight: just prior to travelling (i.e. at the yard on the morning of departure), the horse should be weighed, and this weight compared to its weight on arrival in the host country. This allows fluid losses to be calculated.

Travel

In the Atlanta recommendations, it was suggested that if the journey to the airport was over 5 hours then a recovery period prior to flying of 12–24 hours should be built in, more if the journey was longer. For road journeys in excess of 15 hours, 3 days recovery were recommended prior to flying. This is important to allow the horses to rehydrate and recover from the stress of the road journey. We have already discussed methods of reducing trans-

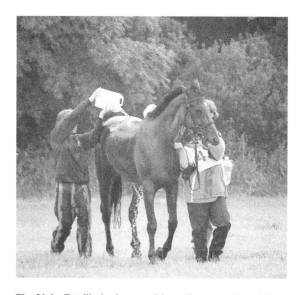

Fig. 21.4 Familiarise horses with cooling procedures before competition.

port stress, and these should be paid particular attention to when embarking on journeys of over 5 hours.

Flying

As far as possible, the hold temperature should be kept to 16–17°C which helps to minimise fluid losses through sweating. The air in flight is often very dry, and this can exacerbate respiratory problems. All bedding (preferably paper) should be kept very clean and dust-free and hay should be soaked. Feeding small, frequent meals from the ground or as low as possible is better in terms of maintaining hydration status (as horses will drink more if they are also eating) and also in encouraging mucociliary clearance (clearance of inhaled debris and mucus from the airways).

Horses should be allowed to drink as and when they require, and so buckets should be kept full and within reach of the horse.

Some horses never travel well, despite all the usual precautions being taken. In some instances, vets may use additional methods of safeguarding the horses well-being, such as administering fluids intravenously or by nasogastric tube, or administering prophylactic antibiotics.

Arrival

Horses should be given a routine veterinary examination on arrival, particularly after long distance flights. They should be weighed, and this weight compared to their pre-travel weight, as described above. The percentage weight loss is important, and can be used to assess how much fluid the horse will require to rehydrate.

The horse should be moved as soon as possible to its destination, but in hot climates it may be advisable to wait until the end of the day or early in the morning when it is cooler to reduce the impact of further travel-induced stress.

Recovery from travelling

The loss of bodyweight during transport is a good indicator of how the horse has been affected. Recovery from transport is considered to have occurred when the horse has resumed its pre-transport bodyweight, judged by weighing the horse at the same time each day. Horses should be weighed as soon as possible after their arrival so that they may be treated appropriately. The recommendations for Atlanta were that horses losing more than 4% bodyweight should be given 8 litres of isotonic fluid by nasogastric tube. For horses losing in excess of 6% bodyweight it was suggested that they be treated with intravenous fluid therapy.

The horse may require up to 5 days to recover from a long haul flight and this must be complete before acclimatisation exercise can begin. Whilst the horse is recovering from transport, only light exercise should be undertaken. In hot and humid climates horses should work at low intensities, and early in the morning to avoid any additional stress due to heat and humidity. After the first five days (or following suitable recovery from transport, whichever is first) horses may resume their normal training programme.

Acclimatisation

A suitable acclimatisation period is necessary as lack of acclimatisation before competition will reduce the horses strength, coordination, concentration and endurance. Horses that are not adequately acclimatised will suffer far more from the effects of heat and humidity and are more likely to be at risk of heat-related illness. Having recovered sufficiently from the flight, training can be resumed as normal, but in a way which produces optimal acclimatisation to the more challenging environment without unnecessary exposure to heat and humidity. Exercise during the hottest part of the day should be avoided initially and limited until the horse is fully acclimatised. Don't forget that horses can also be prone to the effects of sun burn, with potentially disastrous effects on the acclimatisation process. Following a training session, the horse should be returned to the shade and cooled until its respiratory rate and rectal temperature have been significantly reduced. Measurements of weight before and after exercise give a good indication of how well the horse is acclimatising. There is no advantage in increasing the horse's exposure to the hot and humid conditions above that which is necessary in order to exercise the horse. During periods of inactivity, it is best to make the horse as comfortable as possible, even by using fans in the stables to help keep the horses cool.

It is also important to record the horse's water intake, another useful indicator of acclimatisation. More general observations of heat tolerance can also be used, such as maintenance of feed intake, less sweating during exercise, and a general appearance of increased comfort. Based on the research undertaken at the University of Guelph and the Animal Health Trust, it is known that most acclimatisation will be complete after 14 days of daily training in hot humid conditions.

KEY POINTS

- The main effects of transport may include stress, respiratory and gastrointestinal tract disturbance/disease, increased energy expenditure and decreased performance.
- The effort of travelling may be equivalent to walking, and the energy expended during travelling has also been estimated to be twice that for standing in the stable.
- Transport of healthy horses in good conditions for under 3 h is considered to have little or no effect on performance and minimal risks for health.
- Horses lose around 0.4–0.5% body mass per hour of road or air transport in ideal conditions. Losses may be doubled by bad driving, rough roads, turbulence when flying, thermal stress and inadequate space.
- Mass loss during transport can be due to decreased water and feed intake and increased sweat, faecal and insensible water losses (the latter especially during flying).

- Dehydration affects the gastrointestinal tract and may predispose to colic.
- Dehydration affects the respiratory tract and may be a risk factor for the development of shipping fever or exacerbate pre-existing allergic conditions such as RAO (COPD).
- Recovery of body mass loss following transport usually takes much longer than for the same loss of body mass induced by exercise. Complete recovery of 4–5% loss of body mass following transport may take 5–7 days.
- The most common problem affecting transported horses is shipping fever (pneumonia). The risk of shipping fever increases with the duration of transport.
- On the basis of scientific studies, around two-thirds of horses choose to face backwards when travelled loose.

References

Aikawa, K.M., Quintanilha, A.T., de Lumen, B.O., Brooks, G.A. & Packer, L. (1984) Exercise endurance-training alters vitamin E tissue levels and red-blood-cell hemolysis in rodents. *Bioscience Reports*, **4**(3), 253–257.

Ainsworth, D.M., Smith, C.A., Eicker, S.W., Ducharme, N.G., Henderson, K.S., Snedden, K. & Dempsey, J.A. (1997) Pulmonary–locomotory interactions in exercising dogs and horses. *Respiration Physiology*, **110**(2–3), 287–294.

Amis, T.C., Pascoe, J.R. & Hornof, W. (1984) Topographic distribution of pulmonary ventilation and perfusion in the horse. *American Journal of Veterinary Research*, **45**(8), 1597–1601.

Art, T., Anderson, L., Woakes, A.J., Roberts, C., Butler, P.J., Snow, D.H. & Leukeux, P. (1990a) Mechanics of breathing during strenuous exercise in thoroughbred horses. *Respiratory Physiology*, **82**, 279–294.

Art, T., Amory, H., Desmecht, D. & Lekeux, P. (1990b) Effect of show jumping on heart rate, blood lactate and other plasma biochemical values. *Equine Veterinary Journal* (Suppl.), **9**, 78–82.

Attenburrow, D.P. (1976) Respiratory sounds in exercising horses together with some applications. Fellowship thesis, Royal College of Veterinary Surgeons, London.

Attenburrow, D.P. (1982) Time relationship between the respiratory cycle and limb cycle in the horse. *Equine Veterinary Journal*, **14**(1), 69–72.

Audigie, F., Pourcelot, P., Degueurce, C., Denoix, J.M. & Geiger, D. (1999) Kinematics of the equine back: flexion–extension movements in sound trotting horses. *Equine Veterinary Journal* (Suppl.), **30**, 210–213.

Back, W., Barneveld, A., Briun, G., Schamhardt, H.C. & Hartman, W. (1994) Kinematic detection of superior gait quality in young trotting warmbloods. *Veterinary Quarterly*, **16**(Suppl. 2), S91–S96.

Badoux, D.M. (1975) General biostatics and biomechanics. In: *Sisson and Grossman's The Anatomy of Domestic Animals*, 5th edn (ed. R. Getty), pp. 48–83. W.B. Saunders, Philadelphia, PA.

Barrey, E. & Galloux, P. (1997) Analysis of the equine jumping technique by accelerometry. *Equine Veterinary Journal* (Suppl.), **23**, 45–49.

Bernard, S.L., Glenny, R.W., Erickson, H.H., Fedde, M.R., Polissar, N., Basaraba, R., Hlastala, M.P. (1996) Minimal redistribution of pulmonary blood flow with exercise in racehorses. *Journal of Applied Physiology*, **81**(3), 1062–1070.

Birch, H.L., McLaughlin, L., Smith, R.K.W. & Goodship, A.E. (1999) Treadmill exercise-induced tendon hypertrophy: assessment of tendons with different mechanical functions. *Equine Veterinary Journal* (Suppl.), **30**, 222–226.

Buick, F.J., Gledhill, N., Froese, A.B., Spriet, L. & Meyers, E.C. (1980) Effect of induced erythrocythaemia on aerobic work capacity. *Journal of Applied Physiology: Respiratory, Environmental & Exercise Physiology*, **48**(4), 636–642.

Burrell, M.H., Wood, J.L., Whitwell, K.E., Chanter, N., Mackintosh, M.E. & Mumford, J.A. (1996) Respiratory disease in thoroughbred horses in training: the relationships between disease and viruses, bacteria and environment. *Veterinary Record*, **139**(13), 308–313.

Butler, P.J., Woakes, A.J., Anderson, L.S., Smale, K., Roberts, C.A. & Snow, D.H. (1991) The effect of cessation of training on cardiorespiratory variables during exercise. In: *Equine Exercise Physiology*, Vol. 3 (eds S.G.B. Persson, A. Lindholm & L.B. Jeffcott), pp. 71–76. ICEEP Publications, Davis, CA.

Carlson, G.P. (1983) Thermoregulation, fluid and electrolyte balance. In: *Equine Exercise Physiology* (eds D.H. Snow, S.G.B. Persson & R.J. Rose), pp. 291–309. Granta Editions, Cambridge.

Carroll, C.L. & Huntington, P.J. (1988) Body condition scoring and weight estimation of horses. *Equine Veterinary Journal*, **20**(1), 41–45.

Cherdchutham, W., Becker, C., Smith, R.K.W., Barneveld, A. & van Weeren, P.R. (1999) Age-related changes and effect of exercise on the molecular composition of immature equine superficial digital flexor tendons. *Equine Veterinary Journal* (Suppl.), **31**, 86–94.

Clarke, L.L., Roberts, M.C. & Argenzio, R.A. (1990) Feeding and digestive problems in horses: responses to a concentrated meal. In: *Clinical Nutrition, Veterinary Clinics of North America* (ed. H.F. Hintz), pp. 433–450. W.B. Saunders, Philadelphia, PA.

Clayton, H.M. (1989a) Terminology for the description of equine jumping kinematics. *Journal of Equine Veterinary Science*, **9**, 341–348.

Clayton, H.M. (1989b) Time–motion analysis in equestrian sports: the Grand Prix dressage test. *Proceedings of the American Association of Equine Practitioners*, **35**, 367–373.

Clayton, H.M. (1993) Development of conditioning programs for dressage horses based on time–motion analysis of competitions. *Journal of Applied Physiology*, **74**(5), 2325–2329.

Clayton, H.M. (1994a) Comparison of the stride kinematics of the collected, working, medium and extended trot in horses. *Equine Veterinary Journal*, **26**(3), 230–234.

Clayton, H.M. (1994b) Comparison of the collected, working,

medium and extended canters. *Equine Veterinary Journal* (Suppl.), **17**, 16–19.

Clayton, H.M. (1995) Comparison of the stride kinematics of the collected, medium, and extended walks in horses. *American Journal of Veterinary Research*, **56**(7), 849–852.

Clayton, H.M. (1997) Effect of added weight on landing kinematics in jumping horses. *Equine Veterinary Journal* (Suppl.), **23**, 50–53.

Clayton, H.M., Lanovaz, J.L., Schamhardt, H.C., Willemen, M.A. & Colborne, G.R. (1998) Net joint moments and powers in the equine forelimb during the stance phase of the trot. *Equine Veterinary Journal*, **30**(5), 384–389.

Colborne, G.R., Clayton, H.M. & Lanovaz, J.L. (1995) Factors that influence vertical velocity during take-off over a water jump. *Equine Veterinary Journal* (Suppl.), **18**, 138–140.

Colborne, G.R., Lanovaz, J.L., Sprigings, E.J., Schamhardt, H.C. & Clayton, H.M. (1998) Forelimb joint moments and power during the walking stance phase of horses. *American Journal of Veterinary Research*, **59**(5), 609–614.

Cook, W.R. (1974) Epistaxis in the racehorse. *Equine Veterinary Journal*, **6**(2), 45–58.

Couroucé, A., Chatard, J.C. & Auvinet, B. (1997) Estimation of performance potential of standardbred trotters from blood lactate concentrations measured in field conditions. *Equine Veterinary Journal*, **29**(5), 365–369.

Deuel, N. (1995) Dressage canter kinematics and performances in an Olympic three-day event. *Proceedings of the European Association for Animal Production*, **46**, 341–344.

Deuel, N.R. & Park, J. (1990) The gait patterns of Olympic dressage horses. *International Journal of Sports Biomechanics*, **6**, 198–226.

Deuel, N.R. & Park, J. (1991) Kinematic analysis of jumping sequences of Olympic show-jumping horses. *Equine Exercise Physiology*, **3**, 158–166.

Deuel, N.R. & Park, J. (1993) Gallop kinematics of Olympic three-day event horses. *Acta Anatomica*, **146**(2–3), 168–174.

Erickson, H.H., Sexton, W.L., Erickson, B.K. & Coffman, J.R. (1987) Cardiopulmonary response to exercise and detraining in the Quarter horse. In: *Equine Exercise Physiology*, vol. 2 (eds J.R. Gillespie & N.E. Robinson), ICEEP Publications, Davis, CA.

Erickson, H.H., Bernard, S.L., Glenny, R.W., *et al.* (1999) Effect of furosemide on pulmonary blood flow distribution in resting and exercising horses. *Journal of Applied Physiology*, **86**(6), 2034–2043.

Evans, B.A. (1988) Animal Health Trust survey of wastage amongst racehorses in training 1984 and 1985 undertaken at the request of the committee for the coordination of veterinary research requirements for the racing industry. Animal Health Trust, Newmarket.

Evans, D.L., Harris, R.C. & Snow, D.H. (1993) Correlation of racing performance with blood lactate and heart rate after exercise in thoroughbred horses. *Equine Veterinary Journal*, **25**(5), 441–445.

Fedde M.R. (1991) Blood gas analyses on equine blood: required correction factors. *Equine Veterinary Journal*, **23**(6), 410–412.

Fedde, M.R. & Erickson, H.H. (1998) Increase in blood viscosity in the sprinting horse: can it account for the high pulmonary arterial pressure? *Equine Veterinary Journal*, **30**(4), 329–334.

Firth, E.C., Delahunt, J., Wichtel, J.W., Birch, H.L. & Goodship, A.E. (1999) Galloping exercise induces regional changes in bone density within the third and radial carpal bones of Thoroughbred horses. *Equine Veterinary Journal*, **31**(2), 111–115.

Frape, D. (1998) Feeding for performance and the metabolism of nutrients during exercise. In: *Equine Nutrition and Feeding*, 2nd edn (ed. D. Frape), pp. 259–318. Blackwell Science, Oxford.

Garlinghouse, S.E. & Burrill, M.J. (1999) Relationship of body condition score to completion rate during 160 km endurance races. *Equine Veterinary Journal* (Suppl.), **30**, 591–595.

Geor, R.J., McCutcheon, L.J. & Lindinger, M.I. (1996) Adaptations to daily exercise in hot and humid ambient conditions in trained thoroughbred horses. *Equine Veterinary Journal* (Suppl.), **22**, 63–68.

Geor, R.J., Ommundson, L., Fenton, G. & Pagan, J.D. (2001) Effects of a nasal strip and frusemide on pulmonary haemorrhage in Thoroughbreds following high-intensity exercise. *Equine Veterinary Journal*, **33**(6), 577–584.

Gillis, C.L., Meagher, D.M., Pool, R.R., Stover, S.M., Craychee, T.J. & Willits, N. (1993) Ultrasonographically detected changes in equine superficial digital flexor tendons during the first few months of race training. *American Journal of Veterinary Research*, **12**, 877–894.

Goodship, A.E., Cunningham, J.L., Organov, V., Darling, J., Miles, A.W. & Owen, G.W. (1998) Bone loss during long term space flight is prevented by the application of a short term impulsive electrical stimulus. *Acta Astronautica*, **43**(3–6), 65–76.

Harris, P.A. (1990) An outbreak of the equine rhabdomyolysis syndrome in a racing yard. *Veterinary Record*, **127**(19), 468–470.

Henneke, D.R. (1985) A condition score system for horses. *Equine Practice*, **7**(9), 13–15.

Henneke, D.R., Potter, G.D. & Krieder, J.L. (1981) A condition score relationship to body fat content of mares during gestation and lactation. In: *Proceedings of 7th Equine Nutrition and Physiology Symposium*, Warrenton, VA, p. 105.

Herholz, C., Weishaupt, M., Lauk, H., Straub, R. & Leadon, D. (1994) Clinical and submaximal performance parameters in the identification of subclinical pulmonary disease in warmblood competition horses. *Pfereheilkunde*, **10**(6), 419–422.

Hlastala, M.P., Bernard, S.L., Erickson, H.H., *et al.* (1996) Pulmonary blood flow distribution in standing horses is not dominated by gravity. *Journal of Applied Physiology*, **81**(3), 1051–1061.

Hodson, E., Clayton, H.M. & Lanovaz, J.L. (1999) Temporal analysis of walk movements in the Grand Prix dressage test at the 1996 Olympic Games. *Applied Animal Behavioural Science*, **62**, 89–97.

Holcombe, S.J., Jackson, C., Gerber, V., *et al.* (2001) Stabling is associated with airway inflammation in young Arabian horses. *Equine Veterinary Journal*, **33**(3), 244–249.

Holmstrom, M., Magnusson, L.-E. & Philipsson, J. (1990) Variation in conformation of Swedish Warmblood horses and conformational characteristics of elite sport horses. *Equine Veterinary Journal*, **22**, 186–193.

Hornicke, H., Weber, M. & Schweiker, W. (1987) Pulmonary ventilation in Thoroughbred horses at maximum performance. In: *Equine Exercise Physiology*, vol. 2 (eds J.R. Gillespie & N.E. Robinson), pp. 216–224. ICEEP Publications, Davis, CA.

Hoyt, D.F. & Taylor, C.F. (1981) Gait and the energetics of locomotion in horses. *Nature*, **292**, 239.

Ishida, N., Hobo, S., Takahashi, T., *et al.* (1999) Chronological changes in superoxide-scavenging ability and lipid peroxide concentration of equine serum due to stress from exercise and transport. *Equine Veterinary Journal* (Suppl.), **30**, 430–433.

Jeffcott, L.B. (1980) Disorders of the thoracolumbar spine of the horse – a survey of 443 cases. *Equine Veterinary Journal*, **12**, 197–210.

Jeffcott, L. (1996) Recommendations for horses going to the 1996 Atlanta Olympic Games. *Equine Athlete*, **9**(3), 19–25.

Jeffcott, L.B. & Dalin, G. (1980) Natural rigidity of the horse's backbone. *Equine Veterinary Journal*, **12**, 101–108.

Jeffcott, L.B., Rossdale, P.D., Freestone, J., Frank, C.J. & Towers-Clark, P.F. (1982) An assessment of wastage in thoroughbred racing from conception to 4 years of age. *Equine Veterinary Journal*, **14**(3), 185–198.

Kannegieter, N.J. & Dore, M.L. (1995) Endoscopy of the upper respiratory tract during treadmill exercise: a clinical study of 100 horses. *Australian Veterinary Journal*, **72**(3), 101–107.

Karlstrom, K., Essen-Gustavsson, B., Lindholm, A. & Persson, S.G.B. (1991) Capillary supply in relation to muscle metabolic profile and cardiocirculatory parameters. In: *Equine Exercise Physiology*, vol. 3 (eds S.G.B. Persson, A. Lindholm & L.B. Jeffcott), pp. 239–244. ICEEP Publications, Davis, CA.

Kimmich, H.P. & Spaan, J.G. (1980) Combined flow and P_{O_2} sensors for telemetric assessment of oxygen uptake in horses. In: *Biotelemetry*, vol. 5 (eds G. Matsumoto & H.P. Kimmich), pp. 165–168. Matsumoto, Hokkaido.

Kindig, C.A., McDonough, P., Fenton, G., Poole, D.C. & Erickson, H.H. (2001a) Efficacy of nasal strip and furosemide in mitigating EIPH in Thoroughbred horses. *Journal of Applied Physiology* (Suppl.), **91**(3), 1396–1400.

Kindig, C.A., McDonough, P., Finley, M.R., *et al.* (2001b) NO inhalation reduces pulmonary arterial pressure but not hemorrhage in maximally exercising horses. *Journal of Applied Physiology*, **91**(6), 2674–2678.

Kline, H. & Foreman, J.H. (1991) Heart and spleen weights as a function of breed and somatotype. In: *Equine Exercise Physiology*, vol. 3 (eds S.G.B. Persson, A. Lindholm & L.B. Jeffcott), p. 17. ICEEP Publications, Davis, CA.

Kriz, N.G., Hodgson, D.R. & Rose, R.J. (2000) Prevalence and clinical importance of heart murmurs in racehorses. *Journal of the American Veterinary Medical Association*, **216**(9), 1441–1445.

Kubo, K., Senta, T. & Osamu, S. (1974) Relationship between training and heart in the Thoroughbred racehorse. *Experimental Reports of Equine Health Laboratory*, **11**, 87–93.

Kuwahara, M., Hiraga, A., Kai, M., Tsubone, H. & Sugano, S. (1999) Influence of training on autonomic nervous function in horses: evaluation by power spectral analysis of heart rate variability. *Equine Veterinary Journal* (Suppl.), **30**, 178–180.

Langlois, B., Froideveaux, J., Lamarche, L., Legault, P., Tassencourt, L. & Theret, M. (1978) Analyse de liaisons centre la morphologie et l'aptitude au gallop, au trot et au saut d'obstacle chez le cheval. *Annales Genetique et de Selection Animale*, **10**, 443–474.

Langsetmo, I., Weigle, G.E., Fedde, M.R., Erickson, H.H., Barstow, T.J. & Poole, D.C. (1997) $\dot{V}_{O_2}$ kinetics in the horse during moderate and heavy exercise. *Journal of Applied Physiology*, **83**(4), 1235–1241.

Lapointe, J.M., Vrins, A. & McCarvill, E. (1994) A survey of exercise-induced pulmonary haemorrhage in Quebec Standardbred racehorses. *Equine Veterinary Journal*, **26**(6), 482–485.

Leach, D. (1993) Recommended terminology for researchers in locomotion and biomechanics of quadrupedal animals. *Acta Anatomica*, **146**(2–3), 130–136.

Leach, D.H., Ormrod, K. & Clayton, H.M. (1984) Standardised terminology for the description and analysis of equine locomotion. *Equine Veterinary Journal*, **16**(6), 522–528.

Lester, G., Clark, C., Rice, B., Steible-Hartless, C. & Vetro-Widenhouse, T. (1999) Effect of timing and route of administration of furosemide on pulmonary haemorrhage and pulmonary arterial pressure in exercising Thoroughbred racehorses. *American Journal of Veterinary Research*, **60**(1), 22–28.

Lim, A.S. (1981) Bodyweight and performance in racehorses. *Proceedings of the 14th International Conference on Drugs in Racehorses*, p. 93.

Loew, F.M. & Bettany, J.M. (1973) Thiamine concentrations in the blood of Standardbred horses. *American Journal of Veterinary Research*, **34**(9), 1207–1208.

Lovell, D.K. & Rose, R.J. (1991) Changes in skeletal muscle composition in response to interval and high intensity training. In: *Equine Exercise Physiology*, vol. 3 (eds S.G.B. Persson, A. Lindholm & L.B. Jeffcott), pp. 215–222. ICEEP Publications, Davis, CA.

McCutcheon, L.J., Geor, R.J., Hare, M.J., Ecker, G.L. & Lindinger, M.I. (1995) Sweating rate and sweat composition during exercise and recovery in ambient heat and humidity. *Equine Veterinary Journal* (Suppl.), **20**, 153–157.

McKeever, K.H. & Malinowski, K. (1997) Exercise capacity in young and old mares. *American Journal of Veterinary Research*, **58**(12), 1468–1472.

McKeever, K.H., Schurg, W.A., Jarrett, S.H. & Convertino, V.A. (1987) Exercise training-induced hypervolemia in the horse. *Medicine & Science in Sports & Exercise*, **19**(1), 21–27.

McMiken, D.F. (1983) An energetic basis of equine performance. *Equine Veterinary Journal*, **15**(2), 123–133.

Manohar, M., Goetz, T.E., Sulivan, E. & Griffin, R. (1997) Pulmonary vascular pressures of strenuously exercising Thoroughbreds after administration of varying doses of frusemide. *Equine Veterinary Journal*, **29**(4), 298–304.

Marlin, D.J. (2001) Exercise-induced pulmonary haemorrhage: a global review of recent findings. In: *Proceedings of World Equine Airways Symposium and Veterinary and Comparative Respiratory Society*, Edinburgh, 19–23 July 2001. World Equine Airways Society, Canada (http://web.vet.cornell.edu/internet/weaf/ and also available on CD).

Marlin, D.J. (2002) Exercise induced pulmonary haemorrhage (EIPH). In: *Current Therapy in Equine Medicine*, vol. 5 (ed. N.E. Robinson), W.B. Saunders, Philadelphia, PA.

Marlin, D.J. & Allen, J.C.R. (1999) Cardiovascular demands of low-goal (non-elite) polo ponies. *Equine Veterinary Journal*, **31**(5), 378–382.

Marlin, D.J., Scott, C.M., Schroter, R.C., *et al.* (1996a) Acclimation of horses to high temperature and humidity. *Equine Athlete*, **9**, 8–11.

Marlin, D.J., Scott, C.M., Schroter, R.C., *et al.* (1996b) Physiological responses in non-heat acclimated horses performing treadmill exercise in cool (20°C/40% RH), hot dry (30°C/40% RH) and hot humid (30°C/80% RH) conditions. *Equine Veterinary Journal* (Suppl.), **22**, 70–84.

Mason, D.K., Collins, E.A. & Watkins, K.L. (1983) Exercise-induced pulmonary haemorrhage in horses. In: *Equine Exercise Physiology. Proceedings of the First International Conference* (eds D.H. Snow, S.G.B. Persson & R.J. Rose), pp. 57–63.

Morris, E.A. & Seeherman, H.J. (1991) Clinical evaluation of poor performance in the racehorse: the results of 275 evaluations. *Equine Veterinary Journal*, **23**(3), 169–174.

Murray, R.C., Henson, F.M.D., Zhu, C.F., Goodship, A.E., Agrawal, C.M. & Athanasiou, K.A. (1998) The effects of strenuous training on equine carpal articular cartilage mechanical behaviour and morphology. *Transactions, Orthopaedics and Trauma*, **8**, 133–140.

Murray, R.C., Whitton, R.C., Vedi, S., Goodship, A.E. & Lekeux, P. (1999) The effect of training on the calcified zone of equine middle carpal articular cartilage. *Equine Veterinary Journal* (Suppl.), **30**, 274–278.

Muybridge, E. (1899/1957) *Animals in Motion* (ed. L.S. Brown) (Republished 1957). Dover Publications, New York.

Nagata, S., Takeda, F., Kurosawa, M., *et al.* (1999) Plasma adrenocorticotropin, cortisol and catecholamines response to various exercises. *Equine Veterinary Journal* (Suppl.), **30**, 570–574.

Nielan, G.J., Rehder, R.S., Ducharme, N.G. & Hackett, R.P. (1992) Measurement of tracheal static pressure in exercising horses. *Veterinary Surgery*, **21**(6), 423–428.

Novelli, G.P., Bracciotti, G. & Falsini, S. (1990) Spin-trappers and vitamin E prolong endurance to muscle fatigue in mice. *Free Radical Biology and Medicine*, **8**(1), 9–13.

Nunn, J.F. (1993) *Nunn's Applied Respiratory Physiology*, 4th edn. Butterworth-Heinemann, Oxford.

Oikawa, M. (1999) Exercise-induced haemorrhagic lesions in the dorsocaudal extremities of the caudal lobes of the lungs of young thoroughbred horses. *Journal of Comparative Pathology*, **121**(4), 339–347.

Pagan, J.D. & Harris, P.A. (1999) The effects of timing and amount of forage and grain on exercise response in Thoroughbred horses. *Equine Veterinary Journal* (Suppl.), **30**, 451–457.

Pagan, J.D., Essen-Gustavsson, B., Lindholm, A. & Thornton, J. (1987) The effect of dietary energy source on exercise performance in Standardbred horses. In: *Equine Exercise Physiology*, vol. 2 (eds J.R. Gillespie & N.E. Robinson), pp. 686–700. ICEEP Publications, Davis, CA.

Parks, C.M. & Manohar, M. (1983) Distribution of blood flow during moderate and strenuous exercise in ponies (*Equus caballus*). *American Journal of Veterinary Research*, **44**(10), 1861–1866.

Pascoe, J.R., Hiraga, A., Hobo, S., *et al.* (1999) Cardiac output measurements using sonomicrometer crystals on the left ventricle at rest and exercise. *Equine Veterinary Journal* (Suppl.), **30**, 148–152.

Persson, S.G. & Osterberg, I. (1999) Racing performance in red blood cell hypervolaemic standardbred trotters. *Equine Veterinary Journal* (Suppl.), **30**, 617–620.

Preedy, D.F. & Colborne, G.R. (2001) A method to determine mechanical energy conservation and efficiency in equine gait: a preliminary study. *Equine Veterinary Journal* (Suppl.), **33**, 94–98.

Rainger, J.E., Evans, D.L., Hodgson, D.R. & Rose, R.J. (1994) Blood lactate disappearance after maximal exercise in trained and detrained horses. *Research in Veterinary Science*, **57**(3), 325–331.

Rehder, R.S., Ducharme, N.G., Hackett, R.P. & Nielan, G.J. (1995) Measurement of upper airway pressures in exercising horses with dorsal displacement of the soft palate. *American Journal of Veterinary Research*, **56**(3), 269–274.

Reilly, G.C., Currey, J.D. & Goodship, A.E. (1997) Exercise of young Thoroughbred horses increases impact strength of the third metacarpal bone. *Journal of Orthopaedic Research*, **15**(6), 862–868.

Ricketts, S.W., Young, A., Mowbray, J.F., Yousef, G.E. & Wood, J. (1992) Equine fatigue syndrome. *Veterinary Record*, **131**(3), 58–59.

Roberts, C. (1998) Relationship between visible tracheal mucus, EIPH, age and finishing position in Thoroughbred racehorses in the U.K. (abstract). In: *Proceedings of the World Equine Airways Symposium*, p. 4.

Roberts, C.A. & Marlin, D.J. (2001) The diagnostic value of post-racing endoscopy for the detection of EIPH in Thoroughbred racehorses in the UK. *World Equine Airways Symposium and Veterinary and Comparative Respiratory Society*, Edinburgh, 19–23 July 2001, p. 37. World Equine Airways Society, Canada (http://web.vet.cornell.edu/internet/weaf/ and also available on CD).

Roberts, C. & Wright, I. (1999) The use of treadmill exercise to determine the significance of orthopedic conditions in a Thoroughbred racehorse. *Journal of Equine Veterinary Science*, **19**, 559.

Roberts, C., Hillidge, C. & Marlin, D. (1993) Exercise-induced pulmonary haemorrhage in racing Thoroughbreds in Great Britain (abstract). In: *Proceedings of the International EIPH Conference*, p. 11.

Roneus, M., Linholm, A. & Asheim, A. (1991) Muscle characteristics in Thoroughbreds of different ages and sexes. *Equine Veterinary Journal*, 23(3), 207.

Rose, R.J., Hodgson, D.R., Kelso, T.B., McCutcheon, L.J., Reid, T.A., Bayly, W.M. & Gollnick, P.D. (1988) Maximum O_2 uptake, O_2 debt and deficit, and muscle metabolites in Thoroughbred horses. *Journal of Applied Physiology*, 64(2), 781–788.

Rose, R.J., King, C.M., Evans, D.L., Tyler, C.M. & Hodgson, D.R. (1995) Indices of exercise capacity in horses presented for poor racing performance. *Equine Veterinary Journal* (Suppl.), 18, 418–421.

Rossdale, P.D., Hopes, R., Digby, N.J. & Offord, K. (1985) Epidemiological study of wastage among racehorses 1982 and 1983. *Veterinary Record*, 116(3), 66–69.

Sahlin, K. (1985) Metabolic changes limiting muscle performance. In: *Biochemistry of Exercise VI* (ed. B. Saltin), International Series on Sport Sciences 16, pp. 323–344. Human Kinetics Publishers, Champaign, IL.

Schroter, R.C., Marlin, D.J. & Jeffcott, L.B. (1996) Use of the wet bulb globe temperature (WBGT) index to quantify environmental heat loads during three-day-event competitions. *Equine Veterinary Journal* (Suppl.), 22, 3–6.

Schubert, R. (1990) Nutrition of the performance horse. Influence of high vitamin E doses on performance of racehorse. Session II: horse production. *Proceedings of the 42nd Annual Meeting of the European Association for Animal Production*, Berlin, 8–12 September, p. 538.

Schwane, J.A., Johnson, S.R., Vandenakker, C.B. & Armstrong, R.B. (1983) Delayed-onset muscular soreness and plasma CPK and LDH activities after downhill running. *Medicine and Science in Sports and Exercise*, 15, 51–56.

Scott, C., Marlin, D.J. & Schroter, R.C. (1996) Modified ventilated capsule for the measurement of sweating rate in the exercising horse. *Equine Veterinary Journal* (Suppl.), 22, 48–53.

Sewell, D.A. & Harris, R.C. (1992) Adenine nucleotide degradation in the thoroughbred horse with increasing exercise duration. *European Journal of Applied Physiology & Occupational Physiology*, 65(3), 271–277.

Sewell, D.A., Harris, R.C. & Marlin, D.J. (1994) Skeletal muscle characteristics in 2 year-old race-trained thoroughbred horses. *Comparative Biochemistry & Physiology A*, 108(1), 87–96.

Sinha, A.K., Ray, S.P. & Rose, R.J. (1991) Effect of training intensity and detraining on adaptations in different skeletal muscles. In: *Equine Exercise Physiology*, vol. 3 (eds S.G.B. Persson, A. Lindholm & L.B. Jeffcott) pp. 239–244. ICEEP Publications, Davis, CA.

Smith, R.K., Birch, H., Patterson-Kane, J., *et al.* (1999) Should equine athletes commence training during skeletal development? Changes in tendon matrix associated with development, ageing, function and exercise. *Equine Veterinary Journal* (Suppl.), 30, 201–209.

Snow, D.H. & Guy, P.S. (1981) Fibre type and enzyme activities of the gluteus medius in different breeds of horse. In: *Biochemistry of Exercise*, vol. IV-B (eds J. Poortmans & G. Niset), pp. 275–282. University Park Press, Baltimore, MD.

Snow, D.H., Harris, R.C. & Gash, S.P. (1985) Metabolic response of equine muscle to intermittent maximal exercise. *Journal of Applied Physiology*, 58(5), 1689–1697.

Steel, J.D. (1963) *Studies on the Electrocardiogram of the Racehorse*. Australasian Medical Publishing, Sydney.

Stephens, P.R., Nunamaker, D.M. & Butterweck, D.M. (1989) Application of a Hall-effect transducer for measurement of tendon strains in horses. *American Journal of Veterinary Research*, 50(7), 1089–1095.

Thomas, D.P., Fregin, G.F., Gerber, N.H. & Ailes, N.B. (1983) Effects of training on cardiorespiratory function in the horse. *American Journal of Physiology*, 245(2), R160–R165.

Thornton, J., Essen-Gustavsson, B., Lindholm, A., *et al.* (1983) Effects of training and detraining on oxygen uptake, cardiac output, blood gas tensions, pH and lactate concentrations during and after exercise in the horse. In: *Equine Exercise Physiology* (eds D.H. Snow, S.G.B. Persson & R.J. Rose), p. 470. Granta Editions, Cambridge.

Townsend, H.G.G. & Leach, D.H. (1983) Kinematics of the equine thoracolumbar spine. *Equine Veterinary Journal*, 15, 117–122.

Waran, N.K., Robertson, V., Cuddeford, D., Kokoszko, A. & Marlin, D.J. (1996) Effects of transporting horses facing either forwards or backwards on their behaviour and heart rate. *Veterinary Record*, 139, 7–11.

Whitwell, K.E. & Greet, T.R. (1984) Collection and evaluation of tracheobronchial washes in the horse. *Equine Veterinary Journal*, 16(6), 499–508.

Wilson, A.M. (1991) The effect of exercise intensity on the biochemistry, morphology and mechanical properties of a tendon. PhD thesis, University of Bristol, UK.

Wood, J.L., Burrell, M.H., Roberts, C.A., Chanter, N. & Shaw, Y. (1993) *Streptococci* and *Pasteuralla* spp. associated with disease of the equine lower respiratory tract. *Equine Veterinary Journal*, 25(4), 314–318.

Wood, J.L.N., Newton, J.R., Chanter, N., *et al.* (1999) *Equine Infectious Diseases VIII: Proceedings of the Eighth International Conference* (eds U. Wernery, J.F. Wade, J.A. Mumford & O.R. Kaaden), Dubai, 23–26 March 1998, pp. 64–70.

Young, D.R., Richardson, D.W., Markel, M.D. & Nunamaker, D.M. (1991) Mechanical and morphometric analysis of the third carpal bone of Thoroughbreds. *American Journal of Veterinary Research*, 52, 402–409.

Young, L.E. (1999) Cardiac responses to training in 2-year old thoroughbreds: an echocardiographic study. *Equine Veterinary Journal* (Suppl.), 30, 195–198.

Young, L.E. & Wood, J.L. (2000) Effect of age and training on murmurs of atrioventricular valvular regurgitation in young thoroughbreds. *Equine Veterinary Journal*, 32(3), 195–199.

Young, L.E., Marlin, D.J., Deaton, C., Brown-Feltner, H., Roberts, C.A. & Wood, J.L.N. (In press) Heart size estimated by echocardiography correlates with maximal oxygen uptake. *Equine Veterinary Journal*.

Further reading

Back, W., and Clayton, H. M. (2001) *Equine Locomotion*. W.B. Saunders, Philadelphia.

Frape, D. (1998) *Equine Nutrition and Feeding*, 2nd edn. Blackwell Science, Oxford.

Hodgson, D.R. and Rose, R.J. (1994) *Principles and Practice of Equine Sports Medicine: The Athletic Horse*. W.B. Saunders, Philadelphia.

Kohn, C.W. (2000) *Guidelines for Horse Transport by Road and Air*. American Horse Shows Association. ISBN 0-9700169-1-3.

Loving, N.S. and Johnston, A.M. (1995) *Veterinary Manual for the Performance Horse*. Blackwell Science, Oxford.

Marlin, D.J., Schroter, R.C., White, S.L., *et al.* (2001) Recovery from transport and acclimatisation of competition horses in a hot and humid environment. *Equine Veterinary Journal*, **33**(4), 371–379.

Nigg, B.M. and Herzog, W. (1999) *Biomechanics of the musculo-skeletal system*, 2nd edn. John Wiley and Sons, Chichester.

Nunn, J.F. (1993) *Nunn's Applied Respiratory Physiology*, 4th edn. Butterworth-Heinemann, Oxford.

Racklyeft, D.J. & Love, D.N. (1990) Influence of head posture on the respiratory tract health of horses. *Australian Veterinary Journal*, **67**(11), 402–405.

Slade, L.M. (1986) Trailer transportation and racing performance. In: *Proceedings of the 9th Equine Nutrition and Physiology Symposium*, p. 511.

Stryer, L. (1988) *Biochemistry*. 3rd edn. W.H. Freeman and Company, New York.

Wilmore, J.H. and Costill, D.L. (1999) *Physiology of Sport and Exercise*, 2nd edn. Human Kinetics, Leeds.

Index

Note: page numbers in *italics* refer to figures; those in **bold** refer to tables

Printed and bound by CPI Group (UK) Ltd, Croydon, CR0 4YY

27/10/2024

14580396-0003